# Handbook of
# PEDIATRIC OBESITY

## Clinical Management

# Handbook of
# PEDIATRIC
# OBESITY

## Clinical Management

Edited by
Melinda S. Sothern
Stewart T. Gordon
T. Kristian von Almen

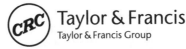

## Taylor & Francis
Taylor & Francis Group

Boca Raton   London   New York

A CRC title, part of the Taylor & Francis imprint, a member of the
Taylor & Francis Group, the academic division of T&F Informa plc.

Published in 2006 by
CRC Press
Taylor & Francis Group
6000 Broken Sound Parkway NW, Suite 300
Boca Raton, FL 33487-2742

International Standard Book Number-10: 1-57444-913-3 (Hardcover)
International Standard Book Number-13: 978-1-57444-913-6 (Hardcover)
Library of Congress Card Number 2005050122

**Library of Congress Cataloging-in-Publication Data**

Handbook of pediatric obesity : clinical management / edited by Melinda Sothern, Stewart T. Gordon,
   T. Kristian von Almen.
     p. ; cm.
   Includes bibliographical references and index.
   ISBN 1-57444-913-3 (alk. paper)
   1. Obesity in children--Treatment--Handbooks, manuals, etc. I. Sothern, Melinda. II. Gordon, Stewart T.
III. Von Almen, T. Kristian.
   [DNLM: 1. Obesity--therapy--Child. 2. Obesity--diet therapy--Child. WD 210  H2368 2005]

RJ399.C6H36 2005
618.92'398--dc22
                                                    2005050122

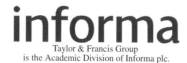

informa
Taylor & Francis Group
is the Academic Division of Informa plc.

Visit the Taylor & Francis Web site at
http://www.taylorandfrancis.com

and the CRC Press Web site at
http://www.crcpress.com

# Preface

We are very pleased and honored to edit the *Handbook of Pediatric Obesity: Clinical Management*. We accept this responsibility with much enthusiasm. We believe that this text will provide a scientifically sound, clinically relevant survey of the available approaches for the treatment of pediatric obesity to pediatric health care and research professionals. In addition, a portion of proceeds of this book will be donated to the Pediatric Obesity Interest Group of the North American Association for the Study of the Obesity (NAASO): The Obesity Society and, thus, will be available to us as a community of researchers and health care providers for the purposes of educational seminars, research opportunities, and future pediatric obesity prevention and treatment projects.

Over the last two decades, we have been privileged to participate in clinical research studies that provided continued opportunities to review the scientific evidence related to pediatric obesity. This experience and knowledge confirmed the complexity of pediatric obesity. It is clear from the scientific literature that the direct causes of pediatric obesity remain undiscovered and that standards for treatment, although desperately needed, are nonexistent.

During this same two decades, we also had the opportunity to provide treatment to thousands of overweight children and their families. We observed over this time that the severity of obesity in these patients has increased and, even more disturbing, that these children have become more and more resistant to traditional treatment approaches. Today's overweight children are very difficult to treat. The sentiment of most clinicians and researchers has become negative and self-defeating. However, rather than assume the position that the only way to curb the current pediatric obesity epidemic is to ignore this generation and focus on prevention in the next, we, along with the contributing authors, accepted the task of compiling the available management, medical, nutrition, psychological, and physical activity facts, models, theories, interventions, and evaluation techniques. Our mission was to provide the most clinically appropriate, scientifically supported source of information to the pediatric health care and research professional. It is our hope we have accomplished our mission. We feel we have produced a comprehensive, state-of-the-art, and easy-to-use reference that can be used by pediatric health care and research professionals to develop programs and provide the best possible care to overweight children in clinical settings.

The introduction provides an overview of the problem of pediatric obesity and includes global options for solutions. Section 1 details pediatric obesity clinical management strategies, challenges, business plans, and evaluation methods. Section 2 discusses the medical aspects of treatment including complications and comorbidities of pediatric obesity and the physician's role in treatment. In Section 3, psychosocial and physical considerations associated with pediatric obesity are discussed, as well as how each affects the treatment process. Section 4 offers the reader a comprehensive survey of pediatric obesity medical, nutrition, behavioral, and exercise evaluation methods and techniques. Options for nutrition intervention in overweight youth are detailed in Section 5, behavioral counseling in Section 6, and methods to increase physical activity and provide exercise training in Section 7. Section 8 discusses Internet-based approaches used in pediatric clinical settings, Section 9, the role of pharmacology as it relates to pediatric obesity treatment, and Section 10, an overview of surgery options for significantly obese adolescents. The final section presents specific techniques and methods for conducting interdisciplinary, interactive group instruction for overweight children and their families. A comprehensive appendix follows Chapter 20 and is divided into three sections: clinical management forms, testing and measurement protocols, and sample intervention materials. Throughout the text, individual chapters discuss management strategies, methods, and techniques that refer to specific forms, protocols, handouts, and sources located in the Appendix. These are practical and applied techniques, information, and tools that may be used, as needed, to develop, modify, implement, and evaluate weight-management programs for children and adolescents in clinical and research settings.

As pediatric health care and research professionals, you have an important responsibility to overweight children and adolescents. Your approach, interaction, and follow-up procedures have a tremendous effect on the physical and emotional health of your patients. When families come to you for help with overweight problems, your initial words, actions, and demeanor will set the stage for weight-management success or failure. We strongly believe that the success or failure of your patients to achieve a healthy weight is a shared responsibility. We encourage you to accept this responsibility and this challenge with an open heart and a positive attitude. We hope you will dedicate the necessary time and energy to providing the most appropriate care to your overweight patients. Your reward will be an unbelievable feeling of accomplishment and self-satisfaction.

Throughout this text we've provided you with the necessary information and tools to do your job well. This knowledge will enable you to become proficient in matching or tailoring the available treatment plans to the medical, physical, and emotional needs of your patient. There are many options, and it is clear that there is no single solution for every overweight child. However, for each child, an individualized plan can be developed that will best manage obesity and enhance his or her emotional and physical health.

**Melinda S. Sothern, Ph.D.**
*Associate Professor and Director*
*Section of Health Promotion*
*School of Public Health*
*Louisiana State University*
*Health Sciences Center*

**T. Kristian von Almen, Ph.D.**
*Research Psychologist,*
*Assistant Clinical Professor in Pediatrics*
*Louisiana State University*
*Health Sciences Center*

**Stewart T. Gordon, M.D., F.A.A.P.**
*Associate Professor of Clinical Pediatrics*
*Louisiana State University of Medicine*
*and*
*Chief of Pediatrics*
*LSU Health Sciences Center/*
*Earl K. Long Medical Center*

# Acknowledgments

We gratefully acknowledge the expert manuscripts provided by all of the contributing authors in this volume, who took time away from their challenging clinical and research obligations to provide this important information. We wish to express our gratitude to Dr. Michael Goran for accepting the challenge of editing *The Handbook of Pediatric Obesity: Epidemiology, Etiology, and Prevention*, which provides essential background information for this volume — *Clinical Management*. Our research associate, Connie VanVrancken-Tompkins, deserves special mention not only for her assistance in editing the chapters and appendix but also for help in writing several chapters. We especially thank our Acquisitions Editor at Dekker/CRC Press, Susan Lee, for her assistance during the proposal process and for believing in this project and providing us with a venue to reach so many health care and research professionals. We wish to also thank Ms. Leslie Capo, whose long hours of hard work as our media coordinator at the Louisiana State University Health Sciences Center (LSUHSC) have provided us with a multitude of opportunities to highlight our academic and clinical successes and translate other important pediatric obesity scientific findings to the public. We appreciate the guidance and support of Dr. Eric Ravussin, Dr. Mark Loftin, Dr. John Udall, Dr. Frank Greenway, and Dr. Claude Bouchard, who are not only mentors but also inspirations and role models for all of us. We are grateful for the help and encouragement of Dr. Elizabeth Fontham, Dr. Charlie Brown, Dr. Donna Ryan, Dr. George Bray, Dr. Keely Carlisle, Dr. Sandra Hunter, Dr. Alphonso Vargas, Dr. Ricardo Sorensen, Dr. Robert Suskind, and Dr. Stuart Chalew. We gratefully acknowledge the editorial, computer, and clerical support of our student worker, Courtney Brooks, and the thoughtful review and helpful comments provided by Dr. David Ludwig and Dr. Cara Ebbeling. We sincerely appreciate the continued support and guidance of LSUHSC, School of Public Health and Department of Pediatrics, the Pennington Biomedical Research Center, The University of New Orleans, and NAASO: The Obesity Society. We are grateful to the American Academy of Pediatrics, the American Dietetic Association, the American College of Sports Medicine, the United States Centers for Disease Control and Prevention, and the U.S. Surgeon General for their continued commitment to pediatric obesity prevention and treatment.

# Contributors

**Oded Bar-Or, M.D., F.A.C.S.M.**
Children's Exercise and Nutrition Centre
McMaster University
Hamilton, Ontario, Canada

**Robert I. Berkowitz, M.D.**
Weight and Eating Disorders Program
University of Pennsylvania School of Medicine
Philadelphia, Pennsylvania

**Courtney Brooks, B.S.**
Louisiana State University Health Sciences
  Center, School of Public Health
New Orleans, Louisiana

**Lauren Keely Carlisle, M.D., M.P.H.**
Department of Pediatrics
Louisiana State University Health Sciences
  Center
New Orleans, Louisiana

**Nancy Copperman, M.S., R.D., C.D.N.**
Division of Adolescent Medicine
Schneider Children's Hospital
New Hyde Park, New York

**Canice E. Crerand, Ph.D.**
Department of Psychiatry Weight and Eating
  Disorders Program
University of Pennsylvania School of Medicine
Philadelphia, Pennsylvania

**Stephen Daniels, M.D., Ph.D.**
Division of Cardiology
University of Cincinnati
Cincinnati, Ohio
and
Comprehensive Weight Management Center
Cincinnati Children's Hospital Medical Center
Cincinnati, Ohio

**Stewart T. Gordon, M.D., F.A.A.P.**
Louisiana State University School of Medicine
and
LSU Health Sciences Center/Earl K. Long
  Medical Center
Baton Rouge, Louisiana

**Thomas Inge, M.D., Ph.D., F.A.C.S., F.A.A.P.**
Department of Surgery, Division of Pediatric
  Surgery
University of Cincinnati
Cincinnati, Ohio
and
Comprehensive Weight Management Center
Cincinnati Children's Hospital Medical Center
Cincinnati, Ohio

**Marc S. Jacobson, M.D.**
Albert Einstein College of Medicine
Yeshiva University
and
Center for Atherosclerosis Prevention, Division
  of Adolescent Medicine
Schneider Children's Hospital Center
New Hyde Park, New York

**Shelley Kirk, Ph.D., R.D., L.D.**
Division of Cardiology
University of Cincinnati
Cincinnati, Ohio
and
Comprehensive Weight Management Center
Cincinnati Children's Hospital Medical Center
Cincinnati, Ohio

**Nancy F. Krebs, M.D., M.S.**
University of Colorado School of Medicine
Denver, Colorado

**Mark Loftin, Ph.D.**
Department of Human Performance and Health
  Promotion
University of New Orleans
New Orleans, Louisiana

**Pamela Davis Martin, Ph.D.**
Pennington Biomedical Research Center
Baton Rouge, Louisiana

**Valerie H. Myers, Ph.D.**
Pennington Biomedical Research Center
Baton Rouge, Louisiana

**Scott Owens, Ph.D.**
Department of Health, Exercise Science, and
  Recreation Management
University of Mississippi
Oxford, Mississippi

**Thomas Rowland, M.D.**
Baystate Medical Center
Springfield, Massachusetts

**Heidi Schumacher, R.D., L.D.N., C.D.E.**
Children's Hospital of New Orleans
New Orleans, Louisiana
and
Louisiana State University Health Sciences
  Center Pediatric Weight Management
  Program
New Orleans, Louisiana

**Jeffrey B. Schwimmer, M.D.**
Department of Pediatrics
University of California, San Diego
San Diego, California
and
San Diego Children's Hospital and Health Center
San Diego, California

**Melinda S. Sothern, Ph.D., C.E.P.**
School of Public Health
Louisiana State University Health Sciences
  Center
New Orleans, Louisiana

**Tiffany M. Stewart, Ph.D.**
Pennington Biomedical Research Center
Baton Rouge, Louisiana

**Dennis M. Styne, M.D.**
University of California Davis
Sacramento, California

**Camille Thélin, B.A.**
Louisiana State University Health Sciences
  Center, School of Public Health
New Orleans, Louisiana

**Connie VanVrancken-Tompkins, M.A.**
Louisiana State University Health Sciences
  Center, School of Public Health
New Orleans, Louisiana

**T. Kristian von Almen, Ph.D.**
Louisiana State University Health Sciences
  Center
New Orleans, Louisiana

**Thomas A. Wadden, Ph.D.**
University of Pennsylvania
Philadelphia, Pennsylvania

**Heather Walden, M.S.**
Pennington Biomedical Research Center
Baton Rouge, Louisiana

**Donald A. Williamson, Ph.D.**
Pennington Biomedical Research Center
Baton Rouge, Louisiana

**Emily York-Crowe, M.A.**
Pennington Biomedical Research Center
Baton Rouge, Louisiana

**Meg Zeller, Ph.D.**
Cincinnati Children's Hospital Medical Center,
  University of Cincinnati
Cincinnati, Ohio

## REVIEWERS

**Cara B. Ebbeling, Ph.D.**
Division of Endocrinology
Children's Hospital
Boston, Massachusetts

**David S. Ludwig, M.D., Ph.D.**
Children's Hospital
Boston, Massachusetts

# Table of Contents

# SECTION 9  Pharmacology

# SECTION 10  Surgery

# SECTION 11  Interdisciplinary, Interactive, Group Instruction

# 1  Clinical Management of Pediatric Obesity: An Overview

*Dennis M. Styne*

## CONTENTS

This second volume of this *Handbook of Childhood Obesity* contains detailed information on all of the approaches to the treatment and management of childhood obesity. This brief introductory chapter aims not to repeat such important information but, rather, to reflect on the role of these approaches in this international epidemic of chronic disease that is occurring as a result of the many factors highlighted in the first volume.

Perhaps there is the danger of our becoming desensitized to the remarkable prevalence of pediatric obesity, as we read about this subject daily in the lay or medical press. As shown in volume one, the prevalence of childhood obesity or overweight (defined as BMI [body mass index] ≥ 95th percentile by the Centers for Disease Control and Prevention) has tripled in the last 20 years to about 31% [1], and the prevalence of those at risk for obesity or at risk for overweight (defined as BMI ≥ 85th < 95th percentile) has increased over 50%, to approximately 26% [1]. Ethnic groups in the U.S. other than Caucasians, i.e., Native Americans, African Americans, Hispanic Americans, and most recently, Asian Americans, are at greater risk than Caucasian Americans, although Caucasians suffer in large numbers as well. These same trends are found around the world with the same rising prevalence. These ethnic tendencies are caused partially by genetic factors and partially by socioeconomic and educational influences. Such health disparities, already well known in the adult population, are more recently recognized in children [2]. Indeed, toddlers are already manifesting remarkable weight gain. Significant political repercussions over and above concerns about the cost to individuals and families in physical and emotional health can arise out of such a situation.

Our goals as medical professionals may differ from those of the lay public, and communication may thus suffer. The laity often focuses on a more "acceptable or pleasing" appearance as the goal for the treatment of obesity. They often take aim at unreachable goals fostered by the remarkably slim figures of media stars. Why do health professionals seek to find a treatment for childhood obesity? Metabolic and emotional health (the latter may itself be affected by the social response to appearance) is the focus of these two volumes and of providers of medical care for those who are overweight. We seek as our primary goal to improve metabolic fitness and body composition and to improve health and emotional status, leaving as a secondary goal the loss of weight or, in younger subjects, the control of its velocity of increase. The successful social marketing techniques that have convinced large numbers of U.S. smokers to cease using tobacco focused not primarily on improvement in health and limitation of the damage caused by smoking to lungs, heart, and offspring, as few smokers seemed to be moved by these goals. The successful approach was to take aim at daily habits rather than loftier goals of health. Can we follow such successes in the reduction of smoking by limiting the prevalence of obesity? Can we encourage individuals to eat healthier diets and decrease inactivity in a supportive and successful manner rather than by more grim pronouncements of the type that have had little effect in the past? Part of the success of antismoking campaigns was to make the very act of smoking socially unacceptable, and there is no direct parallel in the realm of obesity that can be invoked without targeting obese individuals themselves. We must take care to influence the causes and complications of obesity, but not take aim at the obese individuals themselves, lest those affected be made to feel more marginalized than they feel now.

Careful investigation of the understanding and acceptance of our techniques of weight management on the consumer is necessary. For example, we strive to use the euphemistic term "overweight" in place of "obesity" in childhood to limit stigmatization of the latter term. However, there are reports that the public fully understands the term "obesity" but is unclear on the meaning and importance of "overweight." We have sought to convince a generation of children to eat "5 a day" of vegetables and fruit, but we find that parents label these very foods as "not convenient to eat" (perhaps because they need to be washed and sometimes cut and cooked), and children describe them as "messy" (perhaps because they rot when not eaten) [3].

Now the goal of the U.S. Department of Agriculture has been modified, because of increased clinical insight, before we have even successfully reached our earlier target. We must find what will motivate the population by using social marketing techniques to change their habits to achieve metabolic fitness. Simply preaching exercise and a healthier diet has not worked up to now and is unlikely to be successful alone in the future.

Weight acceptance groups speak of being "healthy at any weight"; however, recent studies point out that overweight is itself a risk factor for comorbidities, over and above a lack of fitness [4]. Unfortunately, we cannot yet predict which individual will develop which serious comorbidities as their weight increases. Genetic analysis may ultimately reveal how one individual who has a BMI > 95th percentile does not have diabetes, steatohepatitis, or dyslipidemia, whereas another develops some or all of theses conditions, even though he or she may be thinner. Until such time as these techniques are developed, we have to attend to the general population of obese individuals.

The distribution of adiposity in the population is another concern. The distribution of percentiles of BMI values for age of a child has changed over the last two decades [5]. The newest analysis of BMI values for age does not demonstrate a uniform rise in all values compared with past decades. The lower end of the curve of the lowest BMI values for age has remained relatively stable, whereas the upper end of greater BMI values at a given age has become all the more skewed to the right, indicating a greater prevalence of the highest values in recent decades. It is theorized that an individual who 20 years ago would have had a moderately elevated BMI for age (e.g., above the 85th percentile) in today's world would have a much greater BMI value (e.g., above the 95th percentile) at the same age. This is usually attributed to the effects of today's environment on a stable genetic tendency for some individuals to gain more weight than others. In contrast, those individuals 20 years age who were close to, or less than, appropriate ideal for age would in today's world have a modest increase in BMI values, if any increase at all. These data indicate that the entire population may not be at risk for obesity; rather, those who have an innate tendency toward higher BMI values have developed even greater BMI values in this decade, presumably because of the effects of today's environment. It appears that obesity develops from a certain genetic makeup exposed to an unfortunate environment, so that not all exposed to the environment suffer equally.

There is concern about various features of puberty being affected by obesity [6]. Although it is true that the age of menarche in many studies is lower today in girls who have greater BMI values, mathematical modeling shows that the later age of attainment of menarche in girls studied 20 years ago would, if their BMI was adjusted upward to values found more commonly today, have menarche at a younger age today. We can take some grim solace in the data from the latest Health and Nutrition Evaluation Survey (HANES) survey that indicate that the shift to higher BMI values in the United States may be leveling off, albeit at values higher than seen two decades ago.

What, then, should be done to approach the epidemic of pediatric obesity? An expert panel proposed that attention should first be directed to those whose standard deviation scores of BMI for age is above the 85th percentile. Second, there should be a determination of whether there is a family history of risk factors or the presence of comorbidities in the child [7]. Weight maintenance was recommended for those without comorbidities who could "grow into their weight" as they became taller, whereas weight loss was indicated for those already too old to allow enough growth in stature, as well as for those with significant comorbidities. The recommendation of referral to an "Obesity Treatment Center" must have seemed to be wishful thinking in 1998 when first published. With increased interest in the problem of obesity, however, many larger medical centers now offer a team approach to the evaluation and treatment of obesity, such as detailed elsewhere in the volume.

Having decided who needs to lose or maintain weight as children grow, how shall these goals be accomplished? First, there is consistent agreement among clinicians and researchers that a reasonable diet and level of activity should be reached. No matter what factors are ultimately shown to be the proximate causes of obesity, our stated goals should not awaken controversy in reasonable individuals even if the method to reach these goals is sometimes in question. For example, common sense informs us that highly sweetened beverages and juices increase caloric intake, leading to weight gain; however, although there are compelling data that this is true for sodas, there is less strong evidence that juice consumption has the same effects, even if the caloric content is similar or higher than for soda [8]. Later in the volume, the content of diets (e.g., calories, fat, and carbohydrate) is discussed, but the society of obesity researchers is far from agreement on what modifications should be universal in our attempts to control weight gain. The new discipline of nutrigenomics should give us just such valuable information. Our creative discussions in the scientific community foster confusion — and even disbelief — in the community, at a time when a clear message is all the more important. Perhaps we can at least agree on two statements: fun and safe forms of exercise can be supported by all, and reduced caloric intake in those who consume an excess of calories is a desirable goal.

How can we change behavior in our quest to increase activity and consume a reasonable diet? As you will see later in the volume, there are effective societal, group, and individual approaches to the problem. Many use behavior modification in those who demonstrate that they are ready to accept change in their life. However, it is clear that if either the child or the family is not ready to change, no changes will occur. Because of a high rate of recidivism, constant reinforcement is necessary. The recent rewording of the Medicare guidelines that accept obesity as a chronic disease should remind us that some consistent level of attention is required to lose or maintain weight once obesity develops. Others say that our warnings have made adolescents "afraid to eat" and have driven children to unsafe dieting practices, even as we fail to show widespread success of our behavior modification methods [9].

One of our goals in any program is first to "do no harm." The several-years-long Pathways program addressed the children of the population with the highest prevalence of obesity and its complications — Native Americans. Pathways used the expertise of some of our best researchers to craft a comprehensive curriculum. Still, with such maximal effort, the BMI of the children rose, although much important knowledge was gained through the implementation of the study [10]. This experience further emphasized the difficulty in addressing the problem.

We know that family-centered behavior modification therapy for younger children and individual or family-centered therapy for adolescents can be effective [11]. How can we spread such success to a majority of the pediatric population? The cost in personnel of such measures would likely be staggering, given the numbers of overweight and obese children. Although the cost of such a program depends on numerous details, a 10-week program could be carried out for approximately $100 to $600 per child. Cost reductions might be achieved by using proven, standardized techniques; by the use of specially trained "lay" counselors; by incorporating effective curricula, perhaps in the (admittedly overextended) public school system; or by invoking techniques of extending personnel such as telemedicine, whereby a few providers can reach many more subjects.

These measures can likely be made effective and should be made widely available with adequate support. However, targeted behavior modification techniques could be offered, but the requirement for large numbers of personnel and the expense involved remains an issue.

A few medications are available to address obesity, and more are being developed. The best will focus on our basic understanding of the control of appetite and food intake, as well as energy expenditure. However, at the time of this writing, only orlistat is available for subjects as young as 10 years, although there is a likelihood that sibutramine may soon follow suit. Unfortunately, the mean loss of weight using available medications approximates 5 to 8% over what behavior modification or placebo treatment can accomplish alone. These measures may not be adequate to address the problem of children and adolescents who have BMI values over the 97th percentile, as far more than 10% weight loss may be desirable. Still, the loss of 10% weight in adults does improve their elevated lipid levels, their insulin resistance, and other features of obesity, and it may be a reachable and commendable goal in childhood as well. How long shall we treat these children with medications? Present trials rarely exceed a few months, and there are no large studies with long-term results spanning years as yet. Weight loss medications would be taken for many decades if started in childhood. Of course, there are no presently approved medications approved for use over such long periods. Furthermore, studies demonstrate a form of tachyphylaxis, in which the weight loss "reaches a wall," and weight no longer decreases. Shall we, without adequate study, treat children over four to six decades of their lives with medications? If comorbidities can be reduced in overweight children with moderate weight loss, and if careful study demonstrates long-term safety, perhaps this approach will prove viable, just as insulin or oral hypoglycemic agents are the appropriate treatments for diabetes mellitus over decades. However, once again, the cost for addressing the population will be remarkably high. On the basis of the price of the agents in today's markets, medical therapy approximates $240 per month, depending on the source.

Surgery has, to date, been reported in an anecdotal manner or in small groups of children retrospectively studied [12]. The results of prospective studies are needed, and such studies have already begun. The only proven long-term method of weight control in adults has been bariatric surgery. Perhaps this technique has a role in childhood. First, the long-term safety of these methods must be proven, appropriate bone acquisition and physical (including pubertal) development must be demonstrated, and nutritional status must be evaluated before this approach can be supported. In addition, reports from the adult literature demonstrate the necessity for effective behavior change, as the subject may be able to circumvent the procedure and gain some or all of the weight back. Thus, behavior modification is an essential component to weight loss surgery in children and adolescents. Bariatric surgery programs for youth with comprehensive evaluation and treatment are in progress that will allow the collection of prospective data. The dilemma is that lack of success in changing one's habits is one reason some of the younger candidates were proposed for surgery initially. Surgery will no doubt be invoked in some young subjects who have substantial, life-threatening complications of obesity. However, for practical reasons alone, such as cost and personnel requirements, surgery cannot become the common approach to the problem.

What should the focus be in the arena of childhood obesity? If we accept the concept that our present epidemic is based on environmental effects exerted on a susceptible genetic predisposition, we must address these environmental issues, as manipulation of genes is not yet possible and may not be desirable. Effective prevention of the development of obesity should be the goal. This is emphasized in the Institute of Medicine's recent volume, *Preventing Childhood Obesity: Health in the Balance*, which appropriately emphasizes the importance of prevention of obesity [13]. This volume also lays out goals for industry, government, education, families, and of course, medical professionals. A recent critical review of childhood obesity provides another rich resource of what is known about prevention and treatment of this complex subject [14].

We must find effective methods of turning back the clock to allow children to grow up with BMI values characteristic of past decades as they live in their 21st-century environment. Rather than targeting a portion of the population, the healthy habits that can counteract increased weight gain must be applied to the entire population. If we are fostering healthy habits of diet and exercise in all, all should benefit. Too often politicians or pundits speak of the individual's or parent's responsibility in the development of their obesity, rather than attempting to understand the complex network of social and commercial changes over and above parenting abilities that contribute to this state. Only by applying prevention techniques to all will we reduce or eliminate the social stigma that may develop if we focus only on those who most need to modify their lives with increased activity and a healthy diet. Our goal should be improvement in the habits of the whole population. If we are successful in reducing the portion of the population above the 85th percentile of BMI for age to 15% and above the 95th percentile of BMI for age to 5% by preventative measures, we can then focus our behavior, medial, or invasive techniques on the then smaller numbers needing such interventions.

The role of the readers of these volumes extends further than the development of treatment or research programs. Those interested in this field must lend their expertise and voice to the local, state, and national government agencies that need direction as they confront this epidemic. Lay advocacy must be encouraged. Some actions must be taken to foster prevention even if all the results of studies, performed or planned, are not yet completed. We must reach consensus on promising, even if unproven, commonsense techniques if the likelihood of harm is small in approaches. We must translate that knowledge into action. More important, we must, in addition to being researchers and clinicians, be advocates for healthy habits for all. We have seen failure to modify weight gain patterns in large, carefully thought-out, multisite studies that held promise. This only further emphasizes the fact that we have our work cut out for us as we rise to the challenge.

## REFERENCES

1. Hedley, A. A., C. L. Ogden, C. L. Johnson, M. D. Carroll, L. R. Curtin, and K. M. Flegal. Prevalence of overweight and obesity among U.S. children, adolescents, and adults, 1999–2002. *JAMA,* 291(23):2847–2850, 2004.
2. Styne, D. M. Childhood and adolescent obesity. Prevalence and significance. *Pediatr Clin North Am.* 48:823–854, vii, 2001.
3. Cohen, J. Overweight kids: Why should we care? 2000. California State Library, CRB-00-008.
4. Hu, F. B., W. C. Willett, T. Li, M. J. Stampfer, G. A. Colditz, and J. E. Manson. Adiposity as compared with physical activity in predicting mortality among women. *N Engl J Med.* 351:2694–2703, 2004.
5. Flegal, K. M. and R. P. Troiano. Changes in the distribution of body mass index of adults and children in the U.S. population. *Int J Obes Relat Metab Disord.* 24:807–818, 2000.
6. Styne, D. M. Puberty, obesity and ethnicity. *Trends Endocrinol Metab.* 15:472–478, 2004.
7. Barlow, S. E. and W. H. Dietz. Obesity evaluation and treatment: Expert Committee recommendations. The Maternal and Child Health Bureau, Health Resources and Services Administration and the Department of Health and Human Services. *Pediatrics.* 102:E29, 1998.
8. Ludwig, D. S., K. E. Peterson, and S. L. Gortmaker. Relation between consumption of sugar-sweetened drinks and childhood obesity: a prospective, observational analysis. *Lancet.* 357:505–508, 2001.
9. Berg, F. M. *Children and Teens Afraid to Eat: Helping Youth in Today's Weight-Obsessed World,* 3rd ed. Healthy Weight Publishing Network, 2001, 352.
10. Caballero, B., T. Clay, S. M. Davis, B. Ethelbah, B. H. Rock, T. Lohman, J. Norman, M. Story, E. J. Stone, L. Stephenson, and J. Stevens. Pathways: a school-based, randomized controlled trial for the prevention of obesity in American Indian schoolchildren. *Am J Clin Nutr.* 78:1030–1038, 2003.
11. Epstein, L. H., J. N. Roemmich, and H. A. Raynor. Behavioral therapy in the treatment of pediatric obesity. *Pediatr Clin North Am.* 48:981–993, 2001.
12. Inge, T. H., N. F. Krebs, V. F. Garcia, J. A. Skelton, K. S. Guice, R. S. Strauss et al. Bariatric surgery for severely overweight adolescents: concerns and recommendations. *Pediatrics.* 114:217–223, 2004.
13. Koplan, J. P., C. T. Liverman, and V. A. Krack, Eds., Committee on Prevention of Obesity in Children and Growth. *Preventing Childhood Obesity: Health in the Balance.* Institute of Medicine, Washington, DC: The National Academies Press, 2005, 414.
14. Speiser, B. W., M. C. Rudolf, H. Anhalt, C. Camacho-Hubner, F. Chiarelli, A. Eliakim et al. Childhood obesity. *J Clin Endocrinol Metab.* 90(3):1871–1887, 2005.

# Section 1

## Clinical Management

# 2 The Business of Weight Management

*Melinda S. Sothern*

## CONTENTS

## INTRODUCTION

### ECONOMIC BURDEN OF PEDIATRIC OBESITY

The economic burden of obesity-associated illness during childhood has increased threefold from 35 to 127 million in the last two decades [1,2]. Costs of diseases associated with obesity, including diabetes mellitus, hypertension, heart disease, stroke, gout, arthritis, and cancer, exceed 100 billion dollars per year in the United States, or about 8% of the national health care budget [3]. Insulin resistance, a precursor to type 2 diabetes, has been documented in approximately 25 to 46% [4,5] of overweight adolescents. In one study, 4% of overweight youth had silent type 2 diabetes [4]. In a recent study, it was noted that because of the obesity-related increase in type 2 diabetes, parents of the present generation may outlive their children [6].

### FINANCIAL ASPECTS OF MANAGING PEDIATRIC OBESITY IN THE CLINICAL SETTING

The cost to treat overweight children in clinical settings varies by location, staff expertise, and level of medical care that is provided. Typically, parents bear the burden of cost [7,8]. The few studies available indicate that group treatment programs are more cost-effective than mixed (individual plus group) therapy [9]. In addition, the use of school-based nutrition and physical activity intervention is far less expensive than the cost associated with clinical management and, more important, than the estimated costs associated with adult obesity later in life [2]. Otherwise, there is little information that details the cost of providing clinical treatment to overweight children.

In 1992, Spielman and colleagues [10] reported that the costs to the patient of adult outpatient weight loss programs range from approximately $108 to $2120 per 12-week session. In another study, conducted in 1980, the cost to provide treatment to overweight adults was quoted as $19.05 to $131.20 per week per patient [11]. Cost variations were primarily associated with food products and individual versus group counseling expenses [12]. Surveys of available adult weight loss programs indicate that the costs related to reducing weight by 5 to 10%, the amount recommended to gain health benefits, are reasonable and affordable for most individuals [10].

For many families, the cost of treating obesity is a burden that limits the ability to adhere to dietary recommendations, particularly when it comes to food purchases. This financial burden explains why less disposable income is spent on food, such as lean meats, fish, fresh vegetables, and fruit [13–15]. This is consistent with many studies that believe that more money is needed to attain a healthy diet [13–16]. On the contrary, there is evidence that shows that healthy diets do not increase costs over time [17]. In a study of family-based obesity treatment, the costs of adopting a nutrient-dense diet did not change at 6 months and, in fact, considerably decreased after 1 year, from $6.77 to $5.04 per 1000 kcal of food consumed. A possible explanation for this decrease is that although families purchased more fruits and vegetables, they did not purchase snack food; therefore, the overall food bill decreased [17]. Further research is needed to determine whether these findings can be replicated for their beneficial results. Financial considerations of promoting physical activity and medications costs are also lacking in research.

### CHALLENGES OF PROVIDING CLINICAL MANAGEMENT OF PEDIATRIC OBESITY

In most cases, pediatric obesity is the result of overeating and underactivity. Most scientists and clinicians believe that early intervention addressing these factors, along with family guidance to promote healthy lifestyles, is the key to the successful management of pediatric obesity [18]. The pediatric obesity scientific literature presents strong arguments for encouraging methods to prevent the onset of obesity in youth [19–22]. Unfortunately, for the 10 million children in the United States who are already classified as overweight, prevention is not an option [23]. There are, of course, many challenges to providing weight management interventions to these overweight children, including financial and time limitations. That said, there are also many well-designed studies that document successful weight loss, improvement of chronic disease factors, and long-term weight maintenance in overweight children [24,25]. Cost-effective, targeted family-based dietary and physical activity interventions are available [22]. Physician-supervised individual and group programs that use quality, clinically proven, and scientifically tested approaches should be encouraged for the treatment of pediatric obesity. Many common barriers to providing such treatment can be addressed through education, careful planning, and the application of sound implementation strategies [26].

## MODELS FOR HEALTH EDUCATION, HEALTH PROMOTION AND PROGRAM DEVELOPMENT

Systematic planning models should be consulted before beginning the process of organizing a weight management program. Popular health promotion models include the Predisposing, Reinforcing, and Enabling constructs in Educational/Ecological Diagnosis and Evaluation (PRECEDE)–Policy, Regulatory, and Organizational Constructs in Educational and Environmental Development (PROCEED) model, the Multilevel Approach to Community Health (MATCH) model, the Social Marketing Assesment and Response Tool (SMART), and others [27]. Green and Kreuter [28] detail the PRECEDE-PROCEED model, which was developed over two decades. There are nine phases of this model, which begin with a detailed assessment of social, epidemiological, behavioral, and environmental factors related to the target population. Educational, ecological, and administrative and policy factors are also reviewed. It is only after careful consideration and study of these factors that planners then select the methods and strategies required for implementation of the health promotion program [28]. The MATCH model was developed for use in community settings [29]. It is a multilevel approach that begins with goals selection and intervention planning and places less emphasis on the assessment of target audience needs [30]. Consumer-based planning requires a different approach and uses health communication skills to influence perceptions, social norms, and awareness. SMART is a social marketing planning framework composed of seven phases including consumer analysis, market analysis, and channel analysis [31,32]. SMART is a useful model to refer to when analyzing the needs of the target audience and during the planning of the marketing phase of weight management interventions.

## THE PLANNING PROCESS

Perhaps the most significant step in the planning process is enlisting the support of the organization's administration and decision makers [27]. This requires precise and accurate information concerning the specific health problem, a careful analysis of the needs of the target population, and the identification of common values and benefits. In the case of pediatric obesity treatment, studies indicate that the public, in general, recognizes that pediatric obesity is a significant health problem and is very supportive of interventions to reduce weight in youth [33]. Of particular interest to the public are school-, community-, and media-based approaches that increase healthy nutrition and physical activity. Although the family environment was not considered, 91% of study respondents felt that parents were most responsible for reducing overweight conditions in childhood [33]. This indicates, at least in part, support for family-based educational interventions.

The argument of a reduction in heath care costs is often used to promote pediatric weight management programs to decision makers and high-level administration. As stated earlier, obesity-related chronic diseases significantly affect health care costs not only during childhood [2,4] but also later, during adulthood [3,34,35]. However, a link must be established between the pediatric obesity risk factors that the intervention will modify and the medical expenditures associated with those risks specifically [36]. Wang and colleagues [2] conducted an economic analysis of a school-based program, Planet Health, to assess the cost effectiveness and cost benefit of preventing obesity in youth. They estimated intervention costs to be approximately $14.00 per child and illustrated that if only 2% of children were prevented from developing obesity, the total savings to society would be $7300 per child. These types of analysis are suggested for use in influencing federal and state level health care decision makers [37]. However, many organizations favor programs that promote health care reductions in the short term. Often it is difficult to "sell" downstream benefits to decision makers, and ultimately, the cost to modify behaviors that lower health risks must clearly be below the cost of later treatment [36].

Another approach to gaining the support of decision makers is the presentation of successful program outcomes, both locally and nationally [27]. There are a few studies that demonstrate successful weight loss outcome in individual primary care settings [38–40]. However, the short-term benefits of multidisciplinary treatment programs including dietary, exercise, and behavioral counseling intervention for overweight youth are well established [41–50] (see Appendix A3.1.1). In Chapter 13 of this volume, Martin and Myers detail the results of successful pediatric weight management programs over the last two decades.

## ASSESSING THE NEEDS OF YOUR TARGET POPULATION

### Needs Assessment

The needs assessment determines the health problems of a specific population [51] and what action will resolve the problem. Data can be collected from secondary sources, such as scientific literature searches and government statistics, or from primary sources, such as surveys, focus groups, or observations. Secondary data on the prevalence and progression of pediatric obesity are abundant. Nationally published statistics and reference material may be used to establish program need (see Appendix A3.1.2). For example, the prevalence of obesity in children and adolescents is higher than 20 years ago in all ethnic, age, and gender groups [52–54]. Over 11% of these children are considered overweight or obese, defined as greater than the 95th percentile for age and height (U.S. Centers for Disease Control Body Mass Index Percentiles) [55], and children are becoming obese at younger ages [56]. The prevalence of obesity in teenagers has tripled in the past 40 years. Additional prevalence data and advocacy information can be found in Chapter 1 of this volume by Styne.

The research literature clearly establishes a link between pediatric obesity and a multitude of health problems. This information may be used to further establish the need for the creation of a pediatric weight management program. For example, the escalating rates of adolescent obesity will affect the future health of Americans [57,58]. According to the U.S. Surgeon General, risk factors for heart disease, such as high cholesterol and high blood pressure, occur with increased frequency in overweight children and adolescents compared with children with a healthy weight. At present, 80% of children diagnosed with Blount disease and 50 to 70% of those with slipped capital femoral epiphyses are significantly overweight [1]. There is an 80% correlation between obesity and a very serious neurological disorder called Pseudotumor cerebri. Type 2 diabetes, previously considered an adult disease, has increased dramatically in children and adolescents. Overweight and obesity are closely linked to type 2 diabetes, which has increased 10-fold between 1982 and 1994. Refer to Chapter 3 by Jacobson for more information on the medical complications of childhood obesity.

An example of primary data collection can be found in a recent study by Roux and colleagues [59]. They applied a method called the Discrete Choice Experiment to evaluate a monetary measure of benefit, willingness to pay, to overweight individuals seeking treatment. The willingness to pay factors considered most valuable to consumers were accessibility, individualized or tailored approach specific to their needs, and comprehensive program (including diet, self management, and exercise). Although an adult study, results could be considered in the planning of pediatric weight management programs because it is the parents of overweight children who typically make financial decisions with regard to medical treatment. Service needs and demands must both be considered. Thus, when acquiring needs assessment data, primary source information from the target population is equally as critical as that provided by the planner's survey of secondary sources.

## Site Analysis

As was stated earlier, in adults, one of the most desirable factors in seeking weight management treatment is convenience [59]. Selecting a site for treatment that is within easy reach of families may be important. Care must be taken to ensure that the site has sufficient space and equipment to facilitate the delivery of quality care. Specific space requirements for conducting a pediatric weight management program are detailed in the "Identification and Allocation of Resources" section later in this chapter.

## Learner Analysis

Participants who should be considered eligible for pediatric weight management programs are children ranging in age from 5 to 17 years. Their parents will typically range in age from 25 to 55 years. Participants will be referred to the program by physicians or other health care professionals or may be self-referred after learning of the program through the media. The overweight level of the patients will range from greater than the 85th to greater than the 99th percentile BMI (body mass index; Appendix A1.10). If the program is a private endeavor requiring a self payment, the participants will most likely be from middle- to upper-socioeconomic status households. Government-assisted programs will likely enroll youth from lower-socioeconomic status households. The participants may be from a variety of ethnic backgrounds. For the purposes of designing the program materials for readability, it is usually safe to assume an average eighth-grade level of education for the parents. Because the children range in age from 7 to 17 years, the materials targeting the children should be developed specifically for each age group — elementary, middle, and high school.

The participants' knowledge base of medicine, nutrition, physical fitness, and psychology may be low and obtained primarily from television, radio, and print media and from elementary school courses. For most participants, this may be the first time they have had experience in a formal, medically supervised multidisciplinary setting. The participants will likely arrive at the pediatric weight management program with many misconceptions about health, nutrition, exercise, and appropriate child development.

## Establishing Goals and Objectives

The goals of a pediatric weight management program are to establish an outpatient clinical service to manage pediatric obesity; to provide a quality medical, nutritional, psychosocial, and physical activity/exercise educational intervention to the overweight child or adolescent along with the entire family; to coordinate the clinical intervention with ongoing medical care and research; and to periodically evaluate the intervention and testing methods to improve program quality and effectiveness.

Specific objectives for patients are as follows: (1) children and adolescents completing the pediatric weight management program will become motivated to adopt specific behaviors associated with long-term emotional, physical, and psychological health; (2) from a medical perspective, children will learn to identify safe and effective methods for achieving and maintaining weight loss; (3) concerning nutrition, children will acquire knowledge of the basic principles of sound nutrition and healthy eating patterns; (4) in the realm of behavior modification, children will become aware of their eating behaviors and activity patterns and will learn alternate behaviors to promote long-term health; and (5) in terms of physical activity and exercise, children will gain the physiologic and kinesthetic awareness necessary to adopt activity patterns that promote long-term health.

The main objective of treatment is to improve eating patterns and increase daily energy expenditure to maintain an existing healthy weight; to stabilize the existing weight while growing,

**TABLE 2.1**
**Suggested Objectives of Pediatric Weight Management Program**

**Nutrition Education**

Children will classify foods into the basic food groups.

Children will understand their healthy body weight for age and height.

Children will accurately measure foods and calculate caloric and fat content.

Children will identify foods high in calories, sugar, and saturated fat.

Children will analyze food labels and menus.

**Behavior Modification**

Children will improve their self-esteem, self-efficacy, and self-control.

Children will reduce anxiety and depression associated with obesity.

Children will recognize techniques to alter eating behaviors to promote and maintain weight loss and health.

Children will identify positive behaviors associated with long-term health.

**Exercise and Fitness**

Children will identify the basic components of fitness.

Children will identify the types of exercise appropriate to achieving a healthy body weight.

Children will become aware of body parts and movements that facilitate the acquisition of a balanced, well-trained, and healthy physique.

Children will increase daily activity levels and, therefore, increase daily energy expenditure.

Children will maintain or increase lean muscle tissue.

Children will improve muscular strength and endurance.

Children will improve cardiorespiratory endurance.

Children will improve muscular flexibility.

Children will gain vigor and an overall feeling of well-being.

until a healthy weight is achieved; or to reduce body weight to a healthy level. Specific medical objectives include maintaining or achieving a body weight that corresponds with ≤ 85th percentile BMI, and a reduction in total cholesterol, triglycerides, and percentage body fat while maintaining normal biochemical parameters, thus significantly reducing the present and future risk of chronic disease. Specific nutrition education, behavior modification, and physical activity/exercise objectives are outlined in Table 2.1.

## DESIGNING HEALTH PROMOTION INTERVENTIONS

### APPLYING HEALTH PROMOTION MODELS AND THEORIES TO PRACTICE

It is vital that pertinent models and theories are used when designing health promotion programs. There are numerous health promotion theories and models that have been applied to the planning and implementation of pediatric intervention programs. In Chapters 5, 14, and 20, Schwimmer, Sothern, and von Almen provide detailed descriptions and thorough literature reviews of studies that have successfully incorporated these models and theories. Once an appropriate model or theory has been selected to meet the established goals and objectives, the design of the intervention can begin. Program planners should consider the results of the needs assessment and the different types of intervention activities [51]. They should also refer to standardized guidelines published by public health, medical, research, and educational institutions to ensure that the intervention will be safe, credible, and ethical [19,24,60,61]. There are hundreds of well-established, well-studied programs available for increasing physical activity and promoting healthy nutrition (see Appendix A3.1.1, A3.1.2, and A3.1.3). Many of these programs target children at risk for developing obesity and those who are already considered overweight. Sometimes it may be more advantageous to consider implementing an existing program or adapting the program components of these interventions to the specific needs of your population. In all cases, be aware of the existing copyright and trademark requirements associated with each program.

## MARKETING

The current pediatric epidemic is neither the fault nor the responsibility of any one single sector of society [22]. There are several areas to consider when attempting to change public opinion and behavior concerning healthy nutrition and physical activity. There are five major target areas that can be identified (Table 2.2) [22]. The marketing of these various segments is part of a step-by-step process called audience or market segmentation [27]. This type of marketing approach helps to ensure that programs are specific to the needs of the target consumer group. Consumers typically want to know primarily whether weight management interventions are safe [62]. Second, they seek specific information concerning the type of diet used, a description of the behavior modification component, and the cost. Surprisingly, in one study, the credentials of the staff were not considered important by consumers seeking commercial weight loss treatment [62]. This information is valuable when designing promotions and advertising strategies for weight management programs. There are no specific

---

**TABLE 2.2**
**Target Areas — Obesity Prevention in Children**

**Family and Home Environment**

Parental education and awareness
Neighborhood safety

**Public Educators, Administrators, and School Environment**

Cafeteria
Physical education
Academic classroom
After school and recess
Nonfood incentives for academic achievement and positive behavior

**Health Care (obstetricians, pediatricians, family physicians, dietitians, psychologists, exercise and related health care professionals)**

Patient education
Monitoring of high-risk populations
Referral system
Prevention and treatment programs
Maintenance and relapse prevention programs.

**Public Policy**

Insurance and governmental reimbursement for medical evaluation, monitoring prevention, treatment, and maintenance programs
Food labeling and packaging (portion control)
School nutrition and physical activity policy (cafeteria, vending machines, unstructured physical activity periods [recess], physical education class, limits on homework, grants and funds to schools that promote a healthy school environment)
Work site policy (flex time, home offices, family and medical leave)
Youth media and marketing
Increased funding for childhood overweight research

**Public Awareness**

Community programs
Promotions and social marketing campaigns

*Source:* With permission, Sothern, M. S. Obesity prevention in children: physical activity and nutrition. *Nutrition,* 20:704–708, 2004.

---

studies addressing the needs and concerns of parents of overweight children. Thus, careful application of information gathered from the needs assessment should be included in the marketing process.

Next, it is important to develop informative and persuasive communication flows [27]. Several questions must first be answered: What are the costs of treatment versus the worth? Will the message reach a large proportion of the parents of overweight children? If so, how frequently should it be delivered, and through which channels? Planners should consider the type of product that will meet the needs of the largest proportion of overweight children. They should first determine who is most likely going to pay for the program [27]. Typically, third-party payer reimbursement rates for the treatment of pediatric obesity are very low [8]. Therefore, planners may need to consider a self-pay program, in which case it will be the parents who are responsible for the costs of the pediatric weight management program. "Selling" the program to parents may be quite challenging, especially if they are also overweight. Moreover, adults report that they support school and community intervention for the prevention and treatment of pediatric obesity, which may indirectly indicate a lack of support for programs that target the home environment [33].

### Program Promotion: Getting the Word Out

The participants who successfully complete the weight management program provide "word-of-mouth" advertising and promotion; however, if you are just starting up a program in your area, you will need to let the community know about your services. You should develop two brochures, one aimed at parents and another at referring physicians. Consider the information obtained in your needs assessment when drafting the text for the brochure. The brochures should include details of your program, location, and fees. You may choose to develop and mail a quarterly newsletter to your patients, along with notices of upcoming special events. As the successes of the program accumulate, the local newspapers, magazines, and radio and television reporters, along with institutional public relations departments, may want to offer feature articles on your patients' progress.

## IMPLEMENTING A HEALTH PROMOTION PROGRAM

There are several implementation strategies, including pilot programming, preliminary field testing, and phasing-in approaches [27]. Experienced planners do not recommend a total implementation approach. Rather, a pilot or preliminary test is preferred to gain primary data from participants for the purpose of revising and tailoring the intervention, and to provide marketing information. Borg and Gall's Research and Development Cycle provides a sound, systematic plan to health promotion program implementation that details the use of pilot testing [63].

### CONCERNS OF IMPLEMENTATION

Several medical, legal, and ethical issues must be considered before program implementation. Safety is the primary concern [65,66]. Thorough preliminary testing, along with careful review of the existing medical literature, will ensure that the components of the program are sound. Regardless, interventionists must do everything to reduce the risk of liability associated with treatment. Informed consent must be obtained from the patient and his or her parents [65,66], medical concerns related to the treatment of obesity must be documented [67,68], and staff must be licensed, degreed, and certified professionals who are well trained in all aspects of treatment, including testing and interpersonal skills [69]. These are often standard practices in clinical settings. However, if parts of the program will be delivered outside of the physician's office, care must be taken to ensure that related personnel and sites are well-prepared and safe.

Another concern is sufficient preparation time. Recruiting and training staff, ordering equipment, and marketing takes weeks and often months in large organizations. A suggested timeline for successful implementation is presented in Table 2.3.

**TABLE 2.3**
**Pediatric Weight Management Implementation Flow Chart**

| Time before First Orientation, days | Action |
|---|---|
| 210 | Recruit staff and select intervention site |
| 180 | Attend Pediatric Weight Management Professional Training (Appendix A3.1.1) |
| 150 | Staff meeting to review testing and intervention techniques |
|  | Begin media campaign |
| 120 | Order supplies and equipment |
|  | Mail out physician, school, and community center advertising letters |
| 90 | Mail public service announcements introducing program in your area |
| 60 | Establish patient/parent communication system |
|  | Answer phone and mail inquiries |
|  | Mail out information brochures as necessary |
|  | Enroll and register new patients |
|  | Begin screening of new patients |
| 45 | Mail public service announcement for community/parent information session |
|  | Continue screening and enrollment of new patients |
| 21 | Community/parent information session |
|  | Continue screening and enrollment of new patients |
| 14 | Continue screening and enrollment of new patients |
|  | Staff meeting to finalize intervention schedule |
| 7 | Review intervention materials |
|  | Finalize class roster |
|  | Begin media campaign for next session |

## IDENTIFICATION AND ALLOCATION OF RESOURCES

### Personnel

*Organization of the Pediatric Weight Management Program Staff*

At the center of the pediatric weight management program is the family (Figure 2.1). A family physician or pediatrician leads the team as the medical director. He or she provides medical supervision and guidance for the clinic, performs medical history and physical examinations, and conducts educational sessions on the medical aspects of the program. The remaining staff members include a registered dietician, a behavior specialist, an exercise specialist, and the clinic coordinator. The registered dietitian provides nutritional supervision and guidance for the clinic, conducts weekly

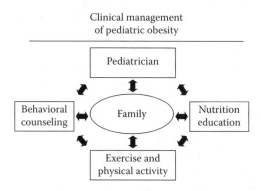

**FIGURE 2.1** Organization of the pediatric weight management program staff.

educational sessions on nutrition topics, and instructs patients in the proper administration of the clinic diet. A dietician with experience in the pediatric setting is desirable. The exercise specialist provides exercise supervision and guidance and conducts weekly educational sessions on the physical fitness aspects of pediatric obesity. The exercise specialist should be a degreed professional with experience in adapting exercise to children of all ages. The behavior specialist provides instruction in behavior-modification skills and techniques and conducts weekly educational sessions on the psychosocial aspects of obesity in children. The behavior specialist should be a degreed and licensed counselor or psychologist with experience in family therapy. The clinic coordinator super-vises patient scheduling and billing for the program and is responsible for day-to-day office and program functions. It is recommended that the coordinator be experienced in health care manage-ment. He or she supervises the secretary-receptionist, who provides clerical support for the clinic and is responsible for communicating with parents and patients. The coordinator also oversees the distribution of information about the clinic to prospective clients, as well as news of upcoming events (see Table 2.3). A sample job description for pediatric weight management clinical coordi-nator may be found in the Appendix A1.1.

## Space

The minimal space requirements to conduct a multidisciplinary intervention in a clinical setting for 10 to 15 families are as follows: meeting room (500 sq. ft.), exercise room (800 sq. ft.), patient examination rooms (2 @ 200 sq. ft.), kitchen or nutrition demonstration area (500 sq. ft.), and clinic waiting area (500 sq. ft.)

Suggested sites for pediatric clinical management programs include hospitals, medical centers, and wellness/fitness centers. The following sites may be used for the delivery of the educational intervention in conjunction with a family physician or pediatrician office: community centers, church activity centers, school auditoriums/cafeterias, recreation centers, and reception halls.

## Scheduling

If there is a large amount of meeting space in the facility, staff expenses can be reduced by scheduling several different groups of families during the same clinic interval. This strategy makes the most efficient use of the clinicians' time, which is especially desirable when part-time clinicians are paid on an hourly basis. However, if full-time staff are employed, but meeting space is limited, several groups can be scheduled into separate clinic intervals, whereby the program is offered several times per day on several days per week. This strategy most fully employs existing full-time staff, with the additional advantage of smaller intervention groups. In all cases, if different groups of families are conducted during one clinic interval, there should be at least a 10- to 20-minute interval of time when all of the members of the intervention team are conducting the session together. This is the time during which the "team" approach is greatly reinforced. Researchers attribute much of the success of multidisciplinary pediatric weight management programs to the peer support and coun-seling the kids receive during these integrated, interactive, multidisciplinary sessions [49,50,70]. A sample pediatric weight management class schedule may be found in Table 2.4. If there are more than two groups of families attending clinic at the same time, the intervention clinicians can alternate between groups during the session (Table 2.5). A blank schedule may be found in Appendix A1.2.

## Intervention Materials, Equipment, and Supplies

The intervention materials, equipment, and supplies required to deliver a pediatric weight manage-ment program can be classified in four different categories: clinical administration, educational, incentive, and marketing. Clinical administration materials include patient charts, record forms, growth charts, etc. and equipment and supplies that are necessary to conduct a medical examination and obesity evaluation (Appendix A1). Refer to the testing protocol in Appendix 2 for descriptions

**TABLE 2.4**
**Pediatric Weight Management Sample Class Schedule**

| Time | Medicine | Nutrition | Behavior | Exercise |
|---|---|---|---|---|
| 4:00-4:30 | | Return calls, set up | | |
| 4:30-4:45 | Nurse supervises weigh-in | Check food records | Talk with parents, review charts | Check exercise cards |
| 4:45-5:00 | Accomplishments | Accomplishments | Accomplishments | Accomplishments |
| 5:00-5:30 | Review charts | Nutrition session | Return calls, review charts | Review charts, return calls |
| 5:30-6:00 | Physician Q&A or session | Clean up | Behavior session | Set up, exercise |
| 6:00-6:30 | Physician Q&A or session | | | Exercise session |
| 6:30-7:00 | Clean up | Clean up | Clean up | Clean up |

**TABLE 2.5**
**Pediatric Weight Management Class Schedule — Two groups**

| Time | Medicine | Nutrition | Behavior | Exercise |
|---|---|---|---|---|
| 4:00-4:30 | Set up | Set up | Set up | Set up |
| 4:30-4:50 | Nurse supervises weigh-in | Check food records | Talk with parents, review charts, return calls | Check exercise cards |
| 4:50-5:00 | Accomplishments | Accomplishments | Accomplishments | Accomplishments |
| 5:00-5:30 | Physician Q&A or session | Nutrition education, group 1 | Behavior session, group 2 | Set-up, exercise |
| 5:30-6:00 | | Review charts, return calls | Behavior session, group 1 | Exercise session, group 2 |
| 6:00-6:30 | | Nutrition education, group 2 | | Exercise session, group 1 |
| 6:30-7:00 | Clean up | Clean up | Clean up | Clean up |

*Note:* The intervention clinicians will alternate between groups during the clinic.

of suitable equipment. Educational materials include books, self-monitoring forms, handouts, pamphlets, and so on. Appendix A3 provides a list of resources for pediatric weight management educational materials and sample handouts and self-monitoring forms. Educational equipment and supplies may include audiovisual items, flip charts, and props for modeling sessions, exercise aids, and games (see Appendix A3). Incentives for participants should be healthy, nonfood items. For example, sports equipment and active play games promote increased physical activity and are typically well-received by program participants. Marketing materials should be developed for your individual program. This is discussed in more detail earlier in this chapter. However, there are dozens of national resource centers that provide, often free of charge, items to assist you with promoting your program (see Appendix A3.1.2).

## Financial Resources

Funding remains the greatest barrier to successful implementation of pediatric weight management programs. Even though there is a consistent message of concern regarding pediatric obesity in the media, clinical weight management programs receive minimal federal funding [7], are often not reimbursed by insurance companies or other third parties [8], and lack understanding by the general

**TABLE 2.6**
**Sample 1-Year, Weekly Outpatient Pediatric Weight Management Budget**

**Income**

| | |
|---|---|
| Patient fees (40 children @ $40/wk [48 wks]) | $76,800 |
| Insurance/government payments | * |
| Other (sponsors, contributions, grants) | **17,168 |
| Total income | $93,968 |

**Expenses**

| | |
|---|---|
| Intervention staff (4 @ $4,992/year [based on $104/session] @ 48 weekly sessions) | $19,968 |
| Blood Tests (40 @ [baseline and 12 weeks] @ $650) | 52,000 |
| Physician examination fees (40 @ $350) | 14,000 |
| Educational supplies (40 @ $200) | 8,000 |
| Total expenses | $93,968 |

* Varies by state, company, and location.
** Amount of additional funding required if medical insurance or government funding is not available.

public [33]. Unless you are able to engage the support of decision makers to provide funding for treatment, you will need to survey the financial resources that are available. The first step in this process is the development of a budget.

## Preparing a Budget

Sponsors ultimately want to know the "bottom line" of pediatric weight management. Will the costs to deliver such a service outweigh the proposed funding? A carefully planned budget will consider the various sources of income, including participant fees, grants, insurance reimbursement, and contributions [27]. Expenses will include personnel, space, medical testing, intervention materials, supplies, marketing, and travel. Table 2.6 describes a typical 1-year budget for a pediatric weight management program enrolling approximately 10 families per session. Carefully consider any additional income sources or expenses specific to your institution before finalizing your budget.

## PEDIATRIC WEIGHT MANAGEMENT PROGRAM: STEP-BY-STEP INSTRUCTIONS

The pediatric weight management program (Table 2.7) emphasizes lifestyle adjustment through behavioral modification of activity level, eating patterns, and family and personal thoughts and attitudes. Only one study, by Saelens and colleagues [38], evaluated the posttreatment and short-term follow-up efficacy of a 4-month behavioral weight control program for overweight adolescents in a primary care setting. The results indicated that a physician-based, individual counseling program including nutrition and physical activity education was superior to a standard care approach in overweight teenagers. However, over 40 evidence-based studies using a multidisciplinary, family-based intervention have been published to date [24]. This multidisciplinary approach has produced some of the most promising results to date in the treatment of pediatric obesity. This section of the chapter provides the supporting materials you will need to implement a group, family-based, multidisciplinary pediatric weight management program that effectively serves the needs of overweight children and adolescents ages 5 to 17 years.

## Referral from Pediatrician, Family Physician, or Phone Inquiry

In step 1, the receptionist discusses the program in detail with parents and referring physicians who have telephoned, inquiring about the program. It is helpful to have a basic information sheet to

**TABLE 2.7**
**Pediatric Weight Management Program:**
**Step-by-Step Instructions**

| Step | Action Item |
| --- | --- |
| 1 | Referral from pediatrician or family physician. |
| 2 | Community/parent information session and registration (optional) |
| 3 | History and physical |
| 4 | Patient screening |
| 5 | Assign patients to the appropriate treatment |
| 6 | Orientation session |
| 7 | Initial evaluation |
| 8 | Initial lesson |
| 9 | Intervention classes |
| 10 | Follow-up evaluation |
| 11 | Registration for incoming participants |
| 12 | Awards, graduation, new goals |

assist the receptionist. He or she fills in the Phone Screening and Information Form (Appendix A1.3) and the Physician Referral Form (Appendix A1.4) completely. These forms are then placed into a collated patient file. A cover letter, program brochure, and Registration Form (Appendix A1.5) are mailed to the patient's address. As a courtesy, program diet and exercise instructions may be mailed to the referring physician also. The patient's insurance company or referring physician is contacted at this time for precertification.

## Parent Information Session and Registration

Two to 3 weeks before the orientation meeting the staff may conduct a 1-hour information session to attract new patients. Media announcements should be mailed at least 2 weeks before the information session. The session may consist of staff introduction, a formal presentation, and a 15-minute question-and-answer session. The session is detailed in full in Chapter 19 by Carlisle and Gordon. Registration forms should be available, and parents may choose to register and pay the appropriate fees at this time or complete at home and mail to the center.

## History and Physical

After receiving the completed registration form and fee deposit from the parent, the receptionist schedules the patient for an appointment with the staff pediatrician or the referring physician. The Medical History and Physical Examination Form (Appendix A1.6), located in the patient file, is completed by the family and the staff pediatrician during this visit. The Clearance Form (Appendix A1.7) is filled in and put into the file, and the file is given back to the receptionist. The receptionist mails the Program Information Letter (Appendix A1.8) and telephones the patient to give instructions.

## Patient Screening

The staff psychologist meets with the family and completes the Initial Parent Questionnaire (Appendix A1.9), which should be located in the patient file. This can be done at the same time as the physical examination or in a separate meeting. However, this must be done before the orientation meeting. The staff dietitian uses the height and weight variables obtained at the physical examination to plot the patient on the Centers for Disease Control and Prevention BMI percentiles also to be housed in the patient file. He or she calculates the BMI and overweight status using the BMI percentiles (Appendix A1.10).

---

**TABLE 2.8**
**Weight Level**

| Level | Status | Percentile |
|-------|--------|------------|
| Level I | Severely overweight | >99th BMI |
| Level II | Overweight | >95th BMI |
| Level III | At risk for overweight | >85th BMI |
| Level IV | Healthy weight | ≤85th BMI |

BMI = body mass index.

---

## Assign Participants to the Appropriate Treatment

Using the Weight Level Form (Table 2.8) and the calculations made by the clinic dietitian of percent overweight (refer to the BMI percentile in the Patient File), the child is assigned to a class roster form in the appropriate level. The receptionist will then mail the parents a letter and telephone them to give the date and the time of the clinic meeting.

## Orientation

The orientation meeting is attended by all the weight management staff members, the patients, and their families. Patients' files should be available. The receptionist should prepare extra patient files and information packets with registration forms for late registrants. Educational materials are handed to each family as they arrive and sign in, provided they are registered and have paid the deposit. The medical or program director introduces the weight management staff and begins the presentation. The other staff members may participate. The Orientation Handout (Appendix A1.11) is discussed. The Class Schedule (Appendix A1.13) and Test Preparation Letter (Appendix A1.16) are distributed and discussed. The clinic coordinator should use the Orientation Checklist (Appendix A1.12) to ensure that all procedures are performed. The orientation session is discussed in more detail in Chapter 19 by Carlisle and Gordon.

## Baseline Evaluation

The initial evaluation session follows the orientation meeting. Weight management staff members should arrive at least 30 minutes before meeting time to set up. Refer to the Evaluation Station Checklist (Appendix A1.18) to direct the staff members to their measurement stations. It is recommended that each station be set up in a separate clinic room. Each patient is then given his or her patient file as he or she reports to the weight and height station. The Evaluation Form (Appendix A1.19) should be located in the patient file. This information will be used to complete the Evaluation Results Form (Appendix A1.20), which will be given to the parents during the next class. The patient then carries the file from one station to the next as the measurements are acquired and recorded. The patients should be directed to stop at the checkout desk before departure, where the clinic coordinator will fill out the final Evaluation Checklist (Appendix A1.17). The evaluation forms are then removed from the patient files and given to the coordinator for processing. After the baseline evaluation, the coordinator will schedule a separate meeting for each patient to participate in a Fitness Evaluation (Appendix A1.21). This can be done before the baseline evaluation, after physician clearance. Detailed protocols for the baseline testing procedures are located in Appendix 2. The staff members should be adequately trained before the baseline evaluation. Staff members should review the clinic testing protocols (Appendix 2) and extensively practice the measurement techniques.

## Initial Lesson

The initial lesson begins with individual weigh-in and medical monitoring. Approximately 20 to 30 minutes is needed for up to 15 patients. Refer to the Weekly Clinic Checklist (Appendix A1.14) to ensure that all procedures are completed. Use the Weight Record and Vital Signs Chart (Appendix A1.15) to record the patient's weight and vital signs. Following this period, the patients and their families sit, auditorium style, with all four clinicians in the front of the room. The behavior specialist leads a discussion of each patient's accomplishments, including weight loss, for the past week, as well as since the patient began the program. Accomplishments such as trying new vegetables or a new exercise activity are also recognized and discussed. Clinicians lead applause after each patient's accomplishment. This period lasts approximately 20 to 30 minutes. Positive reinforcement of healthy eating and exercise behaviors is crucial to the success of the program during this period.

Diet instruction follows for the next 45 to 60 minutes, including questions from the patients and the parents. If time permits, and if they are available, the results of the baseline evaluations may be discussed; otherwise, this discussion can be done during lesson 2. The exercise educational materials are briefly discussed by the exercise physiologist. The behavior specialist briefly discusses self monitoring.

## Intervention Classes

Intervention lessons follow the same general format as lesson 1, which describes a typical setting. However, in lessons 2 through 9, nutrition, behavior, and exercise sessions are conducted over approximately 30 minutes each (Tables 2.4 and 2.5). In addition, the clinicians may structure the group intervention as they feel appropriate. For example, the parents may participate in an activity with the dietitian while the patients participate in an activity with the behavior specialist. Older patients and their families may participate in an exercise activity while younger patients and their families participate in a kitchen activity. Many other combinations may apply. Refer to Chapters 12 by Schumacher et al., 14 by VanVrancken-Tompkins and Sothern et al., 20 by von Almen and Sothern, and Appendix A3 for sample lesson plans. The final lesson follows the same format as lessons 2 through 9, except that a small amount of time either at the beginning or at the end of class is dedicated to preparing the patients for the follow-up evaluations, which should be conducted at the next class meeting.

## Quarterly Evaluation Follow-Up

Interventionists should conduct the quarterly follow-up evaluation in a similar manner as the baseline evaluation. Remember to use the Evaluation Form (Appendix A1.19) to record the measures, which will then be inserted into the Quarterly Evaluation Results Form (Appendix A1.22). Refer to the Protocol descriptions for each of the measures (Appendix 2).

Prior to the last session, Awards, Graduation and New Goals, registration should begin for incoming participants. Repeat steps 1 through 5. The parent information session for incoming participants may be scheduled on the same night as the final lesson directly afterward. The orientation session for incoming participants may be scheduled to run simultaneously with the follow-up evaluation in a separate meeting room. Likewise, the baseline evaluation for incoming participants may be conducted in the clinic rooms on the same day continuing participants are presented with awards in a separate meeting room. Thus, continuing and incoming participants may begin lesson 1 during the next weekly meeting (Table 2.5).

## Awards, Graduation, New Goals

During the class that follows the quarterly evaluations, the parents are again given the results of their child's health and fitness evaluations (Appendix A1.22). These are discussed in the group setting, with particular attention given to the positive changes achieved by the patients over the term of the program. Before this class, the clinicians calculate the new goal weights and current BMI percentile; these are listed on the Quarterly Evaluation Results Form (Appendix A1.22). On the basis of these results, a decision is made whether to "graduate" the patient to the next level. Patients who graduate can be given a certificate. Awards can also be given for perfect attendance (prizes may be T-shirts, inexpensive sports equipment, or similar items). An exercise certificate and award can also be given to the boy and the girl with the highest total number of exercise minutes recorded on the exercise self-monitoring records. Award certificates can also be given for most new vegetables sampled.

## EVALUATING A HEALTH PROMOTION PROGRAM

### EVALUATION APPROACHES

There are several ways to approach the evaluation of your pediatric weight management program. Process evaluation will measure variables associated with the delivery of the intervention such as program times, speakers, and participant attendance and approval ratings [27]. Data gathered will enable the interventionist to assess program compliance and participant adherence and satisfaction. Impact evaluation data measure knowledge, awareness, attitudes, and behaviors. Many of the psychological parameters that are outlined in Chapter 9 by Johnson and von Almen fall into this category (see Appendix 2.5). Outcome evaluation is the most commonly used evaluation in the clinical management of pediatric obesity. This type of evaluation measures the variables that answer the primary goal of the program. Variables typically include morbidity or mortality, vital signs and symptoms, and physiologic and metabolic parameters. Because the primary goal of pediatric weight management is the achievement of a healthy body weight, height and weight indices and anthropometry best determine program success (Appendix 2). By using the baseline and quarterly evaluation results, it is possible to perform simple analyses to determine successful outcome.

### RESULTS AND REPORTING

Data collection, analysis, and reporting are time-consuming, tedious tasks. However, the information gathered from these processes is vital to maintaining a successful program. A sample spreadsheet that can be used to extract data from clinical files is located in Appendix A1.23. This information can easily be transferred to a data management system for further analysis. Many modern computer programs are equipped with systems that can transfer this data into visual presentations for marketing and promotions (Figure 2.2).

## SUMMARY

The business of pediatric weight management, although complex, is doable. The economic effect of reversing obesity during childhood is unknown. However, current costs to treat pediatric obesity–related illness are over $100 million. The cost to provide treatment of pediatric obesity varies, but the short-term positive results of programs using family-based, multidisciplinary approaches are consistent. The task then is to apply sound design principles, health promotion models and theories, and implementation strategies to specific populations and locations. This process requires careful research into the needs of the target audience, the specific health problems surrounding obesity, and the development of goals and objectives. The program must then be organized and structured. Medical, legal, and financial concerns must be addressed. Once this is accomplished, step-by-step implementation will ensure successful outcome, and ongoing program evaluation will maintain program quality.

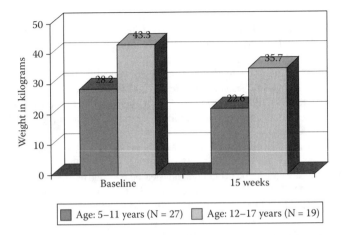

**FIGURE 2.2** Weight change after participation in a pediatric weight management program.

## REFERENCES

1. Must, A. and S. E. Anderson. Effects of obesity on morbidity in children and adolescents. *Nutr Clin Care.* 6:4–12, 2003.
2. Wang, L., Q. Yang, R. Lowry, and H. Wechsler. Economic analysis of a school-based obesity prevention program. *Obes Res.* 11:1313–1324, 2003.
3. Wolf, A. and G. Colditz. Current estimates of the economic cost of obesity in the United States. *Obes Res.* 6:97–106, 1998.
4. Weiss, R., S. Dufour, S. E. Taksali, W. V. Tamborlane, K. F. Petersen, R. C. Bonadonna et al. Prediabetes in obese youth: a syndrome of impaired glucose tolerance, severe insulin resistance, and altered myocellular and abdominal fat partitioning. *Lancet.* 362:951–957, 2003.
5. Viner, R. M., T. Y. Segal, E. Lichtarowicz-Krynska, and P. Hindmarsh. Prevalence of the insulin resistance syndrome in obesity. *Arch Dis Child.* 90:10–14, 2005.
6. Olshansky, S. J., D. J. Passaro, R. C. Hershow, J. Layden, B. A. Carnes, J. Brody et al. A potential decline in life expectancy in the United States in the 21st century. *N Engl J Med.* 352:1138–1145, 2005.
7. Anderson, Z. J. Childhood obesity: assessing the cost. *J Okla State Med Assoc.* 97:418–421, 2004.
8. Tershakovec, A. M., M. H. Watson, W. J. Wenner, Jr., and A. L. Marx. Insurance reimbursement for the treatment of obesity in children. *J Pediatr.* 134:573–578, 1999.
9. Goldfield, G. S., L. H. Epstein, C. K. Kilanowski, R. A. Paluch, and B. Kogut-Bossler. Cost-effectiveness of group and mixed family-based treatment for childhood obesity. *Int J Obes Relat Metab Disord.* 25:1843–1849, 2001.
10. Spielman, A. B., B. Kanders, M. Kienholz, and G. L. Blackburn. The cost of losing: an analysis of commercial weight-loss programs in a metropolitan area. *J Am Coll Nutr.* 11:36–41, 1992.
11. Simko, M. D. and M. T. Conklin. Focusing on the effectiveness side of the cost-effectiveness equation. *J Am Diet Assoc.* 89:485–487, 1989.
12. Witherspoon, B. and M. Rosenzweig. Industry-sponsored weight loss programs: description, cost, and effectiveness. *J Am Acad Nurse Pract.* 16:198–205, 2004.
13. Drewnowski, A., N. Darmon, and A. Briend. Replacing fats and sweets with vegetables and fruits — a question of cost. *Am J Public Health.* 94:1555–1559, 2004.
14. Drewnowski, A. and S. E. Specter. Poverty and obesity: the role of energy density and energy costs. *Am J Clin Nutr.* 79:6–16, 2004.
15. Drewnowski, A. Obesity and the food environment: dietary energy density and diet costs. *Am J Prev Med.* 27:154–162, 2004.
16. Darmon, N., A. Briend, and A. Drewnowski. Energy-dense diets are associated with lower diet costs: a community study of French adults. *Public Health Nutr.* 7:21–27, 2004.

17. Raynor, H. A., C. K. Kilanowski, I. Esterlis, and L. H. Epstein. A cost-analysis of adopting a healthful diet in a family-based obesity treatment program. *J Am Diet Assoc.* 102:645–656, 2002.

18. Batch, J. A. and L. A. Baur. Management and prevention of obesity and its complications in children and adolescents. *Med J Aust.* 182:130–135, 2005.

19. Krebs, N. F. and M. S. Jacobson. American Academy of Pediatrics, Committee on Nutrition. Prevention of pediatric overweight and obesity. *Pediatrics.* 112:424–430, 2003.

20. Baranowski, T., K. W. Cullen, T. Nicklas, D. Thompson, and J. Baranowski. Are current health behavioral change models helpful in guiding prevention of weight gain efforts? *Obes Res.* 11 Suppl:23S–43S, 2003.

21. Davis, K. and K. K. Christoffel. Obesity in preschool and school-age children. Treatment early and often may be best. *Arch Pediatr Adolesc Med.* 148:1257–1261, 1994.

22. Sothern, M. S. Obesity prevention in children: physical activity and nutrition. *Nutrition.* 20:704–708, 2004.

23. Ogden, C. L., K. M. Flegal, M. D. Carroll, and C. L. Johnson. Prevalence and trends in overweight among US children and adolescents, 1999–2000. *JAMA.* 288:1728–1732, 2002.

24. Crawford, P., M., Sothern, D. Hoest. Pediatric overweight: position statement and evidence-based analysis of interventions. *J Amer Diet Assoc.* in press.

25. Epstein, L. H., L. H. Kuller, R. R. Wing, A. Valoski, and J. McCurley. The effect of weight control on lipid changes in obese children. *Am J Dis Child.* 143:454–457, 1989.

26. Trick, J. Effective management of a hospital-based health promotion program: keys to success. *Am J Health Promot.* 4:317–319, 1990.

27. McKenzie, S. J. and J. L. Smeltzer. *Planning, Implementing, and Evaluation Health Promotion Programs,* 3rd ed. Needham Heights, MA: Allyn & Bacon, 2001.

28. Green, I. W. and Kreuter, M.W. *Healtlh Promotion Planning: An Educational and Ecological Approach,* 3rd ed. Mountain View, CA: Mayfield, 1999.

29. Simons-Morton, B. G., W. H. Greene, and N. H. Gottlieb. *Introduction to Health Education and Health Promotion,* 2nd ed. Prospect Heights, IL: Waveland Press, 1995.

30. Simons-Morton, D. G., B. G. Simons-Morton, G. S. Parcel, and J. F. Bunker. Influencing personal and environmental conditions for community health: a multilevel intervention model. *Family Commun. Health.* 11:25–35, 1988.

31. Walsh, D. C., R. E. Rudd, B. A. Moeykens, and T. W. Moloney. Social marketing for public health. *Health Affairs.* 12:104–119, 1993.

32. Neiger, B. L. Social marketing: making public health sense. Paper presented at the annual meeting of the Utah Public Health Association. Provo, UT, 1998.

33. Evans, W., E. Finkelstein, D. Kamerow, and J. Renaud. Public perceptions of childhood obesity. *Am J Prev Med.* 28:26–32, 2005.

34. Thompson, D., J. B. Brown, G. A. Nichols, P. J. Elmer, and G. Oster. Body mass index and future healthcare costs: a retrospective cohort study. *Obes Res.* 9:210–218, 2001.

35. Must, A. Does overweight in childhood have an impact on adult health? *Nutr Rev.* 61:139–142, 2003.

36. Goetzel, R. Z., D. R. Anderson, R. W. Whitmer, R. J. Ozminkowski, R. L. Dunn, and J. Wasserman. The relationship between modifiable health risks and health care expenditures. An analysis of the multi-employer HERO health risk and cost database. The Health Enhancement Research Organization (HERO) Research Committee. *J Occup Environ Med.* 40:843–854, 1998.

37. Ganz, M. L. The economic evaluation of obesity interventions: its time has come. *Obes Res.* 11:1275–1277, 2003.

38. Saelens, B. E., J. F. Sallis, D. E. Wilfley, K. Patrick, J. A. Cella, and R. Buchta. Behavioral weight control for overweight adolescents initiated in primary care. *Obes Res.* 10:22–32, 2002.

39. Schwimmer, J. B. Managing overweight in older children and adolescents. *Pediatr Ann.* 33:39–44, 2004.

40. Pickering, T., L. Clemow, K. Davidson, and W. Gerin. Behavioral cardiology — has its time finally arrived? *Mt Sinai J Med.* 70:101–112, 2003.

41. Hill, J. O. and C. J. Billington. Obesity: its time has come. *Am J Hypertens.* 15(7 Pt. 1):655–656, 2002.

42. Epstein, L., C. Gordy, H. Raynor, M. Beddome, C. Kilanowski, and R. Paluch. Increasing fruit and vegetable intake and decreasing fat and sugar intake in families at risk for childhood obesity. *Obes Res.* 9:171–178, 2001.

43. Edmunds, L., E. Waters, and E. Elliott. Evidence based paediatrics: evidence based management of childhood obesity. *BMJ*. 323:916–919, 2001.

44. Brown, R., M. Sothern, R. Suskind, J. Udall, and U. Blecker. Racial differences in the lipid profiles of obese children and adolescents before and after significant weight loss. *Clin Pediatr* (Phila). 39:427–431, 2000.

45. Ebbeling, C. B., M. M. Leidig, K. B. Sinclair, J. P. Hangen, and D. S. Ludwig. A reduced-glycemic load diet in the treatment of adolescent obesity. *Arch Pediatr Adolesc Med*. 157:773–779, 2003.

46. Epstein, L. H., A. Valoski, R. Koeske, and R. R. Wing. Family-based behavioral weight control in obese young children. *J Am Diet Assoc*. 86:481–484, 1986.

47. Epstein, L. H., A. Valoski, R. R. Wing, and J. McCurley. Ten-year outcomes of behavioral family-based treatment for childhood obesity. *Health Psychol*. 13:373–383, 1994.

48. Sothern, M., J. Udall, R. Suskind, A. Vargas, and U. Blecker. Weight loss and growth velocity in obese children after very low calorie diet, exercise and behavior modification. *Acta Paediatrica*. 89:1036–1043, 2000.

49. Sothern, M. S., M. Loftin, U. Blecker, and J. N. Udall, Jr. Impact of significant weight loss on maximal oxygen uptake in obese children and adolescents. *J Investig Med*. 48:411–416, 2000.

50. Sothern, M. S., H. Schumacher, T. K. von Almen, L. K. Carlisle, and J. N. Udall. Committed to kids: an integrated, 4-level team approach to weight management in adolescents. *J Am Diet Assoc*. 102:S81–85, 2002.

51. McInnis, K. J., B. A. Franklin, and J. M. Rippe. Counseling for physical activity in overweight and obese patients. *Am Fam Physician*. 67:1249–1256, 2003.

52. Falkner, B. and S. Michel. Obesity and other risk factors in children. *Ethn Dis*. 9:284–289, 1999.

53. Hill, J. and F. Throwbridge. The causes and health consequences of obesity in children and adolescents. *Pediatrics*. 101:497–575, 1989.

54. Rippe, J. M. and S. Hess. The role of physical activity in the prevention and management of obesity. *J Am Diet Assoc*. 98:S31–38, 1998.

55. Rosner, B., R. Prineas, J. Loggie, and S. Daniels. Percentiles for body mass index in U.S. children 5 to 17 years of age. *J Pediatrics*. 132:211–222, 1998.

56. Hedley, A., C. Ogden, C. Johnson, M. Carroll, L. Curtin, and K. Flegal. Prevalence of overweight and obesity among US children, adolescents, and adults, 1992–2002. *JAMA*. 291:2847–2850, 2004.

57. Hill, J. and F. Throwbridge. The causes and health consequences of obesity in children and adolescents. *Pediatrics*. 101:497–575, 1998.

58. James, W. P. and A. Ralph. New understanding in obesity research. *Proc Nutr Soc*. 58:385–393, 1999.

59. Roux, L., C. Ubach, C. Donaldson, and M. Ryan. Valuing the benefits of weight loss programs: an application of the discrete choice experiment. *Obes Res*. 12:1342–1351, 2004.

60. American College of Sports Medicine Position Stand. The recommended quantity and quality of exercise for developing and maintaining cardiorespiratory and muscular fitness, and flexibility in healthy adults, *Med Sci Sports Exerc*. 30:975–991, 1998.

61. Ad Hoc Work Group of the American Publish Health Association. Criteria for the development of health promotion and education programs. *Am J Public Health*. 77:89–92, 1987.

62. Wang, S. S., T. A. Wadden, L. G. Womble, and C. A. Nonas. What consumers want to know about commercial weight-loss programs: a pilot investigation. *Obes Res*. 11:48–53, 2003.

63. Borg, W. R., and Gall, M.D. *Educational Research: An Introduction*. 5th ed. New York: Longman, 1989

64. Sothern, M. S. Exercise as a modality in the treatment of childhood obesity. *Pediatr Clin North Am*. 48:995–1015, 2001.

65. Dorn, L. D., E. J. Susman, and J. C. Fletcher. Informed consent in children and adolescents: age, maturation and psychological state. *J Adolesc Health*. 16:185–190, 1995.

66. Susman, E. J., L. D. Dorn, and J. C. Fletcher. Participation in biomedical research: the consent process as viewed by children, adolescents, young adults, and physicians. *J Pediatr*. 121:547–552, 1992.

67. Jelalian, E., J. Boergers, C. S. Alday, and R. Frank. Survey of physician attitudes and practices related to pediatric obesity. *Clin Pediatr* (Phila). 42:235–245, 2003.

68. Daniels, S. R. Obesity in the pediatric patient: cardiovascular complications. *Prog Pediatr Cardiol*. 12:161–167, 2001.

69. Barlow, S. E. and W. H. Dietz. Management of child and adolescent obesity: summary and recommendations based on reports from pediatricians, pediatric nurse practitioners, and registered dietitians. *Pediatrics*. 110:236–238, 2002.

70. Sothern, M. S., S. Hunter, R. M. Suskind, R. Brown, J. N. Udall, Jr., and U. Blecker. Motivating the obese child to move: the role of structured exercise in pediatric weight management. *South Med J*. 92:577–584, 1999.

# Section 2

## Medical Aspects of Treatment

# 3 Medical Complications and Comorbidities of Pediatric Obesity

*Marc S. Jacobson*

## CONTENTS

This chapter reviews the risks and consequences associated with childhood and adolescent obesity. It does not exhaustively list every complication and comorbidity but, rather, focuses on conditions likely to be seen in clinical practice either that are important in the differential diagnosis or that have important acute, immediate, or long-term health consequences. Also emphasized are medical complications that are used in clinical decision making regarding intensity of treatment and in choosing weight goals for children and adolescents [1]. As the number of overweight pediatric patients has increased, so has the incidence and degree of medical complications.

Medical complications of pediatric obesity can be classified as those affecting the child or adolescent in the present and immediate future, or those that have implications primarily for adult health and life span [2]. This distinction has important implications for the motivation of the patient and family, as well as for the practitioner, the third-party payer, and society. Subclassification is by body system, as this method aids in understanding pathophysiology and management.

## GENETIC SYNDROMES ASSOCIATED WITH CHILDHOOD OBESITY

These conditions are rare and are usually associated with an abnormality evident on physical exam, developmental delay, or mental retardation. Many, such as the dysmorphic syndromes, Turner's, and Beckwith–Wiedeman, are generally identified during infancy before the development of obesity. Prader–Willi Syndrome is the best described and most frequent of these syndromes and is associated with hypotonia, poor linear growth, dysmorphic features such as small hands and feet, hypogonadotropic hypogonadism, and developmental delay. It is caused by the loss of paternally expressed genes, including small nuclear ribonucleoprotein, within the critical region of chromosome 15q. The striking hyperphagia associated with high ghrelin levels noted in this syndrome is the syndrome's most difficult management challenge [3]. The Bardet–Biedl syndrome is characterized by mental retardation, retinitis pigmentosa, hypogonadism, and polydactyly. Several chromosome regions have been identified as involved [3]. Pseudohypoparathyroidism, which is so named because of its phenotypic similarity to the features of hypoparathyroidism without the low parathyroid function, consists of short stature, short neck, rounded facies, hypocalcemia, and mental retardation. These syndromes are important to be aware of in the differential diagnosis of pediatric obesity and are more thoroughly discussed in Chapter 7 of Volume 1.

## ENDOCRINE DISORDERS

Taken individually, endocrine disorders are rare causes of obesity in pediatric practice, but as a group they make up an important reversible cause of obesity and have significant morbidity and potential mortality. Recognizing the signs and symptoms is thus important. A general rule is that any child who presents as overweight and is below the 50th percentile of height for age should be screened for an underlying endocrinologic etiology. The yield of endocrine screening tests in taller children will be very low, and without other signs and symptoms, testing should not be done. In the shorter group, it will still be less than 0.5 to 1% in our clinical experience, but high enough to warrant a raised index of suspicion.

### HYPOTHYROIDISM

Congenital hypothyroidism is screened for at birth, but the acquired forms can occur at any age. When it is insidious in onset, it may present as only obesity with hypercholesterolemia. Often the typical growth, metabolic, and intellectual function abnormalities classically described in this condition present subtly, resulting in delayed diagnosis. Screening is therefore warranted, but the specific laboratory investigations for screening should be discussed with a local pediatric endocrinologist because clinical lab specificity and sensitivity may vary considerably from center to center. In our center we screen with a thyroid-stimulating hormone for hypothyroidism among children presenting with short stature or delayed growth, obesity, and hypercholesterolemia [4].

### GROWTH HORMONE DEFICIENCY

Growth hormone–deficient children, in addition to presenting with reduced growth velocity and short stature, have reduced fat-free mass. The metabolic abnormalities in leptin and ghrelin are corrected by growth hormone treatment, but insulin resistance may ensue. Primary growth hormone deficiency is not likely to present as obesity, but growth velocity measures can easily differentiate the two conditions, as in obesity, growth velocity is normal or high.

Hypercortisolism can be either central (adrenocorticotropic hormone [ACTH] excess or Cushing disease), peripheral (ACTH-producing tumor or adrenal adenoma), or iatrogenic in origin. The excess cortisol results in hypertension, glucose intolerance, dyslipidemia, moon facies, decreased muscle mass, broad violaceous stria, visceral adiposity, and poor growth [5]. When history and physical exam warrant screening, an 8 A.M. plasma cortisol test or 24-hour urinary cortisol is indicated.

# CARDIOVASCULAR COMPLICATIONS

## LIPID DISORDERS

The lipid disorders associated with pediatric obesity are among the most frequent, best understood, and most described metabolic abnormalities seen. It has been clear since the beginning of pediatric lipid studies that obesity is associated with lipid abnormalities [6,7]. Recently, with the advent of Centers for Disease Control and Prevention reference data for BMI (body mass index) percentiles, it has become clear that BMI greater than the 95th percentile is a major determinant of hyperlipidemia and dyslipidemia in children [8]. Furthermore, the autopsy data from the PDAY study and from Bogalusa have proved that abnormal lipid patterns in youth are associated with premature atherosclerosis, as measured by fibrous plaque accumulation in aorta and coronary arteries [9,10]. In clinical practice, it has become clear that obesity is the most frequent determinant of abnormal lipids, and in the past decade obesity has become a more common cause than either heterozygous familial hypercholesterolemia or familial combined hyperlipidemia.

Differential diagnosis of lipid disorders in the overweight child includes both primary and secondary causes. They are listed in Table 3.1. Familial hypercholesterolemia is found in 1 in 500 children in the United States and is caused by defects in number or function of the cell surface low-density lipoprotein (LDL) receptors, resulting in impaired LDL clearance and increased intracellular cholesterol synthesis. Associated features of familial hypercholesterolemia include familial history of premature atherosclerosis and findings of peripheral cholesterol deposition, such as tendinous xanthomas, xanthelasma, and corneal arcus in the child or in first-degree relatives. Familial combined hyperlipidemia is found in 1 in 200 to 400 children in the United States. It is caused by hereditary defects in hepatic very low density lipoprotein (VLDL) synthesis and metabolism and is characterized by variable hyperlipidemia patterns in the same family. Children with familial combined hyperlipidemia present with modest elevations of cholesterol and triglycerides, VLDL, and LDL and with depressed levels of high-density lipoprotein cholesterol for age and sex.

Mixed environmental–genetic hyperlipidemia is an imprecise but widely used term that attempts to describe the majority of hyperlipidemia seen in children and adults. These children may or may not initially present as overweight, but they will have no clearly defined genetic abnormality of lipid metabolism. They are more susceptible to raised lipids when they eat diets high in saturated fats or simple carbohydrates. Some of the genetic patterns associated with this type of hyperlipidemia, such as variation in the frequency of apo E isoforms, are well described, but most are not. Excessive adiposity itself is a risk factor for hyperlipidemia in children, as shown most clearly in the Bogalusa data [8]. It is clear though that certain individuals are more susceptible to dietary-induced hyperlipidemia than others and that change in diet and weight loss are sufficient to improve or normalize their lipid patterns.

**TABLE 3.1**
**Differential Diagnosis of Hyperlipidemias in Pediatric Overweight and Obesity**

| Primary | Secondary |
| --- | --- |
| Familial hypercholesterolemia (low-density lipoprotein receptor defect) | Hypothyroidism |
| Familial combined hyperlipidemia (very low density lipoprotein overproduction, decreased metabolism) | Nephrotic syndrome |
| Mixed environmental–genetic hyperlipidemia (apo E) | Hepatitis |
| Dyslipidemia | Diabetes (type I and II) |
| | Connective tissue disorders |

Secondary causes of lipid abnormalities in the overweight child can be ruled out with a careful history, a physical examination, and a few simple laboratory tests. Hypothyroidism has been discussed above, under endocrinopathies. Nephrotic syndrome is characterized by edema and proteinuria, as well as hypercholesterolemia. Hepatitis can be a mild, flulike illness in children and may not demonstrate jaundice; therefore, routine hepatic enzyme testing is warranted. Connective tissue diseases have familial combined hyperlipidemia-like patterns that can be exacerbated by corticosteroid therapy [11,12]. The child treated with prolonged systemic corticosteroids who becomes Cushingoid will present with both elevated cholesterol and triglycerides.

Hypertension is commonly seen in overweight children. Unlike in adults, where the definition and severity of hypertension is independent of age and height, in children, diagnosis of hypertension is based on percentiles adjusted for age, gender, and height percentile. Therefore, it is important to have available up-to-date reference data tables when assessing blood pressure in children [13].

Proper baseline conditions are critical in obtaining accurate and reliable measurement of blood pressure. The child or adolescent should be seated at rest 10 minutes, and an appropriate size cuff should be applied to the right arm. Cuff size is determined by a bladder width that is approximately 40% of the arm circumference, midway between the olecranon and the acromion processes of the humerus. A larger, rather than a smaller, cuff should be chosen if neither is exactly correct. Systolic pressure is recorded as the first sound, and diastolic as the disappearance point, or fifth sound. The average of two measurements is better than one alone.

When an overweight child has been diagnosed with prehypertension or stage 1 hypertension, it is prudent to attempt weight management before pharmacotherapy. If stage 2 hypertension is diagnosed, a pediatric nephrologist should be consulted. There are no data to help us determine how long to prescribe weight management alone before instituting specific antihypertensive therapy; therefore, clinical judgment of whether therapy is working to control weight, as well as twice-monthly measurement of blood pressure, is needed. If stage 1 hypertension persists despite significant weight loss, consultation with a pediatric nephrologist for a renal workup is indicated.

## CARDIAC STRUCTURE AND FUNCTION

It is apparent that a variety of adaptations or alterations in cardiac structure and function occur as excessive adiposity accumulates, even in the absence of comorbidities. When these changes progress, clinical disease ensues. Findings such as left ventricular dilatation, increased wall stress, compensatory left ventricular hypertrophy, and diastolic dysfunction are common [14]. These changes may also occur on the right, where they are associated with sleep apnea, pulmonary hypertension, and hypoventilation. When obesity is longstanding and severe, progressive congestive heart failure and sudden death may result from these hemodynamic alterations. Most of the available pediatric data are from adolescents. Urbina et al. studied 160 healthy 9- to 22-year-old patients from the Bogalusa population to understand the role of weight gain on cardiac structural development [15]. The researchers found that excess weight gain was associated with increased left ventricular mass and systolic blood pressure [15].

Gidding et al. investigated 48 boys and girls aged 8 to 17 with BMI > 40kg/m2 on a graded cycle exercise test [16]. Only 2 had normal fitness. The remainder had various combinations of deconditioning (37/48), upper airway obstruction (7/48), small airway disease (35/48) and left ventricular hypertrophy (8/48). Friberg et al. found left ventricular mass was 16% greater in obese compared with lean adolescents [17]. Giordano et al. found a significant relation of blood pressure, insulin resistance, and left ventricular mass in 24 obese adolescent males compared with controls [18]. Mensah et al. studied 225 adolescents with a family history of hypertension and found that anthropometric indexes of fat mass were significantly correlated measures with left ventricular markers of dysfunction and adverse prognosis [19]. Daniels et al. studied 201 6- to 17-year-old subjects to further understand the relationship of fat and lean mass to hemodynamic determinants of blood pressure [20]. They concluded that lean mass is a more important correlate of blood pressure than fat mass, and that sex and race have significant independent effects on blood pressure in adolescents. Rowland et al. studied adolescent females' (BMI 30 to 40 kg/m$^2$) response to maximal cycle testing. They found that depressed peak VO$_2$ and limited endurance were not associated with decreased cardiac functional capacity [21].

Whether the cardiac changes seen in obesity are reversible was questioned by Humphries et al. [22]. These researchers studied the effect of 4 months of physical training on body composition and left ventricular mass in obese adolescents and found no effect of training on cardiac mass despite a significant reduction in percentage body fat and visceral fat, as measured by magnetic resonance imaging [22]. On a more hopeful note, Uwaifo et al. from the National Institutes of Health reported a case of a 17-year-old obese boy with familial apical hypertrophic cardiomyopathy. After a 1-year program that resulted in a 49-kg weight loss (BMI reduced from 43.6 to 28.1 kg/m$^2$), the patient showed striking improvement in cardiac functional indices [23].

## INSULIN RESISTANCE SYNDROMES

The relative ability of a given amount of insulin secretion to dispose of serum glucose varies as much as sixfold among apparently healthy adults. The highest third of individuals are referred to as insulin resistant, and this resistance is associated with a number of disease states, including cardiovascular disease, hypertension, stroke, type 2 diabetes, nonalcoholic fatty liver disease, and polycystic ovarian syndrome. One fourth to one third of the variance in insulin resistance is related to being overweight, and particularly to abdominal pattern obesity. Although most of the data about the insulin resistance syndromes have been obtained from adults, it is increasingly clear that insulin resistance is present in obese children and adolescents, and that the consequences are increasingly being seen in the pediatric age group. Reinehr et al. were able to show improvement in insulin resistance in 6- to 14-year-old patients over 1 year if treatment resulted in at least a 0.5 decrease in BMI $z$ score [24].

### Metabolic Syndrome or Syndrome X

The Adult Treatment Panel III ([25]) has recently defined the metabolic syndrome (or syndrome X, originally described by Reaven, three decades ago) as having three or more of the following five factors: high BMI (males > 29 kg/m$^2$, females > 25 kg/m$^2$), high glucose (>110 mg/dL), high triglycerides (>150 mg/dL), low high-density lipoprotein cholesterol (males < 40 mg/dL, females < 50 mg/dL), or hypertension (blood pressure > 130/85 mmHg). The importance of diagnosing this syndrome is that it confers a significant burden of cardiovascular disease risk and, for many individuals, is a precursor to type 2 diabetes mellitus.

In a study of 439 obese adolescents, Weiss et al. used three out of the following five items as criteria to diagnose metabolic syndrome: BMI greater than 97th percentile for age and sex, triglycerides greater than 95th percentile, high-density lipoprotein cholesterol below the 5th percentile, systolic or diastolic blood pressure above the 95th percentile, and impaired glucose tolerance. By these criteria, the researchers found metabolic syndrome in 39% of moderately obese adolescents (BMI > 95th percentile) and in 48% of severely obese adolescents (BMI > 2.5 standard deviations above the mean) [26]. The relative risk of metabolic syndrome in that study was increased 1.55 times for each 0.5-unit increase in BMI $z$ score. It is important to realize that although BMI and insulin resistance are related, they are not synonymous. They make independent and different contributions to increasing cardiovascular disease (CVD) risk [27].

### Polycystic Ovarian Syndrome

Polycystic ovarian syndrome consists of hyperinsulinemic hyperandrogenism with anovulation. It is strongly associated with abdominal adiposity, oligomenorrhea, hirsutism, and infertility. These young women can have psychological effects from the constellation of symptoms and signs that often begin during adolescence, when body image concerns are paramount [28]. Risk for diabetes, glucose intolerance, hyperlipidemia, endometrial cancer, infertility, and coronary heart disease are also elevated. One recent study indicates that some young girls at increased risk may be identified and prophylactically treated with insulin-sensitizing agents to prevent polycystic ovarian syndrome. The significant risk factors identified were low birth weight and precocious puberty [29].

## TYPE 2 DIABETES MELLITUS

Type 2 diabetes mellitus, a disease not previously seen in pediatrics, is now recognized as a major concern. It has become common in pediatric diabetes programs in the last decade [30]. The prevalence of this disease is a result of the epidemic of severe obesity and presents a major ongoing challenge to the health care system. It is of so recent an onset that long-term follow-up studies are not available to determine outcome, but most experts are fearful that complications of this epidemic will be formidable. Although routine screening of all overweight children is not indicated, the American Academy of Pediatrics and the American Diabetes Association have guidlines for screening those age 10 years and above who are at high risk by virtue of being overweight and having at least two of the following three findings: family history of diabetes mellitus, signs of insulin resistance, or certain ethnic backgrounds (Native American, African American, Asian-Pacific Islander, Hispanic). The recommended screening test is a fasting glucose or an oral 2-hour glucose tolerance test. Diabetes mellitus is discussed more fully in Chapter 12 of Volume 1.

## GASTROINTESTINAL SYSTEM

### CHOLELITHIASIS (GALLSTONES)

Obesity is a major risk factor for the formation of gallstones, cholecystitis, and cholecystectomy. Any obese child with classic symptoms of right upper quadrant abdominal pain with or without fever, nausea, and vomiting should be carefully evaluated and surgical consultation sought. It is seen mostly in females (70%) and after age 10 years. Cholelithiasis can also be seen following rapid weight loss, particularly on very low calorie diets, as a result of lack of motility of the gallbladder. This can be avoided if sufficient fat is included in the dietary regimen [31].

### HEPATIC STEATOSIS (FATTY LIVER)

Interest in hepatic disorders in obesity has increased as the epidemic of obesity has progressed. As the patients are usually asymptomatic, liver abnormalities are found on routine blood tests of liver enzymes. The concern is that the excess fat storage within the liver will lead to chronic inflammation and eventual cirrhosis, fibrosis, end-stage liver disease, and hepatic failure. The early stage of this problem, known as nonalcoholic fatty liver disease, is associated with the degree of obesity, hypertriglyceridemia, and insulin resistance. It is diagnosed on imaging studies such as ultrasound or computed tomography by evidence of fatty infiltration. Hepatic steatosis is thought to occur initially, through hepatic and peripheral insulin resistance, which leads to altered glucose and free fatty acid metabolism. As much as 77% of pediatric referrals for obesity may have evidence of nonalcoholic fatty liver disease [32]. When the disease progresses, serum chemistries, particularly alanine aminotransferase (ALT) and aspartate aminotransferase (AST), become elevated, showing evidence of inflammation, and the condition becomes known as nonalcoholic steatohepatitis, which has been reported in 5 to 10% of pediatric obesity referrals. The progression, prognosis, and treatment of nonalcoholic fatty liver disease and nonalcoholic steatohepatitis are under active investigation. The work-up for nonalcoholic steatohepatitis should include antibody studies to rule out infectious causes of hepatitis, and enzymes should be monitored during weight management. Drug usage to treat insulin resistance and antioxidant vitamins to reduce inflammation are areas of active investigation.

## PULMONARY COMPLICATIONS OF OBESITY

### GENERAL ALTERATIONS IN PULMONARY FUNCTION

The findings of impaired pulmonary function in overweight children highlight an important concern that decreased lung capacity leads to decreased exercise capacity, followed by decrease in physical activities, leading to a vicious cycle of impaired lifestyle and overweight. Li et al. found reduction in functional residual capacity and diffusion impairment were the most common abnormalities in a cohort of obese patients. Reduction in static lung volume was correlated with the degree of obesity [33]. Lazarus et al., in a randomized population sample of 2500 Australian adolescents, found decreased pulmonary function with increasing adiposity [34]. Because the fall in pulmonary function was severe in obese boys and these falls were correlated with body mass index and skinfolds, it is concluded that diagnosis and management may improve aerobic exercise performance and participation in obese children.

### ASTHMA

Pianosi and Davis studied the pulmonary functions of children with asthma and found that overweight and obese children were more likely to be overmedicated despite similar asthma severity because of their perceived exercise intolerance [35]. The authors concluded that efforts should be directed at understanding the reasons responsible for reduced exercise tolerance before escalating pharmacologic treatment for asthma among the overweight [35]. Tantisira et al. studied pulmonary function in a group of children with asthma and found that the ratio of forced expiratory volume in 1 second to the forced vital capacity was inversely associated with BMI, but that other measures of asthma severity were not independently associated with severity of overweight [36].

### OBSTRUCTIVE SLEEP APNEA HYPOVENTILATION SYNDROME

Obstructive sleep apnea hypoventilation syndrome is associated with obesity in adults. It is characterized by snoring, irregular breathing with long pauses during sleep, and daytime tiredness. In children, it can be confused with attention deficit disorder and other learning problems, as well as depression. Rosen studied a group of 326 children who were referred for sleep studies and found that although obesity was not the only cause of pediatric obstructive sleep apnea hypoventilation syndrome, high BMI was twice as prevalent as expected (28%) in this population [37].

## NEUROLOGICAL

Pseudotumor cerebri (benign intracranial hypertension) presents with headache, dizziness, diploplia, and mild unsteadiness. It generally has a gradual onset and does not show localizing neurological signs. If symptoms begin acutely, or if focal signs are present, other sources of raised intracranial pressure must be sought. Phillips et al. studied the 10-year incidence of this disorder in a hospital-based series of children up to 18 years of age [38]. Obesity was associated with one-third of cases. There was no gender predilection. One third of patients demonstrated some optic atrophy at follow up [38]. Weight loss is recognized as the best treatment.

## ORTHOPEDIC

Two orthopedic conditions are of particular importance in pediatric obesity — Blount disease and slipped capital femoral epiphysis. Both occur primarily in younger adolescents and preteens, and both are disorders of the lower extremity. Both conditions may lead to a vicious cycle of overweight making the orthopedic condition worse, while the raised barrier to physical activity that the conditions present then make the overweight condition worse, and so on. Both should be considered orthopedic emergencies requiring surgical consultation because they can be crippling.

Blount disease (also known as *Tibia vera*, or *Genu varum*) presents as a bowing of the leg with or without pain and limp. It consists of an abnormality in the growth of the medial portion of the proximal tibia. It is unclear whether this abnormality is caused by excess weight placed on the joint at a critical stage in development or whether it is an underlying condition that is aggravated by the excess weight. Plain anterior–posterior x-rays of the leg characteristically show irregularity of the growth of the proximal medial tibial physis, with beaking or a triangulation of the metaphysis. Surgical correction is by osteotomy.

Slipped capital femoral epiphysis occurs when the epiphysis of the proximal femur slips off the metaphysis posteriorly and medially secondary to increased weight on the cartilaginous growth plate of the hip [39]. The classic patient is an overweight, hypogonadal boy with delayed bone age. Symptoms include limp, hip or knee pain, and the typical antalgic gate, with the leg externally rotated and abducted.

## REFERENCES

1. Barlow E, Dietz WH. Obesity evaluation and treatment: Expert Committee recommendations. The Maternal and Child Health Bureau, Health Resources and Services Administration and the Department of Health and Human Services. *Pediatrics* 1998; 102(3): 1–11.
2. Must A, Strauss RS. Risks and consequences of childhood and adolescent obesity. *International J Obes Rel Metab Disord* 1999; 23(Suppl 2): S2–S11.
3. Cummings DE, Clement K, Purnell JQ, Vaisse C, Foster KE, Frayo RS et al. Elevated plasma ghrelin levels in Prader Willi syndrome. *Nat Med* 2002; 8:643–644.
4. Copperman N, Haas T, Arden MA, Jacobson MS. Multidisciplinary intervention in adolescents with cardiovascular risk factors. In: Jacobson MS, ed. *Adolescent Nutritional Disorders: Prevention and Treatment*. New York: Annals of the New York Academy of Sciences. 1997; 817:199–207.
5. Kokkoris P, Pi-Sunyer FX. Obesity and endocrine disease. *Endocrin Metab Clin N Am* 2003; 895–914.
6. Freedman DS, Srinvasan SR, Burke GL. Relation of body fat distribution to hyperinsulinemia in children and adolescents: the Bogalusa Heart Study. *Am J Clin Nutr* 1987; 46:403–410.
7. Lauer RM, Conner WE, Leaverton PE. Coronary heart disease risk factors in school children: The Muscatine study. *J Ped* 1975; 86:967–706.
8. Freedman DS, Dietz WH, Srinivasan SR, Berenson GS. The relation of overweight to cardiovascular risk factors among children and adolescents: the Bogalusa Heart Study. *Pediatrics* 1999 103(6 Pt 1):1175–1182.
9. McGill HC Jr, McMahan CA, Zieske AW, Sloop GD, Walcott JV, Troxclair DA et al. Associations of coronary heart disease risk factors with the intermediate lesion of atherosclerosis in youth. The Pathobiological Determinants of Atherosclerosis in Youth (PDAY) Research Group. *Arterioscler, Thrombo, Vas Biol* 2000; (8):1998–2004.
10. Berenson GS, Srinivasan SR, Bao W, Newman WP, 3rd, Tracy RE, Wattigney WA. Association between multiple cardiovascular risk factors and atherosclerosis in children and young adults. The Bogalusa Heart Study. *NE J Med*1998; 338(23):1650–1656.
13. Blood Pressure Tables for Children and Adolescents. Available at: http://www.nhlbi.nih.gov/guidelines/hypertension/child_tbl.htm.
14. Alpert MA. Obesity cardiomyopathy: pathophysiology and evolution of the clinical syndrome. *Am J Med Sci* 2001; 321(4):225–236.
15. Urbina EM, Gidding SS, Bao W, Pickoff AS, Berdusis K, Berenson GS. Effect of body size, ponderosity, and blood pressure on left ventricular growth in children and young adults in the Bogalusa Heart Study. *Circulation* 1995; 91(9):2400–2406.
16. Gidding SS, Nehgme R, Heise C, Muscar C, Linton A, Hassink S. Severe obesity associated with cardiovascular deconditioning, high prevalence of cardiovascular risk factors, diabetes mellitus/hyperinsulinemia, and respiratory compromise. *J Ped* 2004;144(6):766–769.

17. Friberg P, Allansdotter-Johnsson A, Ambring A, Ahl R, Arheden H, Framme J et al. Increased left ventricular mass in obese adolescents. *Euro Heart J* 2004; 25(11):987–992.

18. Giordano U, Ciampalini P, Turchetta A, Santilli A, Calzolari F, Crino A et al. Cardiovascular hemodynamics: relationships with insulin resistance in obese children. *Ped Cardio* 2003; 24(6):548–552.

19. Mensah GA, Treiber FA, Kapuku GK, Davis H, Barnes VA, Strong WB. Patterns of body fat deposition in youth and their relation to left ventricular markers of adverse cardiovascular prognosis. *Am J Cardo* 1999; 84(5):583–588.

20. Daniels SR, Kimball TR, Khoury P, Witt S, Morrison JA. Correlates of the hemodynamic determinants of blood pressure. *Hypertension* 1996; 28(1):37–41.

21. Rowland T, Bhargava R, Parslow D, Heptulla RA. Cardiac response to progressive cycle exercise in moderately obese adolescent females. *J Adolesc Health* 2003; 32(6):422–427.

22. Humphries MC, Gutin B, Barbeau P, Vemulapalli S, Allison J, Owens S. Relations of adiposity and effects of training on the left ventricle in obese youths. *Med Sci sports Exer* 2002; 34(9):1428–1435.

23. Uwaifo GI, Fallon EM, Calis KA, Drinkard B, McDuffie JR, Yanovski JA. Improvement in hypertrophic cardiomyopathy after significant weight loss: case report. *So Med J* 2003; 96(6):626–631.

24. Reinehr T, Kiess W, Kapellen T, Andler W. Insulin sensitivity among obese children and adolescents, according to degree of weight loss. *Pediatrics* 2004; 114(6):1569–1573.

25. Third report of the National Cholesterol Education Program (NCEP) Expert Panel on Detection, Evaluation, and Treatment of High Blood Cholesterol in Adults (Adult Treatment Panel III) final report. *Circulation* 2002 106:3143–3421.

26. Weiss R, Dziura J, Burgert TS, Tamborlane WV, Taksali SE, Yeckel CW et al. Obesity and the metabolic syndrome in children and adolescents. *NE J med* 2004; 350(23):2362–2374.

27. Reaven G, Abbasi F, McLaughlin T. Obesity, insulin resistance, and cardiovascular disease. *Recent Prog Horm Res* 2004; 59:207–223.

28. Buccola JM, Reynolds EE. Polycystic ovary syndrome: a review for primary providers. *Prim Care* 2003; 30(4):697–710.

29. Ibanez L, Ferrer A, Ong K, Amin R, Dunger D, de Zegher F. Insulin sensitization early after menarche prevents progression from precocious pubarche to polycystic ovary syndrome. *J Ped* 2004;144(1):23–29.

30. Pinhas-Hamiel O, Dolan LM, Daniels SR et al. Increased incidence of non-insulin-dependent diabetes mellitus among adolescents. *J Ped* 1996; 128:608–615.

31. Festi D, Colecchia A, Orsini M, Sangermano A, Sottili S, Simoni P et al. Gallbladder motility and gallstone formation in obese patients following very low calorie diets. Use it (fat) to lose it (well). *International Journal of Obesity and Related Metabolic Disorders* 1998;Jun;22(6):592–600.

32. Chan DF, Li AM, Chu WC, Chan MH, Wong EM, Liu EK et al. Hepatic steatosis in obese Chinese children. *Int J Obes Rel Metabol Disord* 2004; 28(10):1257–1263.

33. Li AM, Chan D, Wong E, Yin J, Nelson EA, Fok TF. The effects of obesity on pulmonary function. *Arch Dis Child* 2003; 88(4):361–363.

34. Lazarus R, Colditz G, Berkey CS, Speizer FE. Effects of body fat on ventilatory function in children and adolescents: cross-sectional findings from a random population sample of school children. *Ped Pulmonol* 1997; 24(3):187–194.

35. Pianosi PT, Davis HT. Determinants of physical fitness in children with asthma. *Pediatrics* 2004; 113:e225–e229.

36. Tantisira KG, Litonjua AA, Weiss ST, Fuhlbrigge AL, Childhood Asthma Management Program Research Group. Association of body mass with pulmonary function in the Childhood Asthma Management Program (CAMP). *Thorax* 2003; 58(12):1036–1041.

37. Rosen CL. Clinical features of obstructive sleep apnea hypoventilation syndrome in otherwise healthy children. *Ped Pulmonol* 1999; 27(6):403–409.

38. Phillips PH, Repka MX, Lambert SR. Pseudotumor cerebri in children. *J AAPOS* 1998; 2(1):33–38.

39. Loder RT, Aronson DD, Greenfield ML. The epidemiology of bilateral slipped capital femoral epiphysis. A study of children in Michigan. *J Bone Joint Surg* 1993;75:1141–1147.

# 4 Medical Aspects of Treatment: The Role of the Physician

*Stewart T. Gordon*

## CONTENTS

## INTRODUCTION

What has led to the current epidemic of childhood obesity? When most of today's parents were growing up, we had more opportunities for free play. Our neighborhoods tended to be safer, and usually someone was at home, supervising our activities. These activities typically did not include the increasing sedentary activities we have today (multiple television stations, computers, Internet, and video games). We spent more of our time engaging in activities that burned more calories — bike riding, playing chase, climbing trees. Most families ate a home-cooked meal every night. The rate of childhood obesity was 5 to 10%. Now, about 15% of children are considered overweight or at risk for overweight.

Environmental factors may contribute as much as 80% to the causes of childhood obesity. These factors include increased caloric and fat intake (e.g., energy-dense foods and beverages, irregular meal patterns, snacking and dining out, and sedentary behaviors, such as television viewing [1,2]) and absence of regular physical activity [3]. Research indicates that obese children demonstrate decreased levels of physical activity and increased psychosocial problems.

It is well accepted that the environment of the family plays a key role in the development of obesity in young children at risk for adult obesity and related diseases such as diabetes [4–7]. Research shows that parent inactivity strongly predicts child inactivity [6]. Moreover, the exercise patterns of parents have a strong influence on the frequency of exercise in their children [8]. Research also shows that parental influences are early determinants of food attitudes and practices in young children [9]. Furthermore, food preferences greatly influence the consumption patterns of young children [10]. Therefore, strategies that positively alter the behaviors and environment of the family may reduce the risk of adult obesity and diabetes by improving physical activity and nutrition. This may prevent the onset of pediatric obesity and the risk of metabolic disease later in life, especially in those children with primary risk factors (at risk). Efforts to halt and reverse obesity and related metabolic disease, therefore, should begin with young children. More important, educational interventions that target the parents of children at risk for obesity should be an integral part of standard pediatric and family medical care.

The health consequences of children's being obese are significant. Obese children are more likely to develop cardiovascular disease (high cholesterol, hypertension), glucose intolerance (which may lead to diabetes), gallstones, and psychological problems, to name a few. The most serious and prevalent long-term consequence of childhood obesity is psychosocial. Obese children are targets of early and systematic discrimination by peers, family members, and others. Obese children frequently have low self-esteem and social isolation and can become depressed. One of the best reasons to treat childhood obesity is to reduce the psychosocial consequences.

## ROLE OF THE PRIMARY CARE PRACTITIONERS

The most successful approach to treating childhood obesity is through a multidisciplinary (medical, nutritional, psychological, physical activity), family-based approach [11]. Such approaches teach both the overweight child and his or her family how to lead a healthier lifestyle to promote the achievement of a healthier weight. Interventions are best delivered in a group family setting. However, the combination of medical supervision, dietary guidance, promoting increased physical activity, and behavioral counseling should be promoted in the individual medical care of overweight youth, as well. Unfortunately, although the number of obese pediatric patients seen by physicians each year is continuously increasing, knowledge of effective treatment techniques is lagging. Recently, Story and others identified a lack of parent involvement and motivation and lack of support services as the most frequent barriers to treatment of pediatric obesity in clinical settings [12].

Even though obesity is recognized by the majority of health care professionals as a serious, chronic disease, they feel unprepared to address the multidimensional aspects of the obesity problem. Studies indicate that health care professionals believe that childhood obesity requires immediate medical attention and treatment [12]. However, many of their treatment practices are not in accordance with current expert recommendations [13]. This was evidenced when a survey of providers identified perceived low proficiency in the use of behavioral management strategies, guidance in parenting techniques, and addressing family conflicts [12]. Moreover, providers feel they lack expertise in motivational skills to promote change in dietary and physical activity patterns [14]. Despite these findings, behavioral therapy has been shown to be effective, even when done briefly. The Worcester Area Trial for Counseling in Hyperlipidemia study is an example of how brief counseling in adults can provide positive results in weight loss [15]. During the study, physicians were given 8 minutes with each patient. Study patients either received counseling alone (control) or counseling combined with handouts and questionnaires concerning dieting (treatment) while in the waiting rooms. A year later, treatment patients were found to have lost 2.3 kg more than the control and, as a benefit of that loss, lowered their cholesterol by 3.8 mg. Still, physicians rarely feel that a great difference can be made in the behavior of the families through the use of individual counseling [15]. This is caused by a lack of both training and experience of physicians in the area of counseling interventions. Another factor affecting this lack of enthusiasm in physicians is that many feel "ill-equipped" to handle behavioral issues [15,16], and that such issues are out of their area of interest [15]. Moreover, because of time constraints, physicians in primary care especially are conflicted, with heavy workloads combining with a strong work ethic to give the best care to their patients. Finally, a lack of incentives offered to physicians is another factor that reduces physician counseling in weight management [15]. However, physicians play a vital role to the safety and effectiveness of weight loss and maintenance interventions in children.

## THE ROLE OF THE PHYSICIAN IN THE TREATMENT OF OVERWEIGHT YOUTH

Initially, physicians are the best source for the diagnosis of pediatric obesity, according to the U.S. Surgeon General. Doctors and other health care professionals are the best source in determining whether a child or adolescent's weight is healthy, and they can help rule out rare medical problems as the cause of unhealthy weight. A body mass index (BMI) can be calculated from measurements of height and weight. Health professionals often use a BMI "growth chart" to help them assess whether a child or adolescent is overweight. A physician will also consider a child or adolescent's age and growth patterns to determine whether his or her weight is healthy. Only providers trained in pediatric medicine possess the level of expertise required to provide an accurate assessment of pediatric obesity. Regardless, studies indicate that pediatric health care providers diagnosed overweight in only one half (53%) of overweight children [17]. We found similar poor rates of diagnosis and referral in a study of Louisiana youth seen in three separate physician's offices [18]. Physicians diagnosed obesity in very few of their patients who were classified as greater than 95th percentile BMI (Table 4.1).

Physicians also provide guidance to parents so that they may best understand the definition of overweight or at risk for overweight in children. The physicians can then, with the parents' input, decide on the best plan of action for the overweight child. Recent studies indicate that at this point, about 75% of physicians will refer patients initially to registered dieticians [14], and only about 20% of patients will be referred to weight management programs. In another study, in those children diagnosed as overweight by their physicians, comprehensive treatment programs were not generally prescribed [17]. In our study, we observed similar low referral rates [18] (Table 4.1). Of more concern is that between 27% and 42% of pediatricians or pediatric health providers report that weight management programs are not available in their area [14].

Several clinical observations [19–26] have detailed an interdisciplinary pediatric weight management intervention in which the physician or pediatric health care provider has an integral role in treatment. He or she is responsible for the overall medical supervision of the program and oversees the diagnosis, evaluation, and dietary and physical activity plan of action. In this chapter, step-by-step details are provided of the medical oversight provided in this approach. Further details may be found in Chapter 2 by Sothern, Chapter 12 by Schumacher et al., Chapter 14 by Sothern, Chapter 19 by Carlisle and Gordon, and Chapter 20 by von Almen and Sothern, and in Appendices A1, A2, and A3.

**TABLE 4.1**
**Patients Diagnosed and Referred for Treatment**

|  | Clinic 1 | Clinic 2 | Clinic 3 |
|---|---|---|---|
| Total number of patients | 552 | 205 | 294 |
| Total number obese | 69 | 30 | 30 |
| Percentage obese | 12.5 | 14.83 | 10.20 |
| Total number diagnosed with obesity | 19 | 12 | 0 |
| Percentage diagnosed | 27.54 | 40.00 | 0 |
| Total number referred for obesity treatment | 6 | 2 | 0 |
| Percentage referred for treatment | 8.70 | 0.667 | 0.00 |

---

**TABLE 4.2**
**Diagnosing Overweight and Risk for Overweight**
**(Initial Medical Evaluation)**

Family/medical history and physical exam
Anthropometric measures
Weight and height
Calculate body mass index (BMI)
Laboratory evaluation (>95th percentile BMI)
Chem 20; CBC w/diff; lipid profile; thyroid profile
Maturation level (Tanner stage)

---

## PERFORMING THE INITIAL MEDICAL EVALUATION (TABLE 4.2)

An initial medical history and a physical examination are performed before enrollment into the treatment program. This medical information is reviewed with the parents and child before entry into the program. Assessment and discussion of the child's growth chart and current weight status occurs at this time. To determine the child's goal weight, the physician observes on the BMI growth chart what weight would match the child's height percentile (Appendix A1.10). This is the child's ideal body weight. The child's goal weight is this weight plus an additional 20%.

## ORDERING AND INTERPRETING LABORATORY BLOOD WORK (TABLE 4.2)

The pediatrician orders an initial battery of blood work that includes a complete blood count, metabolic panel, and lipid profile (Appendix A2.2). These laboratory tests are repeated 3 months into the program and at the end of the program. Other tests may be ordered after the initial medical evaluation as needed.

## PRESCRIBING AN APPROPRIATE DIET IN COORDINATION WITH THE PROGRAM DIETICIAN

The diet will be for either weight loss or weight maintenance. The child's medical history, family health history, age, gender, and current weight status will be considered before prescribing an appropriate diet. In children at risk for overweight, moderate approaches are best. However, in children with clinically significant overweight conditions (BMI > 99th percentile), more aggressive approaches may be necessary. Although the research is limited with respect to such approaches, several clinical observations and a few randomized controlled trials indicate that the use of very low calorie diets, low-carbohydrate diets, and low-glycemic diets may result in short-term weight loss in very overweight youth. In Chapter 11, Sothern and others survey the literature and provide specific guidelines for low glycemic diets. Sample diets are located in Appendix 3.

## PROVIDE ONGOING MEDICAL SUPERVISION (TABLE 4.3)

In group interventions, the pediatrician may choose to attend most of the intervention sessions, especially during the first 3 months of the program. He may elect to weigh the children and check vital signs while discussing their progress and answering questions. This helps to ensure medical safety throughout the course of the program. Whether the physician attends the sessions routinely or not, he or she should be available by phone to address questions or problems that arise between weekly sessions. In overweight and normal-weight children with parental obesity frequent monitoring, reduced television viewing, and increased opportunities for unstructured active play are typically recommended by the physician (Table 4.4).

## FOLLOW-UP (TABLE 4.5)

At the beginning of treatment for pediatric obesity, and every 3 months afterward, patients undergo a comprehensive evaluation. The results of the evaluations are distributed to the children and parents

## TABLE 4.3
## Medical Supervision

Quarterly anthropometric measurements
    Document and follow height growth
    Biolectrical impedance, body mass index, circumferences, skinfolds
Physician is available by phone/beeper during the week
Active weekly participation by the physician
    Get to know the children personally
    Present for questions from kids and family
    Participate in activities with kids

## TABLE 4.4
## Normal and Overweight Children 6 Years or Younger, with Parental Obesity

Regular visits with the pediatrician to monitor growth and development
Parent training and fitness education
Limit access to television/video/computer
Increased opportunities for unstructured physical activity — free play
    Create an environment inside the home that promotes active play
    Create an environment outside the home that promotes active play

## TABLE 4.5
## Childhood Obesity Treatment Quarterly Evaluation

Body composition
    Dual energy x-ray absorptiometry
    Skinfolds
    Bioelectrical impedance
Dietary history
Physical activity rating
Psychological measures
    Self-esteem
    Depression
    Self-efficacy

and are discussed with the family as necessary. In some cases, the physician may choose to refer the family to a staff psychologist, if available, or other appropriate mental health professional. A registered dietician or exercise professional should also be available to assist with interpretation and to answer questions as well. These evaluations consist of the following 10 items. Appendix 2 contains detailed measurement protocols.

## Height and Weight Measurement

The measurement of height or stature is a major indicator of bone length and general body size. The recommended technique for height measurement includes the use of a vertical board with an attached metric rule and horizontal headboard, collectively known as a stadiometer. The standard measure of weight should be recorded using a calibrated electronic scale. The kilograms should be recorded in the patient's chart. For both height and weight measures, the patient should remove shoes and heavy clothing/objects before the measurement.

## BMI and CDC Percentiles

The BMI, the calculated number that adjusts weight for height, uses the following formula:

$$BMI = \text{weight (kilograms)/height (meters}^2).$$

The Centers for Disease Control define at risk of overweight as a BMI between the 85th and 95th percentile for age. Children are considered overweight or obese if the BMI is greater than the 95th percentile for age. In adults, a BMI value greater than or equal to 25 but less than 30 is considered overweight, and a BMI value greater than or equal to 30 defines obesity or severe overweight [27]. However, these BMI cutoffs are not appropriate for classifying children's weight status. First, childhood mortality is not likely to be related to body composition, so it is not possible to develop risk-based criteria [28]. Second, BMI typically varies with age, decreasing in the preschool years, and then increasing after about 6 years of age. Because of these changes in BMI with growth, age-specific criteria are needed. Gender-specific criteria are also needed as a result of differences in body composition and timing of growth patterns in adolescence for boys and girls [29]. Revised growth charts with smoothed age and sex-specific BMI percentile curves were developed by the National Center for Health Statistics for children aged 2 to 17 years [28]. According to current standards, youths with a BMI greater than or equal to the 95th percentile for age and sex are considered overweight, and those with a BMI falling between the 85th and 95th percentiles for age and sex are considered at risk for overweight [30–32].

It is recommended that children with a BMI at the 85th or higher percentile be further evaluated for complications associated with overweight and for recent excessive weight gain. Assessments should include the evaluation of potential genetic, endocrine, or psychological syndromes [30,33–36]. Family medical, diet, and physical activity history should be considered to identify primary risk factors for overweight, such as parental obesity, sedentary behaviors, early feeding practices, metabolic or hormonal stress, socioeconomic factors, and ethnicity [5–7,9,34,37–41].

## Circumference Measurements

An additional method of assessing body composition is the measurement of girth of various body sections [42]. From the sum of the measurements, percentage body fat is determined from equations, tables, or nomograms. A metal or fiberglass measuring tape with a metric scale is used to measure the circumference of the waist and hip. The waist circumference is a useful indicator for determining reduction in fat weight after treatment.

## Blood Pressure and Heart Rate

Resting blood pressure (BP) measurement is taken as a measure of the force of the heart's pumping action. Hypertension in children and adolescents continues to be defined as systolic BP or diastolic BP that is, on repeated measurement, above the 95th percentile. BP between the 90th and 95th percentile in childhood had been designated "high normal." To be consistent with the Seventh Report of the Joint National Committee on the Prevention, Detection, Evaluation, and Treatment of High Blood Pressure [43], this level of BP will now be termed "prehypertensive" and is an indication for lifestyle modifications [43]. Pediatric hypertension is often observed in overweight children, especially those with severe conditions.

## Laboratory Blood Work (Baseline, 3 Months and 1 Year)

Biochemical markers, total cholesterol, triglycerides, high-density lipoproteins, and low-density lipoproteins should be examined by drawing 10 to 20 cc of whole blood in a certified laboratory. Children should be required to fast for 12 hours before the test.

## Body Composition Analysis (Estimate of Percentage Body Fat [Table 4.5])

Skinfold analysis measures the thickness of a double fold of skin and subcutaneous adipose tissue at various body locations [44]. The use of skinfold calipers is the most widely used method for determining obesity. The advantages of this method are its relative simplicity, quickness, and nonevasive nature. In addition, very little space is needed. Various equations have been developed in the prediction of body composition [45–52]. In overweight children, a two-site formula using triceps and subscapular developed by Slaughter et al. [53] has been used and shown to be highly correlated with both underwater weighing and dual-energy x-ray absorptiometry (DEXA) measurements [54].

Bioelectrical impedance may be used to measure the density of lean and adipose tissue in relation to hydration [49,51,52,55]. Studies have shown total body water (TBW) and electrical impedance to be related [56,57]. Further studies also report the utility and reliability of body impedance measurements in the assessment of total body fat [55,58]. Both bioelectrical impedance and skinfolds provide a reasonably accurate, time- and cost-effective method of assessing body fat in overweight children [49–51]. However, care should be taken to select a formula specific to the age, race, and gender of the child, as accuracy varies by study [54,59,60]. More accurate methods are available but are typically reserved for severe overweight conditions or research studies. These include underwater weight and DEXA.

For many years, underwater, or hydrostatic, weighing has been the "gold standard" for the measurement of body fat [44]. The use of underwater weighing is based on Archimedes' principle. Simply stated, Archimedes reasoned that an object submerged in water is buoyed up by a counterforce equaling the weight of the displaced water. An object "loses weight in water." Therefore, if an object weighs 50 kg in air and 3 kg when submerged, the loss of weight in water, 47 kg, equals the weight of displaced water. We can then calculate the volume of water displaced because the density of water at any temperature is known. More recently, DEXA has been used to determine percentage of fat, lean body mass, and bone mineral density in overweight children [49,51,52,61]. DEXA uses an x-ray source to generate photons to scan subjects [62]. Bone-mineral content measurements previously calibrated against secondary standards with ashed bone sections are used to help calculate fat-free mass [63,64]. Percentage of fat and fat-free body can be predicted with accuracy by observing the ratio of absorbance of the different-energy-level photons, which are linearly related to the percentage of fat in the soft tissues of the body [64]. The coefficient of variation of fat-free tissue measurement has been calculated at 2%, which is comparable to that obtained by hydrodensitometry [65].

## Measurement of Physical Activity Level and Fitness (Tables 4.6 and 4.7)

The measurement of the patient's physical activity level provides important clues regarding behaviors that may contribute to the overweight condition. Sedentary behaviors are highly associated with childhood obesity. There are very accurate laboratory procedures that can be used to determine

---

**TABLE 4.6**
**Physical Activity Rating**

Accelerometry
    Intensity-weighted minutes of physical activity
    Records acceleration/deceleration of movement
    Objective measure that provides activity counts and intensity
Heart rate monitoring
    Uses heart rate values to determine amount and intensity of physical activity
Self-report questionnaires
    Godin Leisure Time, 7-day recall, self-administered physical activity checklist (SAPAC)
Direct observation
    System for observing fitness instruction time (SOFIT)

---

---

**TABLE 4.7**
**Metabolic Testing**

Maximal oxygen uptake ($VO_2$ max)
  Graded treadmill test
  Indirect calorimetry
  Heart rate and blood pressure
Resting metabolic rate (RMR) or resting energy expenditure (REE)
  Indirect calorimetry hood system
Respiratory quotient (RQ) or resting energy rate (RER)
  Ratio of oxygen to carbon dioxide
  Indicates fuel source (oxidation)
Total energy expenditure
  Stable isotopes (doubly labeled water)

---

physical activity level. These include accelerometry, total energy expenditure by doubly labeled water, $VO_2$ portable equipment, heart rate monitoring by telemetry, time lapse or video photography, and others [66]. However, the use of such methods is not feasible or cost-effective in primary care settings. Likewise, direct observation techniques such as SOFIT and SOPLAY are impractical in clinical settings. Several self-report questionnaires have been validated in youth 10 years of age or older and are shown to be good predictors of physical activity level (Table 4.6). Samples of these questionnaires may be found in Appendix A2.4.1.

Maximal oxygen uptake ($VO_2$ max) is an indicator of physical fitness level in both adult and youth populations [67–71]. The maximal oxygen uptake indicates the functional capacity of the heart, lungs, and skeletal muscle and is generally assumed to be the single best indicator of physical fitness [69]. The $VO_2$ max is determined by exercising a subject and determining $O_2$ intake and $O_2$ and $CO_2$ concentrations in expired air. All $VO_2$ max tests should be supervised by trained and certified exercise physiologists. Assessing cardiopulmonary fitness in the pediatric population has become the focus of recent research in pediatric medicine and exercise science [72–76], Cardio-vascular responses to exercise stress can be evaluated by obtaining a value for submaximal steady-state or peak or max exercise value (Peak or Max $VO_2$). Maximal oxygen consumption ($VO_2$ max) has been used as an indicator of health related physical fitness [77]. The criteria for achieving a Peak $VO_2$ response in the pediatric population may not be similar to that of adults [78]. Obtaining a plateau in oxygen consumption in children can oftentimes be difficult. However, there have been several protocols that have been used and validated for pediatric exercise testing. In Chapter 10, Rowland and Loftin detail appropriate fitness testing for overweight youth. Detailed exercise testing protocols are also located in Appendix A2.4.2.

## Psychological Testing

Because overweight children are at increased risk for depression, low self-esteem, and other related psychological disorders, it is important that they be screened by an appropriate mental health professional before treatment. Chapter 9 details the appropriate testing procedures for overweight children. Sample referral forms and detailed psychological testing protocols are located in Appendix A1 and A2.5.

## Tanner Staging

Growth and development are affected by many complex factors. Various outcome measures could reflect innate physiological factors rather than our proposed intervention outcome. To assess the effects of nonmodifiable factors such as age and gender on measurement of growth (weight, height), and body composition (lean body mass, percentage of fat), the sexual maturity rating may be determined using methods from Falkner and Tanner [79] on all subjects at fixed intervals (baseline, 10 weeks, 6 months, and 12 months). Sexual maturity ratings (Tanner staging) should be performed during the physical examination by a physician who is specially trained in adolescent medicine (see Appendix A2.6). Alternatively, a self-report tool is available that allows the patient to self-examine his or her level of maturation [80].

## CONCLUSION

The current environmental experience of young children includes few opportunities for physical activity [81] and an overabundance of high-calorie foods. Sedentary lifestyles and poor nutrition challenge children who are genetically predisposed to diabetes, heart disease, and other chronic diseases. Obesity is a logical response to this challenge. Therefore, in predisposed children (e.g., those with obese parents and diabetes history), sedentary, nonnutritious environments challenge their physiologic and metabolic capacity and promote overweight conditions, reduced fitness, further inactivity, and increased sedentary behaviors (television watching and snacking). This results in a clinically significant overweight condition (>95th BMI), reduced insulin sensitivity, and an increased risk of type 2 diabetes and heart disease later in adulthood. Research indicates that increasing physical activity and improving nutrition may significantly affect this series of events [82–84].

The current childhood overweight epidemic is neither the fault nor the responsibility of any one single sector of society. All must work together to develop strategies to change public opinion and behavior concerning healthy nutrition and physical activity across the life span. Because children who are at risk for overweight at 7 years of age or older become increasingly more susceptible as they mature, appropriate, targeted family-based dietary and physical activity interventions should be made available in clinical settings. The economic burden of obesity-associated illness during childhood in the United States has increased by 43% in the last two decades [85]. Cost-effective individual and group approaches are available and should be both encouraged and financially supported by the medical community. More funds are needed for programs that work simultaneously to conduct research and provide ongoing interventions to prevent and treat overweight children in clinical settings. Physicians play a key role in these efforts to prevent and treat overweight conditions, as the epidemic of childhood obesity is the most critical challenge facing the medical community today.

## REFERENCES

1. Taras, H. L., J. F. Sallis, P. R. Nader, and J. Nelson. Children's television-viewing habits and the family environment. *Am J Dis Child*. 144:357–359, 1990.
2. Nguyen, V. T., D. E. Larson, R. K. Johnson, and M. I. Goran. Fat intake and adiposity in children of lean and obese parents. *Am J Clin Nutr*. 63:507–513, 1996.
3. Gill, T. P. Key issues in the prevention of obesity. *Br Med Bull*. 53:359–388, 1997.
4. Strauss, R. S. and J. Knight. Influence of the home environment on the development of obesity in children. *Pediatrics*. 103:e85, 1999.
5. Dietz, W. H. and S. L. Gortmaker. Preventing obesity in children and adolescents. *Annu Rev Public Health*. 22:337–353, 2001.
6. Fogelholm, M., O. Nuutinen, M. Pasanen, E. Myohanen, and T. Saatela. Parent-child relationship of physical activity patterns and obesity. *Int J Obes Relat Metab Disord*. 23:1262–1268., 1999.
7. Dowda, M., B. E. Ainsworth, C. L. Addy, R. Saunders, and W. Riner. Environmental influences, physical activity, and weight status in 8- to 16-year-olds. *Arch Pediatr Adolesc Med*. 155:711–717, 2001.
8. Gottlieb, N. H. and M. S. Chen. Sociocultural correlates of childhood sporting activities: their implications for heart health. *Soc Sci Med*. 21:533–539, 1985.
9. Birch, L. L. and K. K. Davison. Family environmental factors influencing the developing behavioral controls of food intake and childhood overweight. *Pediatr Clin North Am*. 48:893–907, 2001.

10. Birch, L., C. Zimmerman, and H. Hind. The influence of social-affective context on the formation of children's food preferences. *Child Development*. 51:856–861, 1980.

11. Batch, J. A. and L. A. Baur. Management and prevention of obesity and its complications in children and adolescents. *Med J Aust*. 182:130–135, 2005.

12. Story, M. T., D. R. Neumark-Stzainer, N. E. Sherwood, K. Holt, D. Sofka, F. L. Trowbridge, and S. E. Barlow. Management of child and adolescent obesity: attitudes, barriers, skills, and training needs among health care professionals. *Pediatrics*. 110:210–214, 2002.

13. American Academy of Pediatrics, Committee on Nutrition. Prevention of pediatric overweight and obesity. *Pediatrics*. 112:424–430, 2003.

14. Barlow, S. E., F. L. Trowbridge, W. J. Klish, and W. H. Dietz. Treatment of child and adolescent obesity: reports from pediatricians, pediatric nurse practitioners, and registered dietitians. *Pediatrics*. 110:229–235, 2002.

15. Pickering, T., L. Clemow, K. Davidson, and W. Gerin. Behavioral cardiology — has its time finally arrived? *Mt Sinai J Med*. 70:101–112, 2003.

16. Price, J. H., S. M. Desmond, E. S. Ruppert, and C. M. Stelzer. Pediatricians' perceptions and practices regarding childhood obesity. *Am J Prev Med*. 5:95–103, 1989.

17. O'Brien, S. H., R. Holubkov, and E. C. Reis. Identification, evaluation, and management of obesity in an academic primary care center. *Pediatrics*. 114:e154–e159, 2004.

18. Carlisle, L. K., S. T. Gordon, and M. S. Sothern. Can obesity prevention work for our children? *J La State Med Soc*. 157(Spec No 1):S34–S41, 2005.

19. Brown, R., M. Sothern, R. Suskind, J. Udall, and U. Blecker. Racial differences in the lipid profiles of obese children and adolescents before and after significant weight loss. *Clin Pediatr* (Phila). 39:427–431, 2000.

20. Sothern, M., J. Udall, R. Suskind, A. Vargas, and U. Blecker. Weight loss and growth velocity in obese children after very low calorie diet, exercise and behavior modification. *Acta Paediatrica*. 89:1036–1043, 2000.

21. Sothern, M. S. Exercise as a modality in the treatment of childhood obesity. *Pediatr Clin North Am*. 48:995–1015, 2001.

22. Sothern, M. S., B. Despinasse, R. Brown, R. M. Suskind, J. N. Udall, Jr., and U. Blecker. Lipid profiles of obese children and adolescents before and after significant weight loss: differences according to sex. *South Med J*. 93:278–282, 2000.

23. Sothern, M. S., S. Hunter, R. M. Suskind, R. Brown, J. N. Udall, Jr., and U. Blecker. Motivating the obese child to move: the role of structured exercise in pediatric weight management. *South Med J*. 92:577–584, 1999.

24. Sothern, M. S., J. M. Loftin, J. N. Udall, R. M. Suskind, T. L. Ewing, S. C. Tang, and U. Blecker. Safety, feasibility, and efficacy of a resistance training program in preadolescent obese children. *Am J Med Sci*. 319:370–375, 2000.

25. Sothern, M. S., M. Loftin, U. Blecker, and J. N. Udall, Jr. Impact of significant weight loss on maximal oxygen uptake in obese children and adolescents. *J Investig Med*. 48:411–416, 2000.

26. Sothern, M. S., H. Schumacher, T. K. von Almen, L. K. Carlisle, and J. N. Udall. Committed to kids: an integrated, 4-level team approach to weight management in adolescents. *J Am Diet Assoc*. 102:S81–S85, 2002.

27. Hubbard, V.S. Defining overweight and obesity: what are the issues? *Am J Clin Nutr*. 72:1067–1068, 2000.

28. Troiano, R. P. and K. M. Flegal. Overweight children and adolescents: description, epidemiology, and demographics. *Pediatrics*. 101:3, 1998.

29. Troiano, R. P. and K. M. Flegal. Overweight prevalence among youth in the United States: why so many different numbers? *Int J Obes Relat Metab Disord*. 23:S22–S27, 1999.

30. Barlow, S. E. and W. H. Dietz. Obesity evaluation and treatment: Expert Committee recommendations. The Maternal and Child Health Bureau, Health Resources and Services Administration and the Department of Health and Human Services. *Pediatrics*. 102:E29, 1998.

31. Himes, J. and W. J. Dietz. Guidelines for overweight in adolescent preventive services: recommendations from an expert committee. The Expert Committee on Clinical Guidelines for Overweight in Adolescent Preventive Services. *Am J Clin Nutr*. 59:307–316, 1994.

32. Bellizi, M. C. and W. H. Dietz. Workshop on childhood obesity: summary of the discussion. *Am J Clin Nutr*. 70:173S–175S, 1999.

33. Caprio, S. Insulin resistance in childhood obesity. *J Pediatr Endocrinol Metab*. 15(Suppl 1):487–492, 2002.

34. Arslanian, S. A. Metabolic differences between Caucasian and African-American children and the relationship to type 2 diabetes mellitus. *J Pediatr Endocrinol Metab*. 15:509–517, 2002.

35. Zannolli, R., A. Rebeggiani, F. Chiarelli, and G. Morgese. Hyperinsulinism as a marker in obese children. *Am J Dis Child*. 147:837–841, 1993.

36. Brown, R., M. Sothern, R. Suskind, J. Udall, and U. Blecker. Racial differences in the lipid profiles of obese children and adolescents before and after significant weight loss. *Clin Pediatr* (Phila). 39:427–431, 2000.

37. Hill, J. and F. Throwbridge. The causes and health consequences of obesity in children and adolescents. *Pediatrics*. 101:497–575, 1998.

38. Law, C. M., D. J. Barker, C. Osmond, C. H. Fall, and S. J. Simmonds. Early growth and abdominal fatness in adult life. *J Epidemiol Community Health*. 46:184–186, 1992.

39. Steinbeck, K. The importance of physical activity in the prevention of overweight and obesity in childhood: a review and an opinion. *Obes Rev*. 2:117–130, 2001.

40. Micic, D. Obesity in children and adolescents — a new epidemic? Consequences in adult life. *J Pediatr Endocrinol Metab*. 14:1345–1352, 2001.

41. Dietz, W. H. Critical periods in childhood for the development of obesity. *Am J Clin Nutr*. 59:955–959, 1994.

42. Lohman, T., A. A. Roche, and R. Martorell, Eds. *Anthropometric Standardization Reference Manual*. Champaign, IL: Human Kinetics, 1988.

43. Chobanian, A. V., G. L. Bakris, H. R. Black, W. C. Cushman, L. A. Green, J. L. Izzo, Jr. et al. The Seventh Report of the Joint National Committee on Prevention, Detection, Evaluation, and Treatment of High Blood Pressure: the JNC 7 report. *JAMA*. 289:2560–2572, 2003.

44. Roche, A., S. B. Heymsfield, and T. G. Lohman, Eds. *Human Body Composition*. Champaign, IL: Human Kinetics, 1996.

45. Durnin, J. V. and J. Womersley. Body fat assessed from total body density and its estimation from skinfold thickness: measurements on 481 men and women aged from 16 to 72 years. *Br J Nutr*. 32:77–97, 1974.

46. Jackson, A. S. and M. L. Pollock. Generalized equations for predicting body density of men. *Br J Nutr*. 40:497–504, 1978.

47. Lohman, T. G. Skinfolds and body density and their relation to body fatness: a review. *Hum Biol*. 53:181–225, 1981.

48. Sloan, A. W. Estimation of body fat in young men. *J Appl Physiol*. 23:311–315, 1967.

49. Goran, M. I., P. Driscoll, R. Johnson, T. R. Nagy, and G. Hunter. Cross-calibration of body-composition techniques against dual-energy X-ray absorptiometry in young children. *Am J Clin Nutr*. 63:299–305, 1996.

50. Cameron, N., P. L. Griffiths, M. M. Wright, C. Blencowe, N. C. Davis, J. M. Pettifor, and S. A. Norris. Regression equations to estimate percentage body fat in African prepubertal children aged 9 y. *Am J Clin Nutr*. 80:70–75, 2004.

51. Bray, G., J. P. DeLaney, D. W. Volaufova, D. W. Harsha, and C. Champaign. Prediction of body fat in 12-y-old African American and white children: evaluation of methods. *Am J Clin Nutr*. 76:980–990, 2002.

52. Gutin, B., M. Litaker, S. Islam, T. Manos, C. Smith, and F. Treiber. Body-composition measurement in 9-11-y-old children by dual-energy x-ray absorptiometry, skinfold-thickness measurements, and bioimpedance analysis. *Am J Clin Nutr*. 63:287–292, 1996.

53. Slaughter, M. H., T. G. Lohman, R. A. Boileau, C. A. Horswill, R. J. Stillman, M. D. Van Loan, and D. A. Bemben. Skinfold equations for estimation of body fatness in children and youth. *Hum Biol*. 60:709–723, 1988.

54. Boye, K. R., T. Dimitriou, F. Manz, E. Schoenau, C. Neu, S. Wudy, and T. Remer. Anthropometric assessment of muscularity during growth: estimating fat-free mass with 2 skinfold-thickness measurements is superior to measuring midupper arm muscle area in healthy prepubertal children. *Am J Clin Nutr*. 76:628–632, 2002.

55. Fors, H., L. Gelander, R. Bjarnason, K. Albertsson-Wikland, and I. Bosaeus. Body composition, as assessed by bioelectrical impedance spectroscopy and dual-energy X-ray absorptiometry, in a healthy paediatric population. *Acta Paediatr*. 91:755–760, 2002.

56. Hoffer, E. C., C. K. Meador, and D. C. Simpson. Correlation of whole-body impedance with total body water volume. *J Appl Physiol*. 27:531–534, 1969.

57. Eisenkolbl, J., M. Kartasurya, and K. Widhalm. Underestimation of percentage fat mass measured by bioelectrical impedance analysis compared to dual energy X-ray absorptiometry method in obese children. *Eur J Clin Nutr*. 55:423–429, 2001.

58. Casanova Roman, M., I. Rodriguez Ruiz, S. Rico de Cos, and M. Casanova Bellido. [Body composition analysis using bioelectrical and anthropometric parameters]. *An Pediatr* (Barc). 61:23–31, 2004.

59. Parker, L., J. J. Reilly, C. Slater, J. C. Wells, and Y. Pitsiladis. Validity of six field and laboratory methods for measurement of body composition in boys. *Obes Res.* 11:852–858, 2003.

60. Morrison, J. A., S. S. Guo, B. Specker, W. C. Chumlea, S. Z. Yanovski, and J. A. Yanovski. Assessing the body composition of 6-17-year-old Black and White girls in field studies. *Am J Hum Biol.* 13:249–254, 2001.

61. Ogle, G. D., J. R. Allen, and I. R. Humphries. Body-composition assessment by dual-energy x-ray absorptiometry in subjects aged 4-26 y. *Am J Clin Nutr.* 61:746–753, 1995.

62. Pietrobelli A., C. Formica, Z. Wang, and S. Heymsfield. Dual-energy X-ray absorptiometry body composition model: review of physical concepts. *Am J Physiol.* 271:E941–E951, 1996.

63. Friedl, K. E., J. P. DeLuca, L. J. Marchitelli, and J. A. Vogel. Reliability of body-fat estimations from a four-compartment model by using density, body water, and bone mineral measurements. *Am J Clin Nutr.* 55:764–770, 1992.

64. Mazess, R. B., H. S. Barden, J. P. Bisek, and J. Hanson. Dual-energy x-ray absorptiometry for total-body and regional bone-mineral and soft-tissue composition. *Am J Clin Nutr.* 51:1106–1112, 1990.

65. Ellis, K. J., R. J. Shypailo, A. Pratt, and W. G. Pond. Accuracy of dual-energy x-ray absorptiometry for body-composition measurements in children. *Am J Clin Nutr.* 60:660–665, 1994.

66. Bar-Or, O. A., T. W. Rowland, and W. Thomas. *Pediatric Exercise Medicine: From Physiologic Principles to Health Care Application.* Champaign, IL: Human Kinetics, 2004.

67. McArdle, W. D. and J. R. Magel. Physical work capacity and maximum oxygen uptake in treadmill and bicycle exercise. *Med Sci Sports.* 2:118–123, 1970.

68. Casaburi, R., S. Spitzer, R. Haskell, and K. Wasserman. Effect of altering heart rate on oxygen uptake at exercise onset. *Chest.* 95:6–12, 1989.

69. Astrand, P. O., E. Hultman, A. Juhlin-Dannfelt, and G. Reynolds. Disposal of lactate during and after strenuous exercise in humans. *J Appl Physiol.* 61:338–343, 1986.

70. Mitchell, J. H. and G. Blomqvist. Maximal oxygen uptake. *N Engl J Med.* 284:1018–1022, 1971.

71. Rowell, L. B., H. L. Taylor, and Y. Wang. Limitations to prediction of maximal oxygen intake. *J Appl Physiol.* 19:919–927, 1964.

72. Greiwe, J. S., L. A. Kaminsky, M. H. Whaley, and G. B. Dwyer. Evaluation of the ACSM submaximal ergometer test for estimating VO$_2$ max. *Med Sci Sports Exerc.* 27:1315–1320, 1995.

73. American College of Sports Medicine Position Stand. The recommended quantity and quality of exercise for developing and maintaining cardiorespiratory and muscular fitness, and flexibility in healthy adults, 30(6):975–991, 1998.

74. Rowland, T., R. Bhargava, D. Parslow, and R. A. Heptulla. Cardiac response to progressive cycle exercise in moderately obese adolescent females. *J Adolesc Health.* 32:422–427, 2003.

75. Rowland, T., L. Koenigs, and N. Miller. Myocardial performance during maximal exercise in adolescents with anorexia nervosa. *J Sports Med Phys Fitness.* 43:202–208, 2003.

76. Bar-Or, O., Foreyt, J., Bouchard, C. et al. Physical activity, genetic and nutritional considerations in childhood weight management. *Med Sci Sports Exerc.* 30:2–10, 1998.

77. Astrand, P. O. and B. Saltin. Maximal oxygen uptake and heart rate in various types of muscular activity. *J Appl Physiol.* 16:977–981, 1961.

78. Rowland, T., G. Kline, D. Goff, L. Martel, and L. Ferrone. One-mile run performance and cardiovascular fitness in children. *Arch Pediatr Adolesc Med.* 153:845–849, 1999.

79. Falkner, F. and J. Tanner. *Human Growth.* London: Baillier Tindall, 1979.

80. Carskadon, M. A. and C. Acebo. A self-administered rating scale for pubertal development. *J Adolesc Health.* 14:190–195, 1993.

81. Falkner, B. and S. Michel. Obesity and other risk factors in children. *Ethn Dis.* 9:284–289, 1999.

82. Rippe, J. M. and S. Hess. The role of physical activity in the prevention and management of obesity. *J Am Diet Assoc.* 98:S31–S38, 1998.

83. Epstein, L. H. and G. S. Goldfield. Physical activity in the treatment of childhood overweight and obesity: current evidence and research issues. *Med Sci Sports Exerc.* 31:S553–S559, 1999.

84. Gortmaker, S. L., K. Peterson, J. Wiecha, A. M. Sobol, S. Dixit, M. K. Fox, and N. Laird. Reducing obesity via a school-based interdisciplinary intervention among youth: Planet Health. *Arch Pediatr Adolesc Med.* 153:409–418, 1999.

85. Wang, L., Q. Yang, R. Lowry, and H. Wechsler. Economic analysis of a school-based obesity prevention program. *Obes Res.* 11:1313–1324, 2003.

# Section 3

## Psychosocial and Physical Considerations

# 5 Psychosocial Considerations during Treatment

*Jeffrey B. Schwimmer*

## CONTENTS

## INTRODUCTION

Psychosocial factors influence the development of obesity, its comorbidities, and the ability to follow clinical recommendations for therapies, including lifestyle modification. The key components from a psychosocial perspective are to conduct a focused yet complete assessment, to consider psychosocial status as an important clinical outcome, and to successfully use psychosocial tools to enhance the efficacy of weight management [1–3].

Behavioral therapy provides tools to overcome barriers in making lasting dietary and activity changes. Although not effective in isolation, behavioral therapy has been shown to be an important component of successful weight management. There are many psychosocial factors that clinicians must consider when administering behavioral therapy to overweight children and their families. These factors can include underlying/comorbid psychopathologies, family psychosocial issues, and psychosocial consequences. These factors will be discussed in this chapter, in addition to psychosocial tools that may be employed while administering behavioral therapy to these overweight children and families.

## UNDERLYING/COMORBID PSYCHOPATHOLOGY

Psychopathology has been indicated as a possible contributing factor in the development of pediatric obesity [4]. Psychopathological symptoms often found in conjunction with pediatric obesity include depression, anxiety, and eating disorders. Although psychopathology may be more common in overweight children [4], it has been identified as the key cause of obesity in only a small number of overweight children.

Clinicians should be aware of some of the more common symptoms associated with psychopathology, such as poor concentration, low motivation, and social withdrawal [1]. Aggression and behavioral problems are also commonly witnessed with these mental disorders [4]. In a study conducted by Erermis et al. [4], 27% of clinically obese and non-clinically obese adolescents were diagnosed with depressive disorders, compared with only 6% of the normal-weight control group. In general, the frequency of diagnosis of various mental disorders such as depression, anxiety, binge eating, and hyperactivity was significantly higher in the obese adolescents than the youths of normal weight [4].

### DEPRESSION

Depressed mood among adolescents is a risk factor for the development and persistence of obesity. However, the relationship between obesity and depression remains controversial. Whether one condition directly contributes to the other or whether they co-exist due to overlapping but non-causal mechanisms remains unresolved. It is clear, however, that the treatment of one condition can affect the other. The successful treatment of obesity can lead a decrease in symptoms of depression. In contrast, medications used to treat depression have the potential to produce weight gain. In cases of major depression it is usually necessary to adequately treat depression before a patient is able to successfully participate in a program of lasting lifestyle modification for weight management.

### ANXIETY

Anxiety in overweight children is often observed in conjunction with more common psychological disorders such as depression, poor self-esteem, and social isolation/withdrawal. Situations or events that may trigger anxiety in overweight children are not easily identified. In a study conducted by Morgan et al. [7], overweight children who reported episodes of uncontrollable eating were found to have much higher levels of anxiety. Binge eaters also displayed increased feelings of depression and poor self-esteem compared with overweight children who did not report binge-eating episodes [5].

Although anxiety is not currently identified as a sole contributing factor in pediatric obesity, a common test that can be used for screening is the Revised Children's Manifest Anxiety Scale [6].

Of additional concern is that overweight children are more likely to engage in risky behaviors and to experience psychosocial distress. This detrimental behavior may be associated with the consequences of being overweight. These consequences include weight discrimination, negative stereotyping, and pressure to conform to certain body ideals [7]. In extreme cases, overweight children may develop eating disorders.

### EATING DISORDERS

Eating disorders are associated with cycles of weight loss and regain and are considered the exhibition of extreme weight behavior [8]. Disorders include anorexia nervosa, bulimia, and binge eating [8]. These types of extreme dieting can be devastating to a child's life. The child can often experience both physical and psychological consequences. These include menstrual irregularities for girls, decrease in self-esteem, poor concentration, growth retardation, delayed sexual maturation, and disturbed sleep patterns [8]. As with many other comorbid psychosocial factors, eating disorders can also predispose the child to other risky behaviors: alcohol and drug abuse, smoking, promiscuity, autoaggression, and suicide [9].

Eating disorders are an expression of psychosocial factors rather than an expression of how a child feels about his or her body [8]. It is thought that lack of family support and connectedness contribute to this behavior [10]. In a study by Fairburn et al. [10], families of bulimic patients were found to exhibit abusive tendencies. Another study by Hodges et al. [11] determined that families of binge-eating patients scored high in family conflict. In short, family dysfunction has been found to increase the tendency for children to develop negative self-esteem, which may lead to extreme weight behaviors [12].

The link between family dysfunction and unhealthy weight behavior was identified in a study by Fonseca and colleagues [8]. The study consisted of 9402 students, 12 to 18 years of age. Of that number, 4625 were girls, and 4417 were boys. Adolescents with body mass index (BMI) values of less than 10 or more than 50 were excluded, as well as any who were of significantly short stature. These students were asked to complete a survey comprising questions about health, risky behaviors, and protective factors. Health factors included dieting and exercising. Risky behaviors included vomiting; taking diet pills, laxatives, or diuretics; and excessive exercise. Protective factors included family communication, parental supervision and monitoring, family connectedness, and perceived caring and communication with other adults and friends. Behaviors were assessed over a 1-week period, during which each question began with: "During the last week …". Overall, 38.2% of girls versus 12.4% of boys reported dieting in that past week. In addition, girls exceeded boys in trying to lose weight through exercise: 61.1% versus 42.8%. Likewise, more girls were found vomiting (4.0% vs. 1.7%) and using diet pills (3.8% vs. 1.1%). Gender did not, however, affect the use of laxatives and diuretics. Interestingly, it was also found that risk factors included high parental supervision/monitoring. Both groups had a high risk factor when linked with sexual abuse histories [8].

In a study by Grignard et al. [13], a group of 31 obese adolescents were administered a questionnaire and a body dissatisfaction test and were interviewed regarding weight and body image. Although a relationship between weight and self-image was established, the direction of causality was not determined [13]. Therefore, the results did not confirm whether weight loss improves the body image or improving self-esteem results in weight loss.

Although psychopathological problems are more prevalent in overweight children, not all overweight children experience these problems. Clinicians may wish to use some common psychiatric screening methods, including the Child Behavior Checklist, Children Depression Inventory, Rosenberg Self-Esteem Scale, and Eating Attitude Tests [4]. A description of these tools and methods of application is given by Johnson and von Almen in Chapter 9 of this volume.

## FAMILY PSYCHOSOCIAL ISSUES

The family serves as the foundation for the development of a child's mental well-being. Problems within the home environment may manifest through eating disorders and excessive weight gain. In a study by Epstein et al. [14], the mental health of the parent and stability of family relationships were some of the strongest predictors of the child's mental health. Myers et al. [3] supported this view in a study that particularly focused on the mother–child relationship. This study found a reciprocal relationship between the psychological health of the mother and that of the child, with psychological improvement in either case resulting in benefits to the other.

Stradmeijer and colleagues [15] evaluated 143 children and their parents — 73 overweight and 70 normal weight — to examine the relationship between family functioning and psychosocial adjustment. Results indicated that the older overweight girls displayed a lower self-esteem than the younger girls. In contrast, the boys' self-esteem improved with age. In addition, the parents of overweight children reported more negative behavior issues than those of normal weight children. Excessive parental attention was cited as a potential reason for children to develop this negative behavior. More research is needed to determine the relationship between "parental over-concern" and the social and emotional issues of overweight children [15].

## FAMILY STRUCTURE

It was previously mentioned in the chapter that environmental factors have a large effect on unhealthy weight behavior. One such important factor is family structure, as it relates to eating behavior. In a recent study [16], the relationship of family structure and frequency of fast food restaurant use was examined. The results indicated that family structure affects young women more than young men. Specifically, females of single-parent families more often indulged in fast food restaurant dining [16]. By the year 1998, 27% of all households with children were single-parent homes. This higher frequency of fast food visits by females may be attributed to the fact that more women are working, and therefore, less time is available to them for food preparation. As a consequence, because of this larger number of working, single-family households with children, an increasingly larger portion of children are consuming fast food on a regular basis [16], which may indirectly contribute to pediatric obesity.

## CHILD–PARENT CONFLICTS

The relationship between a parent and child can have a significant effect on the behaviors of that child. Mellin et al. [7] compared overweight and nonoverweight adolescents on selected physical activity and dietary behaviors. They also compared the adolescents' behaviors with their family relationships. The overweight girls and boys both engaged in significantly higher levels of unhealthy behaviors compared with the normal-weight children. In addition, an inverse relationship was observed between family connectedness and unhealthy behaviors.

Fonseca et al. [8] examined the association between familial factors and extreme weight control in adolescents. It was observed that family connectedness served as a protective factor for girls displaying extreme weight behaviors. In addition, connectedness to not only parents but also other adults and friends served as a protective factor for boys. In girls, high levels of parental guidance and supervision accounted for protection against extreme weight behaviors; in boys, the opposite was observed [8].

Parental conflicts, including a lack of parental-expressed empathy/affection, were found to be a factor in binge eating relapse [17]. In addition, adolescents exhibiting hostile attitudes toward their family also were found to experience relapses in binge eating [17]. To reduce behavioral and psychological risk factors that lead to pediatric obesity, a healthy parent–child relationship is essential during childhood.

## RELATIONSHIPS BETWEEN CHILD ABUSE AND OBESITY

Abuse significantly affects the behavior patterns of developing children. Both physical and emotional abuse can lead to unhealthy habits. Although some children and adolescents are able to look to friends or family for assistance, others seek to control themselves through extreme dieting or obsession with food [8]. In a recent review article, Gustafson and Sarwer [18] found that childhood sexual abuse may lead to depression, anxiety, substance abuse, and eating disorders. Few studies have concentrated on the relationship between sexual abuse and pediatric obesity.

Childhood sexual abuse has been linked to adult weight problems that may be a result of binge-eating disorders (BED). Williamson et al. [19] investigated the associations between self-reported abuse in childhood and adult body weight and risk of obesity. In those who experienced physical and verbal abuse, body weight and obesity were strongly related. Moreover, as the severity of the abuse increased, so did the risk for obesity. Thus, targeting or preventing abuse during childhood may potentially decrease the progression of obesity into adulthood.

Grilo and Masheb [20] examined the relationship of maltreatment and BED in 145 diagnosed adults. Subjects were administered a childhood trauma questionnaire [20] to assess emotional, physical, and sexual abuse as well as emotional and physical neglect. A total of 83% reported some form of maltreatment during childhood, and the results did not differ by gender or current obesity status. Emotional abuse was the only form of maltreatment that was significantly associated with psychological variables such as greater body dissatisfaction, higher depression, and lower self-esteem. The findings of Grilo and Masheb were consistent with previous studies. Childhood maltreatment is associated with psychological distress in general. However, whether there is a specific association with weight or eating disorder symptomatology in children is unknown.

## CULTURE AS IT INFLUENCES BODY TYPE IMAGES AND DIETARY PREFERENCES

Many cultures set standards as to what they believe defines beauty in individuals. Often, body type images are unrealistic and harmful. Research indicates that those who try to conform to their culture's idea of body image will be more prone to developing eating disorders. Perez and Joiner [21] examined body image dissatisfaction and disordered eating in a small group of both black and white college women based solely on their self-perceptions. Of the women surveyed, the ideal body image size was larger for black women than for white women. The results also indicated that white women reported themselves to be overweight, whereas black women reported being underweight compared with ideal body image size. These perceptions indicate that dissatisfaction with body size may result in differing eating disorders. Although white women may binge and purge, black women may only binge, resulting in malnourishment and obesity, respectively. This is not to say that white women are more likely to have eating disorders compared with black women, but each group may develop eating disorders to either lose or gain weight to fit their culture's mold. To combat these problems, cultures need to encourage realistic and healthy body images [21].

An individual's perception of an ideal body image is greatly influenced by television and advertisements. The public connects with the characters on television and looks to them as role models for how they should appear. A study conducted by Greenberg et al. [22] used an evaluation of prime-time television to identify body type characteristics. The study found that 14% of the female and 24% of the male characters viewed were overweight or obese. These characters were most commonly considered less attractive and unlikely to have romantic partners or show physical affection, and they were shown eating more than the normal-weight characters. On the contrary, 87% of the women viewed during the study were of average weight or underweight. In reality, however, only about half of all women in the United States are average weight or underweight. In real life men are three times more likely to be obese than their television peers; male television characters were six times more likely to be underweight than their counterparts in real life. These findings illustrate that television may promote a negative self-concept in overweight individuals. When overweight individuals compare themselves with television characters, they may incorrectly associate large body types with negative appearance status and behavior.

## PSYCHOSOCIAL CONSEQUENCES

### PEER TEASING

Peer teasing is a problem that affects all children, not just the overweight or obese. It is estimated that up to three-quarters of children suffer from some type of peer teasing [23]. Peer teasing is characterized by the domination of one person over another, with the intent to harm repeatedly [24]. Specifically, peer teasing is usually referred to as bullying, harassment, or victimization [23]. In the case of the overweight or obese, it is referred to as weight-based teasing [13,25]. Grignard and colleagues [13] use the term "peer mockery" to define a psychosocial consequence resulting from weight.

In U.S. culture, there is a strong emphasis placed on body size and shape. This emphasis may explain why overweight children are commonly victims of weight-based teasing [25]. Weight-based teasing is the means by which peers expose the physical differences of overweight and obese individuals, particularly in children [26]. Inevitably, weight-based teasing can become harmful to an child's well-being [25]. Little public attention has been given to weight-based teasing; however, with the increase of obesity in children [23,25,26], more research is dedicated to examining the potentially harmful effects of weight-based teasing. Janssen et al. (2004) [28] examined the association between weight-based teasing and weight status (BMI) in children 11 to 16 years of age. It was observed that as teasing increased, BMI increased.

Social problems, such as self-induced isolation, are associated with psychosocial factors of being overweight or obese [23,25,26]. These factors include low body satisfaction, self-esteem issues, and comorbidities, such as depressive tendencies. Thus, weight-based teasing may increase loneliness, sadness, and unhappiness about weight [23]. Possibly, because of a resulting low-body image, overweight children seek isolation [26]. This self-induced isolation leads to ineffective bonding, which leads to separation from peers [26]. Combined, weight-based teasing and a depressive state can lead to suicidal thoughts or attempts [23,25]. This occurrence was noted in a study by Eisenberg and Aalsma [23], who reported that weight-based teasing increased suicidal attempts to two to three times higher in adolescents who were teased compared with those who were not.

Psychosocial problems associated with weight-based teasing intensify negative short-term and long-term outcomes for overweight and obese adolescents. Short-term outcomes include low academic success and poor high school performance. Long-term outcomes include lower marriage rates and lower income [7,23,26,27].

## SCHOOL

In the school environment, overweight children may be victims of negative stereotyping. These negative stereotypes include inaccurate perceptions by peers, teachers, and administrators that overweight children are lazy, stupid, and lack motivation [28]. In turn, this leads to a stronger expectation for slimmer, fit individuals to achieve high scores in intelligence testing and education [29]. Overweight children and adolescents are found to be four times more likely than healthy children and adolescents to report impaired school function [30]. These results were substantiated by a study in Thailand, which reported that overweight children and adolescents in grades 7 through 9 were twice as likely to have low grades in math and language as healthy children and adolescents [31].

Poor academic success includes poor grades, poor attitude toward school, and poor attendance [23]. It is plausible that weight-based teasing contributes to the development of poor academic success by causing overweight children to further develop low self-esteem [23]. In turn, low self-esteem may further perpetuate poor academic performance, which includes poor grades, poor attitude toward school, and poor attendance [23]. Low self-esteem promotes poor academic performance because the child may come to believe less and less in his or her abilities. Therefore, it is imperative to intervene and address weight-based teasing as soon as possible [7,23,25,26]. Intervention can include alteration of school rules, peer-teasing training for teachers, open forums and discussions in classrooms on the subject, individual meetings, and extracurricular activities to enhance bonding [23]. Other extreme measures, such as legislation, should also be considered, especially when efforts to communicate with school administration have failed.

In a recent study, Latner and Stunkard [32] reported that the stigmatization of obese children has significantly increased over the last 40 years. The overt discrimination of obese youth may limit both their educational aspirations and achievements [7]. Research indicates that overweight children assess their school performance and educational futures lower than do normal-weight children [7]. This perceived low expectation may influence school attrition. We recently reported [30] that obese children and adolescents involved in our study missed a mean of 4.2 days of school in the month before the study. These missed days of school could lead to decreased school performance, with possible long-term consequences. Research has also linked overweight adolescents, especially girls, with fewer years of school completed [27]. Missed school days may subsequently lead to decreased school performance. The negative impact of educational disturbances may be long lasting. Overweight adolescent girls are less likely to attend college and as adults go on to have lower household income than their peers who were normal weight as adolescents. The implications of not attending college and not achieving higher-education status may also serve to explain why overweight adolescents, as adults, have lower household income than adults who were normal weight as adolescents [26,27].

## QUALITY OF LIFE

In the last few years, research has shown that overweight children and adolescents experience a lower health-related quality-of-life (HRQL) [30,33,35]. Quality of Life includes the social, emotional, and physical functioning of a person [36].

Recently, we reported [30] that severely obese children and adolescents had a lower HRQL than healthy children and adolescents. We also compared these severely obese children and adolescents with children and adolescents with cancer because cancer is a chronic health condition with known impaired HRQL. We observed that the severely obese children and adolescents had a similar HRQL as the children and adolescents diagnosed with cancer. Although obese children and adolescents may also experience physical limitations and teasing from peers, they are often not exposed to the intense medical interventions (and subsequent adverse effects) that are common in pediatric cancer. Thus, the impaired HRQL of the obese sample was an unexpected and significant finding [30]. This impaired HRQL can cause difficulties in keeping up with peers and maintaining normal activities [37] and can also result in teasing and withdrawal from peers at school [36]. Such changes can be seen in school-aged children with mild obesity.

## PSYCHOSOCIAL TOOLS

### COGNITIVE BEHAVIORAL THERAPY

The comprehensive framework of a cognitive-behavioral weight management program involves understanding health-related behaviors and modifying those behaviors that are linked to adverse health effects [38]. Behavioral treatments for pediatric obesity should focus on modifying behaviors that bear on health and illness. These can involve issues such as improving dietary choices, decreasing sedentary behaviors, and increasing habitual physical activity and exercise. It is important to focus on the patient's attitudes and beliefs about weight loss while building a partnership with the patient. The physician or health professional should assist the patient in modifying current behaviors and setting achievable goals. As with other behavior therapies, the patient's readiness to change should be assessed and discussed, in addition to identifying potential variables associated with weight loss. Several concepts should be discussed with the patient, in particular, body image and unrealistic weight loss expectations. Cognitive-behavioral treatment can also be used to help overweight children become more assertive in coping with the adverse social stigma of being overweight. This can not only enhance their self-esteem but also reduce their dissatisfaction with their body image, regardless of their weight loss [38]. In a recent study, Warschburger et al. developed and evaluated a cognitive-behavioral training program for obese children and adolescents. The training program was effective in teaching the children and adolescents ways to manage their weight status and to deal with associated psychosocial problems [39].

### KNOWLEDGE AND SELF-EFFICACY

Knowledge has not been shown to be sufficient as a motivating tool when trying to change a behavior [40]. This is particularly important when attempting to change diet and become physically active [41]. In this case, simply providing the patient with information that will help him or her lose weight, or handing out pamphlets with sample exercises to undertake, has not been shown to successfully alter behavior [41]. There are several factors that contribute to this lack of success.

One such barrier is the "cognitive barrier." In the cognitive barrier, a lack of knowledge, low self-efficacy, and a limited acceptance of personal risk can greatly affect a person's desire to change [41].

Environment is also important in behavior change and can many times lead to program failure. For example, an overweight child will likely fail if the parents are not supportive and continue to stock the house with high-fat foods. There are also environments outside of the home that offer cheap convenience food, such as movie theaters and shopping malls [41]. The suburban and urban way of life demands the use of a car for transportation to be able to function. Other environmental barriers to successful implementation include lack of access to care and social support for change, and social and cultural factors such as fast food, sedentary lifestyles, and food preferences [41].

A lack of motivation can also prevent the obese patient from changing his or her behavior. Many times this motivational barrier is deep-set in emotional fears. The fear of giving up a "behavioral crutch" can sometimes limit a person who is trying to change his or her lifestyle. Relapses are also cause for emotional/motivational barriers to behavioral changes. A person may feel that "this is hopeless" because instead of losing weight, he or she has gained weight, or perhaps has put on several pounds after having lost a solid amount. This failure to change may lead to shame, demoralization, and helplessness [41].

## Behavioral Counseling

There are several health behavioral change models that are currently practiced. These change models can be applied to altering behavior in physical activity and diet. One such model is the social learning model, which is concerned with a person's attitude toward change. This change model has been found to have an effect on cognitive, interpersonal, and environmental factors, which in turn have influenced behavior [42].

To apply this change model to physical activity and diet behavior, individuals proceed through a series of steps: self-monitoring, self-analysis, self-management, and replacement of unhealthy behavior [41]. The self-monitoring step typically includes keeping a food diary. The self-analysis step includes the discussion of reasons for amounts of food intake during the day. During the self-management step, the individual identifies certain moods and clues that indicate a need for excess food. The last step — the replacement of unhealthy behavior, such as eating high-fat foods — is the most challenging step. During this last step, adding incentives to replacing the unhealthy behavior is shown to increase success.

Another factor addressed in the social learning model is the management of stress. With successful management of eating and physical activity, overweight individuals increase self-confidence in their ability to gain control over specific behaviors [41]. This would, in turn, reduce their stress level. Self-efficacy states that the greater the perceived ability to maintain a behavior, the greater the actual occurrences of that healthy behavior. Thus, positive self-efficacy with diet and physical change is a very important factor in weight management. Self-efficacy also influences the treatment of depression and the reduction of stress — both psychosocial factors that affect obesity.

Behavioral therapy has been shown to be effective even when done briefly [41]. The Worcester Area Trial for Counseling in Hyperlipidemia study is an example of how brief counseling can provide positive results in weight loss [41]. During the study, physicians were given 8 minutes with each patient. Study patients received either counseling alone (control) or counseling combined with handouts and questionnaires concerning dieting (treatment) while in the waiting rooms [6]. A year later, treatment patients were found to have lost 2.3 kg more than the control and, as a benefit of that loss, to have lowered their cholesterol by 3.8 mg [41].

Several other techniques, such as contracting, have been identified to improve self-care and manage weight. Contracting is the actual writing down of patient goals. Also, providing the patient with small, controllable tasks is another way to allow for success that helps sustain motivation. Finally, it is extremely important to give feedback to the patient, to establish a social support group, and to keep track of the patient's commitment [41]. Remember, though, that the key is to identify the patient's specific problems to correctly assess which techniques to employ. It is the physician's responsibility to ask the patient to identify barriers to changing eating or physical activity behaviors.

Along with social support, another important aid is using a team approach in physician intervention. Not only should the primary care physician be involved but also nurses, psychologists, dietitians, and social workers. Such a team is necessary because behavioral interventions tend to require relatively large amounts of professional time [41].

## MOTIVATIONAL INTERVIEWING

Motivational interviewing (MI) is a technique that originated in the field of substance abuse treatment [43]. The foundation of MI is a nonconfrontational, patient-based counseling approach to behavior change [44], rather than a provider-directed approach [45]. Although MI has been used mainly in the substance abuse realm, MI employs techniques that may be applicable to a variety of behavior changes [43]. Recent studies have suggested the use of MI in health promotion and disease management [46].

VanWormer and Boucher [46] suggest four guiding principles of MI. The first principle is to *express empathy*. The health professional should listen to the patient with respect and expect ambivalence and reluctance to change [43]. The second guideline involves *discrepancy development* [48]. Developing discrepancy involves reviewing the pros and cons of behavior change [43]. The health professional should call attention to a current behavior pattern and future goals, thus increasing motivation from the patient for a lifestyle change [46]. The third principle is *rolling with resistance* [46]. Although resistance should be expected, the health professional should try to steer this resistance to motivation [43]. The health professional should try to provoke a new perspective from the patient [46]. The fourth and final guideline is to *support self-efficacy* [46]. Because a patient's self-efficacy is one of the greatest predictors of treatment outcome [46], the patient's autonomy and confidence should be encouraged and supported by the health professional [43]. Some of the same principles addressed earlier in this chapter and in Chapter 14, such as self-efficacy and readiness to change assessments, can be employed in MI.

To successfully use MI, the health professional should develop his or her interaction techniques. These involve such skills as asking open-ended questions, affirming statements of recognition, and reflective listening [43]. These techniques will help create an environment in which the patient feels at ease to discuss what is important to him or her [45]. MI may be particularly useful in the medical setting because it offers a briefer, alternative approach for intervening with patients (with some meetings as brief as 20 minutes), compared with psychotherapy (typically a series of 50-minute settings) [43].

## CONCLUSION

Consideration of psychosocial factors is a common recommendation in a comprehensive approach to pediatric weight management. This chapter provides a framework for thinking about the different elements encompassed within the psychosocial domain. A challenge is to appreciate that common themes are present among many obese children presenting for weight management but that for any one child the specific set of contributing factors is unique. Furthermore, the resources available to make lifestyle changes as well as the barriers to change that are present must be appropriately identified. The high prevalence of pediatric obesity and the tremendous diversity of the clinical population require both a structured and flexible approach at the same time. Herein lies the foundation of patient-centered care as well as a broad opportunity for future research addressing fundamental unanswered questions.

## REFERENCES

1. Fabricatore, A. N. and T. A. Wadden. Psychological aspects of obesity. *Clin Dermatol.* 22:332–337, 2004.
2. Zeller, M., S. Kirk, R. Claytor, P. Khoury, J. Grieme, M. Santangelo, and S. Daniels. Predictors of attrition from a pediatric weight management program. *J Pediatr.* 144:466–470, 2004.
3. Myers, M. D., H. A. Raynor, and L. H. Epstein. Predictors of child psychological changes during family-based treatment for obesity. *Arch Pediatr Adolesc Med.* 152:855–861, 1998.
4. Erermis, S., N. Cetin, M. Tamar, N. Bukusoglu, F. Akdeniz, and D. Goksen. Is obesity a risk factor for psychopathology among adolescents? *Pediatr Int.* 46:296–301, 2004.
5. Morgan, C. M., S. Z. Yanovski, T. T. Nguyen, J. McDuffie, N. G. Sebring, M. R. Jorge et al. Loss of control over eating, adiposity, and psychopathology in overweight children. *Int J Eat Disord.* 31:430–441, 2002.
6. Strauss, R. S., D. Rodzilsky, G. Burack, and M. Colin. Psychosocial correlates of physical activity in healthy children. *Arch Pediatr Adolesc Med.* 155:897–902, 2001.
7. Mellin, A. E., D. Neumark-Sztainer, M. Story, M. Ireland, and M. D. Resnick. Unhealthy behaviors and psychosocial difficulties among overweight adolescents: the potential impact of familial factors. *J Adolesc Health.* 31:145–153, 2002.
8. Fonseca, H., M. Ireland, and M. D. Resnick. Familial correlates of extreme weight control behaviors among adolescents. *Int J Eat Disord.* 32:441–448, 2002.
9. Kiess, W., A. Galler, A. Reich, G. Muller, T. Kapellen, J. Deutscher et al. Clinical aspects of obesity in childhood and adolescence. *Obes Rev.* 2:29–36, 2001.
10. Fairburn, C. G., S. L. Welch, H. A. Doll, B. A. Davies, and M. E. O'Connor. Risk factors for bulimia nervosa. A community-based case-control study. *Arch Gen Psychiatry.* 54:509–517, 1997.
11. Hodges, E. L., C. E. Cochrane, and T. D. Brewerton. Family characteristics of binge-eating disorder patients. *Int J Eat Disord.* 23:145–151, 1998.
12. Leung, F., A. Schwartzman, and H. Steiger. Testing a dual-process family model in understanding the development of eating pathology: a structural equation modeling analysis. *Int J Eat Disord.* 20:367–375, 1996.
13. Grignard, S., Bourguignon, J., Michel, B., Philippe, M., and Chantal, V. *Characteristics of Adolescent Attempts to Manage Overweight.* Elsevier Science Ireland, 2002.
14. Epstein, L. H., K. R. Klein, and L. Wisniewski. Child and parent factors that influence psychological problems in obese children. *Int J Eat Disord.* 15:151–158, 1994.
15. Stradmeijer, M., J. Bosch, W. Koops, and J. Seidell. Family functioning and psychosocial adjustment in overweight youngsters. *Int J Eat Disord.* 27:110–114, 2000.
16. French, S. A., M. Story, D. Neumark-Sztainer, J. A. Fulkerson, and P. Hannan. Fast food restaurant use among adolescents: associations with nutrient intake, food choices and behavioral and psycho-social variables. *Int J Obes Relat Metab Disord.* 25:1823–1833, 2001.
17. Strober, M., R. Freeman, and W. Morrell. The long-term course of severe anorexia nervosa in adolescents: survival analysis of recovery, relapse, and outcome predictors over 10–15 years in a prospective study. *Int J Eat Disord.* 22:339–360, 1997.
18. Gustafson, T. B. and D. B. Sarwer. Childhood sexual abuse and obesity. *Obes Rev.* 5:129–135, 2004.
19. Williamson, D. F., T. J. Thompson, R. F. Anda, W. H. Dietz, and V. Felitti. Body weight and obesity in adults and self-reported abuse in childhood. *Int J Obes Relat Metab Disord.* 26:1075–1082, 2002.
20. Grilo, C. M. and R. M. Masheb. Childhood psychological, physical, and sexual maltreatment in outpatients with binge eating disorder: frequency and associations with gender, obesity, and eating-related psychopathology. *Obes Res.* 9:320–325, 2001.
21. Perez, M. and T. E. Joiner, Jr. Body image dissatisfaction and disordered eating in black and white women. *Int J Eat Disord.* 33:342–350, 2003.
22. Greenberg, B. S., M. Eastin, L. Hofschire, K. Lachlan, and K. D. Brownell. Portrayals of overweight and obese individuals on commercial television. *Am J Public Health.* 93:1342–1348, 2003.
23. Eisenberg, M. E. and M. C. Aalsma. Bullying and peer victimization: position paper of the Society for Adolescent Medicine. *J Adolesc Health.* 36:88–91, 2005.
24. Camodeca, M. and F. A. Goossens. Aggression, social cognitions, anger and sadness in bullies and victims. *J Child Psychol Psychiat.* 46:186–197, 2005.

25. Eisenberg, M. E., D. Neumark-Sztainer, and M. Story. Associations of weight-based teasing and emotional well-being among adolescents. *Arch Pediatr Adolesc Med.* 157:733–738, 2003.

26. Janssen, I., W. M. Craig, W. F. Boyce, and W. Pickett. Associations between overweight and obesity with bullying behaviors in school-aged children. *Pediatrics.* 113:1187–1194, 2004.

27. Gortmaker, S. L., A. Must, J. M. Perrin, A. M. Sobol, and W. H. Dietz. Social and economic consequences of overweight in adolescence and young adulthood. *N Engl J Med.* 329:1008–1012, 1993.

28. Wang, S. S., K. D. Brownell, and T. A. Wadden. The influence of the stigma of obesity on overweight individuals. *Int J Obes Relat Metab Disord.* 28:1333–1337, 2004.

29. Halkjaer, J., C. Holst, and T. I. Sorensen. Intelligence test score and educational level in relation to BMI changes and obesity. *Obes Res.* 11:1238–1245, 2003.

30. Schwimmer, J. B., T. M. Burwinkle, and J. W. Varni. Health-related quality of life of severely obese children and adolescents. *JAMA.* 289:1813–1819, 2003.

31. Mo-suwan, L., L. Lebel, A. Puetpaiboon, and C. Junjana. School performance and weight status of children and young adolescents in a transitional society in Thailand. *Int J Obes Relat Metab Disord.* 23:272–277, 1999.

32. Latner, J. D. and A. J. Stunkard. Getting worse: the stigmatization of obese children. *Obes Res.* 11:452–456, 2003.

33. Friedlander, S. L., E. K. Larkin, C. L. Rosen, T. M. Palermo, and S. Redline. Decreased quality of life associated with obesity in school-aged children. *Arch Pediatr Adolesc Med.* 157:1206–1211, 2003.

34. Swallen, K. C., E. N. Reither, S. A. Haas, and A. M. Meier. Overweight, obesity, and health-related quality of life among adolescents: the National Longitudinal Study of Adolescent Health. *Pediatrics.* 115:340–347, 2005.

35. Hesketh, K., E. Waters, J. Green, L. Salmon, and J. Williams. Healthy eating, activity and obesity prevention: a qualitative study of parent and child perceptions in Australia. *Health Promot Int.* 20:19–26, 2005.

36. Varni, J. W., M. Seid, and P. S. Kurtin. PedsQL 4.0: reliability and validity of the Pediatric Quality of Life Inventory version 4.0 generic core scales in healthy and patient populations. *Med Care.* 39:800–812, 2001.

37. Spirito, A., D. DeLawyer, and L. Stark. Peer relations and social adjustment of chronically ill children and adolescents. *Psychol Rev.* 11:539–564, 1991.

38. Wisotsky, W. and C. Swencionis. Cognitive-behavioral approaches in the management of obesity. *Adolesc Med.* 14:37–48, 2003.

39. Warschburger, P., C. Fromme, F. Petermann, N. Wojtalla, and J. Oepen. Conceptualisation and evaluation of a cognitive-behavioural training programme for children and adolescents with obesity. *Int J Obes Relat Metab Disord.* 25(Suppl 1):S93–S95, 2001.

40. Baranowski, T., K. W. Cullen, T. Nicklas, D. Thompson, and J. Baranowski. Are current health behavioral change models helpful in guiding prevention of weight gain efforts? *Obes Res.* 11(Suppl):23S–43S, 2003.

41. Pickering, T., L. Clemow, K. Davidson, and W. Gerin. Behavioral cardiology — has its time finally arrived? *Mt Sinai J Med.* 70:101–112, 2003.

42. Bandura, A. *Social Foundations on Thought and Action: A Social Cognition Theory.* Englewood Cliffs, NJ: Prentice-Hall, 1986.

43. Sindelar, H. A., A. M. Abrantes, C. Hart, W. Lewander, and A. Spirito. Motivational interviewing in pediatric practice. *Curr Probl Pediatr Adolesc Health Care.* 34:322–339, 2004.

44. Channon, S., M. V. Huws-Thomas, S. Rollnick, and J. W. Gregory. The potential of motivational interviewing. *Diabet Med.* 22:353, 2005.

45. Ossman, S. S. Motivational interviewing: a process to encourage behavioral change. *Nephrol Nurs J.* 31:346–347, 2004.

46. VanWormer, J. J. and J. L. Boucher. Motivational interviewing and diet modification: a review of the evidence. *Diabetes Educ.* 30:404–406, 408–410, 414–416 passim, 2004.

# 6 Weaknesses and Strengths in the Response of the Obese Child to Exercise

*Connie VanVrancken-Tompkins, Melinda S. Sothern, and Oded Bar-Or*

## CONTENTS

## INTRODUCTION

The clinical management of obese children continues to be a frustrating experience for most families and pediatric health care professionals [1]. This may, in part, be a result of the lack of consistent professional guidelines for nutrition and — especially — exercise therapy. To date, no one professional medical organization provides specific recommendations for intensity, duration, frequency, or modality of exercise for the management of pediatric obesity [2–7]. Pediatric health care professionals must thus rely on the available scientific literature when determining initial exercise recommendations for obese children.

Pediatric exercise science research indicates that there are both advantages and disadvantages to the obese child during physical activity [8]. Obese children typically display advanced physical (bone age and density [9]) and sexual maturation (increased sexual hormone levels [9,10]), promoting increased body mass and height [11]. This may provide a technical advantage during physical activities and sports in which enhanced height and arm span provide an advantage, such as in football, shot put, volleyball, and basketball [8]. In addition, because of their higher ratio of fat to lean body mass, obese children are more buoyant than their healthy-weight peers. This provides an advantage during water-based games and other swimming activities. Furthermore, obese children are more thermally insulated and, therefore, are able to perform for longer durations in cooler water. Despite these advantages, obesity in children is associated with low levels of physical fitness [12] and reduced speed and agility. Thus, obese children are often unable to perform certain physical activities as well as their normal weight peers.

## RESPONSES OF THE OBESE CHILD TO EXERCISE

### AEROBIC PERFORMANCE

Research indicates that overweight children respond differently both physically and emotionally to exercise than do children classified as normal weight [13–17]. Excess body fat confounds the relationship between aerobic fitness, which is measured by maximal oxygen consumption ($VO_2$ max) and age in both male and female children [15]. Thus, excess fat weight serves as a deterrent to exercise and body movement in general [18–22]. When overweight children are compared with normal-weight children during submaximal exercise, they exhibit higher cardiopulmonary values for a given work rate. It is not well understood whether this increase in cardiopulmonary stress per given work rate is a result of reduced physical activity patterns in obese children, the metabolic consequences of the excess weight, or the effect of the additional weight on the modality of exercise. Maffeis and others [14] reported that the cardiopulmonary responses were significantly lower in 17 nonoverweight children than in 23 overweight children during walking and running on a treadmill at different intensities. This study used the measure of percentage of ideal body weight (%IBW) to classify subjects as overweight or nonoverweight. The average %IBW was 138.3% in the overweight children and 95.5% in the nonoverweight children. The study concluded that walking and running demanded greater energy expenditure in overweight children when compared with non-overweight children, and more importantly, that overweight children expended more energy moving their bodies than did nonoverweight subjects. However, this finding differed from the results in a study by Rowland and others [23]. In this study, heart rate values were not significantly different between the nonoverweight and overweight subjects while walking at 3.2 mph, 8% grade, and approximately 97% of $VO_2$ max. Because the intensity of exercise was so close to maximal levels, these results should be interpreted as such. Interestingly, Loftin and others reported that increased body mass was associated with lower maximal heart rate in youth [24].

Studies using cycle (non-weight bearing) as opposed to treadmill (weight bearing) ergometry have yielded conflicting results. Cooper et al. [25] examined the oxygen uptake response in a sample of 18 overweight children ranging in age from 9 to 17 years during cycle ergometry. The authors reported normal $0_2$ kinetic responses when moving from rest to exercise. However, the overweight children had significantly prolonged response kinetics when ventilation (VE) and carbon dioxide output ($VCO_2$) were observed. The authors concluded that overweight children might have normal fitness levels for their individual stages of development. Their findings should be interpreted cautiously, however, because responses may be different during cycle ergometry, as opposed to treadmill, when the excess body weight of the overweight subject is supported. This is evident when the results of Maffeis and colleagues are considered [26]. They reported that $VO_2$ max expressed in absolute values in overweight children was significantly greater than in non-overweight children during treadmill testing, but not significantly different during cycle ergometry. However, when $VO_2$ max was expressed relative to fat-free mass, no differences were observed between overweight and nonoverweight subjects during either walking or cycling protocols [14]. The authors suggested that overweight children experienced no limitation in maximal aerobic power during weight-bearing or non-weight-bearing exercise. However, submaximal exercise results were not discussed [21].

Zanconato et al. [27] reported that $VO_2$ max expressed in milliliters per kilogram per minute was significantly greater in nonoverweight than in overweight children. However, in absolute terms, $VO_2$ max L/min was not significantly different between the two groups. In the same study, the performance run time and maximal work rate were also significantly lower in the overweight compared with the nonoverweight. Loftin and colleagues previously reported that when $VO_2$ max values are adjusted for total body weight in children a significant bias results [28]. Thus, reporting

$VO_2$ max in absolute values or per kilogram of lean body weight reduces this bias. Allometric scaling techniques may also be applied to reduce weight bias. As a result of this bias, and because more research is needed on the obese child's response to aerobic exercise, pediatric health care professionals should use caution when interpreting exercise testing results.

## ENERGY COST OF LOCOMOTION

The energy cost of locomotion can be described as the metabolic cost or actual energy expenditure needed to complete a task. As a result of their excess weight, obese children may have a greater metabolic cost or energy expenditure for executing the same physical activity than does a normal-weight child. This greater cost of locomotion may explain why obese children may not perform as well as nonobese children during aerobic tasks [8]. In a study by Volpe and Bar-Or [29], the energy cost of walking was examined in obese and lean adolescent boys who were matched for total body mass. At the slow and moderate speeds, the obese and lean boys displayed similar energy cost. At the fastest speed, however, the obese adolescents displayed an energy cost that was 12% higher than the lean adolescents. Moreover, total body mass rather than adiposity explained a higher percentage of the variance in energy cost during all the walking speeds.

Wasteful movements, particularly observed in the gait patterns of obese children, also increase the energy cost of locomotion [8]. Hills and Parker [30] observed the gait patterns of normal weight and obese prepubertal children while walking at different velocities on a level surface. Even when the velocity was set at a comfortable pace, the obese children displayed a significantly lower cadence of steps per minute compared with the normal weight children. During the faster, and especially slower, speeds, obese children had even more difficulty walking.

McGraw et al. [31] examined differences in gait patterns and postural stability in obese and nonobese prepubertal boys. Similar to the study by Hills and Parker [30], the obese boys displayed a significantly lower cadence, slower gait cycle, and reduced time in the swing phase, compared with the nonobese boys. With regard to postural stability, greater sway areas were observed, especially in the medial/lateral direction, in the obese boys. The authors concluded that this greater sway area was a result of the excess weight rather than postural instability [31]. Although these studies demonstrate that abnormal gait patterns may increase energy cost during exercise in obese children, it is unknown whether weight loss will reverse this observation.

## MUSCLE STRENGTH

Strength training is defined as the use of a series of progressive resistance exercises to improve an individual's ability to exert muscular force against a resistance [32]. Investigators suggest that if properly administered, resistance-training programs may not only be safe but may also help reduce the risk of injury during other physical activities in children [3,32–35]. In addition, a safe resistance-training program will develop and prepare the muscles for sport and competition [32,36]. However, few studies have examined the obese child's response to strength training. Sothern and colleagues have shown that the inclusion of regular resistance training in a program to prevent and treat pediatric obesity in preadolescent children is not only feasible but also safe and may contribute to increased retention at 1 year [33,34]. In another report, a meta-analysis examined 30 childhood obesity treatment studies that included an exercise intervention [37]. Significant improvements in body composition were associated with programs including high-repetition strength training in conjunction with moderate intensity aerobic exercise. Thus, the combination of high-repetition resistance training, moderate aerobic exercise, and behavioral modification may be most efficacious for reducing body fat variables in overweight children. However, pediatric health care providers should be careful when recommending strength training to obese children. The American Academy of Pediatrics separates the terms *resistance* and *strength training* from the terms *weight lifting*, *power lifting*, and *body building* [4,35] and supports properly supervised strength/resistance training programs as safe methods for strength development in preadolescent children. The developing

**TABLE 6.1**
**Guidelines for Resistance Training**

1. Check for physical and medical contraindication.
2. Ensure experienced supervision, preferably by an adult, when using free weights or training machines.
3. Ascertain proper technique.
4. Warm up with calisthenics and stretches.
5. Begin a program with exercise that uses body weight as resistance before progressing to free weights or weight training machines.
6. Individualize training loads whether using free weights or machines.
7. Train all major muscle groups and both flexors and extensors.
8. Exercise the muscles through their entire range of motion.
9. Alternate days of training with rest days, limiting participation to no more than three times a week.
10. When using free weights or machines, progress gradually from light loads, high repetitions (>15), and few sets (two to three) to heavier loads, fewer repetitions (six to eight), and three to four sets.
11. Cool down after training, using stretch exercises for major joints and muscle groups.
12. When selecting equipment, check for durability, stability, sturdiness, and safety.
13. Consider sharp or persistent pain as a warning, and seek medical advice.

Reprinted with permission from Bar-Or, O. and Rowland, T. *Pediatric Exercise Medicine: From Physiologic Principles to Health Care Application.* Champaign, IL: Human Kinetics, 2004.

---

musculoskeletal system of the preadolescent child must be considered when designing resistance-training programs. The intensity and duration of an individual resistance exercise bout (set) must be appropriate to the level of maturity of the growing bones and muscles [33]. Pediatric obesity is associated with advanced bone age and increased bone and muscle density [10]. This may provide an advantage to obese children when participating in strength training, especially as research indicates that the enhancement of strength associated with resistance training is not accompanied by increased muscle size in prepubertal children [38].

Several agencies have published resistive training guidelines for preadolescent children [3,4,34,35,39,40]. Trained professionals should consult these guidelines before designing a program specific to their patients' or students' needs. Table 6.1 provides general guidelines for resistance training in children and adolescents [8].

Strength training may provide additional benefits and advantages to obese children. Most strength exercises are performed while the body weight is supported. In especially severely over-weight youth, this may enhance performance because although the excess fat weight is supported, the accompanying increased muscle and bone weight will enable more force to be generated. More research is needed; however, it appears that strength/resistance training may be used safely to enhance the efforts to prevent and reverse childhood obesity in clinic-based interventions.

## MOTOR PERFORMANCE

Fundamental motor skills (FMS) are critical to participation in most physical activities [41]. Okely and others [41] examined the association between FMS proficiency and body composition among children and adolescents. The following six FMS measurements were assessed: run, vertical jump, catch, overhand throw, forehand strike, and kick. Body composition was assessed by waist circumference and body mass index. An inverse linear association was observed between the overweight youth's ability to perform FMS and degree of overweight. Moreover, the overweight youth were twice as likely as the nonoverweight ones to be in the lowest FMS quintile [41]. Similar results were also observed when Graf and colleagues [42] examined the correlation between body mass index and gross motor development in first-grade children (mean age 6.7 years). In the overweight/obese children, body mass index was inversely correlated with gross motor development and endurance performance. Thus, excess fat weight may negatively affect the fundamental motor skill performance of some children. Pediatric health care professionals should provide opportunities for obese children to participate in activities that both consider and improve impaired fundamental motor skills.

## RATING OF PERCEIVED EXERTION

The rating of perceived exertion (RPE) scale designed by Borg [43] is a method of determining the intensity of subjective effort. Using a number scale from 6 to 20, individuals can rate their feeling of exertion. For instance, 6 is no exertion at all, whereas 20 is maximal exertion. Marinov et al. [44] examined ventilatory efficiency and the rate of perceived exertion in obese and nonobese children during standardized exercise testing. Sixty children, 30 obese and 30 nonobese, ages 6 to 17 years, matched by age, sex, and height, participated in a modified Balke treadmill test. During standardized work rates, the obese children noted RPEs significantly higher than the nonobese children. This higher RPE may be attributed to a higher aerobic cost of exercise, which was also displayed [44]. Bar-Or and colleagues have also observed similar results in work not yet published [Bar-Or, unpublished].

Ward and Bar-Or examined the use of the Borg scale in exercise prescription for obese children. The authors [45] found that obese children were able to reproduce exercise intensities when prescribed to them as numbers on the RPE scale. They did, however, use a narrower range of prescribed intensities than those available to them. On the cycle, the children overestimated their choice of low intensities and underestimated their choice of high intensities. During the walking/running exercises, the children overestimated their choice of all the prescribed intensities [47]. These studies indicate that obese children may perceive that certain exercises are difficult and perhaps too challenging. This may, in turn, inhibit their motivation to increase physical activity. However, more research is needed to support these observations.

## IMPLICATIONS OF EXERCISE PRESCRIPTION

Previous reports show that encouraging overweight children to adhere to exercise programs is difficult because of the greater cardiopulmonary and biomechanical strain associated primarily with weight-bearing activity [14,15,22,46]. The discomfort associated with transporting an overweight body may result in pain in the lower extremities, breathing difficulty, and premature fatigue, especially in severe conditions of obesity [21,22]. In addition, there are emerging data to indicate that childhood obesity impairs fundamental motor skills. This, combined with a higher-energy cost of locomotion, alters the obese child's perception of exercise difficulty. Therefore, obese children may experience negative consequences to participation in activities considered appropriate for normal-weight children. Although walking looks relatively easy, it is an extremely complex biomechanical process [47]. The excess weight that overweight children carry may affect their gait pattern and posture. Therefore, the child's gait pattern and posture should also be considered because overweight children experience more gait and postural problems compared with normal-weight children [47]. Exercises to improve their gait pattern, posture, and balance should be considered when prescribing a physical activity program to overweight children [30].

### ACTIVITIES SUITABLE FOR THE OBESE CHILD

Most, but not all, physical activities if properly dosed and of appropriate intensity may be performed safely and successfully by obese children. However, several factors inhibit obese children during physical activity, including awkwardness around normal-weight peers and limited speed and agility resulting from carrying excess fat weight. Therefore, it is important to consider the following factors when prescribing exercise to obese children. First, obese children are often inhibited when expected to exercise together with normal-weight peers. In contrast, when their peers are all (or mostly) obese, overweight children play and exercise with little or no inhibition. In settings in which exercise apparel is revealing, such as swimming activities, this is especially evident. Second, obese children are taller than their peers (especially during pre-, early-, and midpubertal years), and although this gives them some advantage in sports where height and arm span are important (e.g., basketball, volleyball, shot put, discus, defensive or offensive line in football), their relative slowness and clumsiness limit their ability to excel in these competitive settings. However, in many cases they can still be useful to their team. Third, another type of activity in which the obese child can perform well is strength training. This may be a result of advanced muscle development and bone age. However, many strength exercises require the body to assume positions in which overall body weight is supported. In this case, obese children's performance will be equal, if not superior, to normal-weight peers. Finally, obese children have two advantages for water-based activities: they are more buoyant and better thermally insulated. The buoyancy gives them a definite advantage in moving or floating in water, which may boost their success in swimming and water games — a major contradistinction to land-based activities. In addition, the better subcutaneous insulation is a definite advantage when the water is cool. In this environment, lean children will lose heat (and feel the cold) much faster than those with more fat [48].

Several steps can be followed to motivate the obese child to be physically active. Chapter 14 examines various motivational theories and models; however, there are specific physical factors that can be addressed as well. Both parents and health professionals can help make physical activity enjoyable for the obese child. They can help identify local facilities for physical activity, including parks, swimming pools, and community walking groups. Health professionals should teach the children how to listen to their bodies and exercise at their own pace [49]. Pacing skills may not be inherent. Therefore, instruction should include methods to help children identify moderate versus vigorous activity and the resulting heat rate and breathing responses (see Chapter 20).

Weight-bearing activities should be limited at the start of a weight-loss program for obese children [8,50]. Deforche et al. [51] reported that obese youth have poorer performances during weight-bearing tasks compared with the nonobese children [51]. Swimming is an ideal, non-weight bearing activity for obese children [8]. Swimming is ideal for obese children not only because of their higher buoyancy and thermal comfort but also because their bodies are completely submerged, therefore avoiding exposure to their nonobese peers.

## ACTIVITIES LESS SUITABLE FOR THE OBESE CHILD

Physical activities that require repeated attempts to lift the entire body weight are not suitable for obese children. Activities in which the obese are unlikely to do well (and therefore should not be part of the initial general prescription) are those that require speed, quickness, and lifting of their own weight. For example, obese children will do poorly in sprinting and jumping. Their poor ability to lift their own body presents a major handicap in routines such as pull-ups and in dips on the parallel bars. Activities such as stair climbing, jogging, and running should also be given a low priority. The lower joints are under a considerable load during these activities. This can pose a threat to the child's joints, posture, and gait pattern [47]. In addition, because obese children will expend more energy performing physical activities of the same intensity as normal-weight children, they should not be prescribed running activities in which they must compete with normal-weight youth [8,22].

## SUMMARY

Exercise alone is not typically accepted as a tool for promoting the achievement of a healthy weight in youth. A large quantity of physical activity is required to reduce body fat [8]. For example, to metabolize just 1 pound of fat, which is equivalent to 3500 calories of energy expenditure, a healthy-weight adult male or an obese child with equivalent body mass must run approximately 30 miles. But the benefits of exercise to the management of pediatric obesity are cumulative. Over time, consistent physical activity will result in a multitude of metabolic and physiologic benefits [36,52].

---

**TABLE 6.2**
**Components of an Optimal Enhanced Activity Program for Juvenile Obesity**

Use large muscle groups (to achieve high-energy expenditure).

Move the whole body over distance (e.g., walking, skating, dancing, swimming).

Emphasize duration; deemphasize intensity.

Aim at energy equivalent of 10–15% total daily expenditure (e.g., 200–300 kcal) per session.

Include resistance training (particularly if program includes low-energy dieting).

Gradually increase frequency and volume (strive for daily activity, 30–45 min per day).

Consider the child's preference for activities.

Emphasize water-based sports and games.

Consider lifestyle changes, not merely regimented activities.

Let parents contract with the child to reduce sedentary activities (e.g., television).

Build in token remuneration.

Include other obese children in group activities (this reduces inhibition).

Remember, key to compliance is fun, fun, fun!

Reprinted with permission from Bar-Or, O. and Rowland, T. *Pediatric Exercise Medicine: From Physiologic Principles to Health Care Application.* Champaign, IL: Human Kinetics, 2004.

---

In particular, frequent vigorous physical activity periods are shown to be associated with decreased abdominal fat in male adolescents [53]. And the adult research literature indicates that regular exercise training (> 6 months) improves fat oxidation (increased oxidative enzymes), glucose metabolism (increased number of glucose transporters and glucose into triglycerides), mitochondrial function, sympathetic nervous system activity (improved catecholamine stimulation response), and lipoprotein lipase activity, which may, indirectly, positively affect metabolic profiles [36,54–56]. Together, these changes and resulting benefits will not only enhance dietary efforts during weight loss but also promote long-term weight maintenance. Unfortunately, the positive effects of exercise training will only be realized if the obese child complies with the prescribed physical activities. Therefore, it is imperative that careful consideration be given to selecting the most appropriate intensity, frequency, duration, and modality of exercise for each obese child. Table 6.2 provides physical activity recommendations for obese children that may be safely and effectively used in the pediatric clinical setting.

## REFERENCES

1. Kiess, W., A. Galler, A. Reich, G. Muller, T. Kapellen, J. Deutscher et al. Clinical aspects of obesity in childhood and adolescence. *Obes Rev.* 2:29–36, 2001.
2. Cabana, M. Barriers to guideline adherence. *Am J Manag Care.* 4:S741–S744, 1998.
3. Pollock, M., Gaesser, G., Butcher, J., Despres, J., Dishman, R., Franklin, B. et al. American College of Sports Medicine Position Stand. The recommended quantity and quality of exercise for developing and maintaining cardiorespiratory and muscular fitness, and flexibility in healthy adults, *Med Sci Sports Exerc.* 30:975–991, 1998.
4. American Academy of Pediatrics Committee on Sports Medicine: Strength training, weight and power lifting, and body building by children and adolescents. *Pediatrics.* 86:801–803, 1990.
5. Krebs, N. F. and M. S. Jacobson. American Academy of Pediatrics, Committee on Nutrition. Prevention of pediatric overweight and obesity. *Pediatrics.* 112:424–430, 2003.
6. Barlow, S. E. and W. H. Dietz. Management of child and adolescent obesity: summary and recommendations based on reports from pediatricians, pediatric nurse practitioners, and registered dietitians. *Pediatrics.* 110:236–238, 2002.
7. Washington, R. L., D. T. Bernhardt, J. Gomez, M. D. Johnson, T. J. Martin, T. W. Rowland et al. Organized sports for children and preadolescents. *Pediatrics.* 107:1459–1462, 2001.

8.  Bar-Or, O. and T. W. Rowland. *Pediatric Exercise Medicine: From Physiologic Principles to Health Care Application*. Champaign, IL: Human Kinetics, 2004.

9.  De Simone, M., G. Farello, M. Palumbo, T. Gentile, M. Ciuffreda, P. Olioso et al. Growth charts, growth velocity and bone development in childhood obesity. *Int J Obes Relat Metab Disord*. 19:851–857, 1995.

10. Austin, H., J. M. Austin, Jr., E. E. Partridge, K. D. Hatch, and H. M. Shingleton. Endometrial cancer, obesity, and body fat distribution. *Cancer Res*. 51:568–572, 1991.

11. Frisch, R. E. and R. Revelle. Height and weight at menarche and a hypothesis of menarche. *Arch Dis Child*. 46:695–701, 1971.

12. Nemet, D., P. Wang, T. Funahashi, Y. Matsuzawa, S. Tanaka, L. Engelman, and D. M. Cooper. Adipocytokines, body composition, and fitness in children. *Pediatr Res*. 53:148–152, 2003.

13. French, S. A., M. Story, and C. L. Perry. Self-esteem and obesity in children and adolescents: a literature review. *Obes Res*. 3:479–490, 1995.

14. Maffeis, C., Y. Schutz, F. Schena, M. Zaffanello, and L. Pinelli. Energy expenditure during walking and running in obese and nonobese prepubertal children. *J Pediatr*. 123:193–199, 1993.

15. Sothern, M. S., J. Loftin, R. M. Suskind, J. N. Udall, and U. Blecker. Physiologic function and childhood obesity. *Int J Pediatr*. 14:135–139, 1999.

16. Schwimmer, J. B., T. M. Burwinkle, and J. W. Varni. Health-related quality of life of severely obese children and adolescents. *JAMA*. 289:1813–1819, 2003.

17. Latner, J. D. and A. J. Stunkard. Getting worse: the stigmatization of obese children. *Obes Res*. 11:452–456, 2003.

18. Bray, G. The role of exercise in obesity: a personal view. In: Wahlwqvist, M., Ed. *Exercise and Obesity*. London: Smith-Gordon, 1994, pp. 7–9.

19. Davis, M. A., W. H. Ettinger, and J. M. Neuhaus. Obesity and osteoarthritis of the knee: evidence from the National Health and Nutrition Examination Survey (NHANES I). *Semin Arthritis Rheum*. 20:34–41, 1990.

20. Hills, A. Locomotor characteristics of obese children. In: Wahlwqvist, M., Ed. *Exercise and Obesity*. London: Smith-Gordon, 1994, pp. 141–150.

21. McGoey, B. V., M. Deitel, R. J. Saplys, and M. E. Kliman. Effect of weight loss on musculoskeletal pain in the morbidly obese. *J Bone Joint Surg Br*. 72:322–323, 1990.

22. Sothern, M. S., S. Hunter, R. M. Suskind, R. Brown, J. N. Udall, and U. Blecker. Motivating the obese child to move: the role of structured exercise in pediatric weight management. *South Med J*. 92:577–584, 1999.

23. Rowland, T. W., M. R. Varzeas, and C. A. Walsh. Aerobic responses to walking training in sedentary adolescents. *J Adolesc Health*. 12:30–34, 1991.

24. Loftin, M., M. Sothern, C. VanVrancken, A. O'Hanlon, and J. Udall. Effect of obesity status on heart rate peak in female youth. *Clin Pediatr* (Phila). 42:505–510, 2003.

25. Cooper, D. M., J. Poage, T. J. Barstow, and C. Springer. Are obese children truly unfit? Minimizing the confounding effect of body size on the exercise response. *J Pediatr*. 116:223–230., 1990.

26. Maffeis, C., F. Schena, M. Zaffanello, L. Zoccante, Y. Schutz, and L. Pinelli. Maximal aerobic power during running and cycling in obese and non-obese children. *Acta Paediatr*. 83:113–116., 1994.

27. Zanconato, S., E. Baraldi, P. Santuz, F. Rigon, L. Vido, L. Da Dalt, and F. Zacchello. Gas exchange during exercise in obese children. *Eur J Pediatr*. 148:614–617, 1989.

28. Loftin, M., M. Sothern, L. Trosclair, A. O'Hanlon, J. Miller, and J. Udall. Scaling VO(2) peak in obese and non-obese girls. *Obes Res*. 9:290–296, 2001.

29. Volpe, A. and Bar-Or, O. Energy cost of walking in boys who differ in adiposity but are matched for body mass. *Med Sci Sports Exerc*. 35:669–674, 2003.

30. Hills, A. P. and A. W. Parker. Locomotor characteristics of obese children. *Child Care Health Dev*. 18:29–34, 1992.

31. McGraw, B., B. A. McClenaghan, H. G. Williams, J. Dickerson, and D. S. Ward. Gait and postural stability in obese and nonobese prepubertal boys. *Arch Phys Med Rehabil*. 81:484–489, 2000.

32. Metcalf, J. A. and S. O. Roberts. Strength training and the immature athlete: an overview. *Pediatr Nurs*. 19:325–332., 1993.

33. Sothern, M. S., J. M. Loftin, J. N. Udall, R. M. Suskind, T. L. Ewing, S. C. Tang, and U. Blecker. Inclusion of resistance exercise in a multidisciplinary outpatient treatment program for preadolescent obese children. *South Med J*. 92:585–592., 1999.

34. Sothern, M. S., J. M. Loftin, J. N. Udall, R. M. Suskind, T. L. Ewing, S. C. Tang, and U. Blecker. Safety, feasibility, and efficacy of a resistance training program in preadolescent obese children. *Am J Med Sci*. 319:370–375, 2000.

35. Bernhardt, D. T., J. Gomez, M. D. Johnson, T. J. Martin, T. W. Rowland, E. Small et al. Strength training by children and adolescents. *Pediatrics*. 107:1470–1472, 2001.

36. Sothern, M. S., M. Loftin, R. M. Suskind, J. N. Udall, and U. Blecker. The health benefits of physical activity in children and adolescents: implications for chronic disease prevention. *Eur J Pediatr*. 158:271–274, 1999.

37. LeMura, L. M. and M. T. Maziekas. Factors that alter body fat, body mass, and fat-free mass in pediatric obesity. *Med Sci Sports Exerc*. 34:487–496, 2002.

38. Blimkie, C. J. Resistance training during preadolescence. Issues and controversies. *Sports Med*. 15:389–407, 1993.

39. Hass, C. J., M. S. Feigenbaum, and B. A. Franklin. Prescription of resistance training for healthy populations. *Sports Med*. 31:953–964, 2001.

40. Pescatello, L. S., B. A. Franklin, R. Fagard, W. B. Farquhar, G. A. Kelley, and C. A. Ray. American College of Sports Medicine position stand. Exercise and hypertension. *Med Sci Sports Exerc*. 36:533–553, 2004.

41. Okely, A. D., M. L. Booth, and T. Chey. Relationships between body composition and fundamental movement skills among children and adolescents. *Res Q Exerc Sport*. 75:238–247, 2004.

42. Graf, C., B. Koch, E. Kretschmann-Kandel, G. Falkowski, H. Christ, S. Coburger et al. Correlation between BMI, leisure habits and motor abilities in childhood (CHILT-project). *Int J Obes Relat Metab Disord*. 28:22–26, 2004.

43. Borg, G. and H. Linderholm. Exercise performance and perceived exertion in patients with coronary insufficiency, arterial hypertension and vasoregulatory asthenia. *Acta Med Scand*. 187:17–26, 1970.

44. Marinov, B., S. Kostianev, and T. Turnovska. Ventilatory efficiency and rate of perceived exertion in obese and non-obese children performing standardized exercise. *Clin Physiol Funct Imaging*. 22:254–260, 2002.

45. Ward, D. S. and O. Bar-Or. Use of the Borg scale in exercise prescription for overweight youth. *Can J Sport Sci*. 15:120–125, 1990.

46. Huttunen, N. P., M. Knip, and T. Paavilainen. Physical activity and fitness in obese children. *Int J Obes*. 10:519–525, 1986.

47. Hills, A. P., E. M. Hennig, N. M. Byrne, and J. R. Steele. The biomechanics of adiposity — structural and functional limitations of obesity and implications for movement. *Obes Rev*. 3:35–43, 2002.

48. Sloan, R. E. and W. R. Keatinge. Cooling rates of young people swimming in cold water. *J Appl Physiol*. 35:371–375, 1973.

49. Hills, A. P. and N. M. Byrne. Physical activity in the management of obesity. *Clin Dermatol*. 22:315–318, 2004.

50. Sothern, M. S. Exercise as a modality in the treatment of childhood obesity. *Pediatr Clin North Am*. 48:995–1015, 2001.

51. Deforche, B., J. Lefevre, I. De Bourdeaudhuij, A. P. Hills, W. Duquet, and J. Bouckaert. Physical fitness and physical activity in obese and nonobese Flemish youth. *Obes Res*. 11:434–441, 2003.

52. Gutin, B., M. Litaker, S. Islam, T. Manos, C. Smith, and F. Treiber. Body-composition measurement in 9-11-y-old children by dual-energy x-ray absorptiometry, skinfold-thickness measurements, and bioimpedance analysis. *Am J Clin Nutr*. 63:287–292, 1996.

53. Dionne, I., N. Almeras, C. Bouchard et al. The association between vigorous physical activities and fat deposition in male adolescents. *Med Sci Sports Exerc*. 32:392–395, 2000.

54. Tonkonogi, M., A. Krook, B. Walsh, and K. Sahlin. Endurance training increases stimulation of uncoupling of skeletal muscle mitochondria in humans by non-esterified fatty acids: an uncoupling-protein-mediated effect? *Biochem J*. 351(Pt 3):805–810, 2000.

55. Tonkonogi, M., B. Walsh, M. Svensson, and K. Sahlin. Mitochondrial function and antioxidative defence in human muscle: effects of endurance training and oxidative stress. *J Physiol*. 528(Pt 2):379–388, 2000.

56. Horowitz, J. F., T. C. Leone, W. Feng, D. P. Kelly, and S. Klein. Effect of endurance training on lipid metabolism in women: a potential role for PPARalpha in the metabolic response to training. *Am J Physiol Endocrinol Metab*. 279:E348–E355, 2000.

# Section 4

*Clinical Evaluation*

# 7 Clinical Evaluation: Diagnosis, Medical Testing, and Follow-up

*Nancy F. Krebs and Melinda S. Sothern*

## CONTENTS

## PREVALENCE

The rapid rise in the prevalence of childhood overweight and obesity is occurring in both industrialized and developing countries all over the world. Pediatricians and other pediatric health care providers will play an increasingly important role in the early identification and prevention of childhood obesity and its associated comorbid conditions [1,2]. Because obesity is usually established at a young age, the pediatric primary care office is critical to national efforts to reverse the pediatric obesity epidemic [3]. According to the 1999–2000 National Health and Nutrition Examination Survey, the prevalence of childhood obesity (at or above the 95th percentile for body mass index [BMI] on standard reference growth charts) in the United States has grown to 15.3% of 6 to 11 year olds and 15.5% of 12 to 19 year olds [2,4]. Obesity prevalence has been found to be even higher among minority and economically disadvantaged populations [2,4,5].

## CAUSES/RISK FACTORS

Lower levels of daily physical activity by children in the United States have lead to a greater number of health problems in children than in previous generations. Sedentary lifestyles increase the risk of childhood medical conditions such as obesity, hypertension, hyperinsulinemia, hypercholesterolemia, and dyslipidemia [2,6]. Studies show that parent inactivity strongly predicts child inactivity [7,8]. A recent study examined the self-reported physical activity and dietary intake patterns of parents and changes in weight status over 2 years in offspring [9]. Girls of parents with high dietary intake and low physical activity (obesogenic) had significantly greater increases in weight status. Thus, in addition to family history of obesity, the environment of the home may equally contribute to the risk for developing obesity in childhood. However, there are also strong arguments for the effect of the genetic profile and the early nutritional environment on the risk for developing obesity during childhood [10–15]. Jackson and colleagues provide a strong argument for nutrition-induced changes in the hypothalamic–pituitary–adrenal axis in the mother and the fetus [10]. It is suggested that the local availability of nutrients during pregnancy, especially in relation to protein intake, may negatively affect future metabolic health. Adjustments may occur to protect brain tissue preferentially over visceral and somatic growth, resulting in an altered metabolic profile [10]. Thus, nutrition during pregnancy may have strong implications for future obesity and related chronic disease.

Infancy is also considered a critical period for obesity development. A high protein intake at the age of 2 years was shown to promote increased fatness at 8 years of age, suggesting that a high-protein diet early in life could promote an increased risk of obesity later in childhood, but findings in this area are limited and have not been consistent [16]. Moreover, research generally supports that children who were breastfed have a lower risk of obesity than those who were formula-fed [17–20]. In addition, those infants who breastfed for longer durations showed an even lower risk of childhood obesity [21]. Differences in feeding between breastfed and formula fed infants may also have a critical influence on infant weight gain. Therefore, low birth weight and breast-feeding history should be considered factors in obesity development in young children (Table 7.1). In addition, children with such risk factors may be predisposed genetically and behaviorally to the early manifestation of subtle, nonsymptomatic metabolic abnormalities that lead to childhood obesity and related chronic disease [22–28]. Therefore, strategies that positively alter the nutrition

---

**TABLE 7.1**
**Risk Factors for Pediatric Obesity**

Socioeconomic status
Ethnicity
Parental obesity — under 6 years of age
Body mass index — over 6 years of age
Critical development periods
   Birth (low/high birth weight)
   5–6 years of age (adiposity rebound)
   Puberty (12–15 years of age)
Infant formula feeding
Poor nutrition, food preferences
Excessive sedentary behaviors

---

and physical activity behaviors and environment of the family may reduce the risk of obesity in young children, especially in those with one or more risk factors. A recent publication of the American Academy of Pediatrics offers pediatric obesity prevention guidelines for medical professionals, which include increased monitoring of at-risk children and parent education [2].

Pediatric health care providers should recognize that environmental factors may greatly affect physical activity patterns. Unsafe neighborhoods and lack of adult supervision after school may increase time spent in sedentary behavior such as watching television and playing DVDs or video or computer games [29].

## COMORBIDITIES

Pediatric obesity is associated with many significant health problems and is strongly linked to increased risks for adult obesity, related comorbid diseases, and shortened life expectancy [2,6]. Growing numbers of obese children exhibit early signs of diseases that were once found only in adult populations including type 2 diabetes mellitus, high blood pressure, and abnormal lipid profiles [3]. Obese children are at an increased risk for diseases that can affect the cardiovascular, pulmonary, endocrine, and gastrointestinal systems, as well as orthopedic conditions and psychological health problems [2,6]. Comorbidities affecting the cardiovascular system include hypercholesterolemia, hypertension, and dyslipidemia [2,6a,30]. Endocrine system comorbidities include hyperinsulinemia, insulin resistance, impaired glucose tolerance, type 2 diabetes mellitus, and menstrual irregularity [2]. Common pulmonary and gastrointestinal comorbidities include sleep apnea, asthma, obesity hypoventilation syndrome, and nonalcoholic steatohepatitis [2,29]. Common orthopedic comorbidities include slipped capital femoral epiphysis, Blount disease (tibia varia), and genu varum. Mental health problems may include depression and low self-esteem [2,6,29].

## TREATMENT APPROACHES

Several weight loss approaches can be considered when choosing a treatment plan for an overweight or obese patient. Because obesity is a multifactorial disease, treatment of the disease is approached from many angles including diet modification, increased physical activity, psychological intervention, pharmacotherapy, and surgery. Reduction of energy intake is a mainstay of treatment, but the ideal approach will vary with the skills and motivation of the family, the severity of the overweight status, and the age of the child. Caution should be used in prescribing "diets" for children, except under well-supervised conditions because of the risks associated with overly restrictive access to food. This has been associated (in young children) with decreased ability to self-regulate energy intake [31,32]. In adolescents, dieting was inversely associated with BMI [33]. Several dietary approaches can be considered including low fat, low carbohydrate, high protein, and low glycemic index. The Traffic Light Diet (see Appendix A3.3B), which applies principles of foods with high versus low caloric density, has been shown to be easy for children to understand and successfully follow [34]. Other popular treatments focus on psychological and family therapy, including behavioral modification [35]. Behavioral modification has been shown to increase the success of obesity treatment and includes such elements as goal setting, maintaining a food diary, reducing availability of high-calorie stimulus foods, positive reinforcement, and parental support [34]. Health providers should seek training in health behavior change techniques, parent limit-setting strategies and reinforcement skills, and family conflict awareness [36]. Dietary treatment should be accompanied by efforts to emphasize increased physical activity [34,35]. However, exercise alone is generally not sufficient to promote significant weight loss without diet modification [34]. Physical activity provides additional health benefits and is linked to successful maintenance of weight-loss. Reduction of sedentary activities such as television viewing, video games, and computer time may be especially effective targets for behavior change [6a,37,38].

Pharmacotherapy is sometimes a useful adjunct to diet, activity, and behavioral change strategies. Examples specific for obesity treatment include sibutramine and orlistat, but each has significant potential side effects, and efficacy data are limited. Bariatric surgery has been successfully performed on severely obese adolescents. Guidelines for patient and site selection have been published [39]. Criteria include a BMI of at least 40, accompanied by significant comorbidities such as obstructive sleep apnea, type 2 diabetes mellitus, and pseudotumor cerebri. This treatment is best undertaken in a center that has surgeons with experience with the procedure in adolescents, and at which a multidisciplinary team is available. The procedure appears to be safe in the short term, and weight loss is typically substantial, with improvement in comorbidities. There are currently few data on long-term outcomes and complications [34,35,40].

## DIAGNOSIS

Early diagnosis and treatment of obesity in children is crucial for the successful management of pediatric health [2,41,42]. Unfortunately, although childhood obesity has now reached epidemic levels, this disease is still under-recognized by the health care community [43]. In addition, underdiagnosis is generally more prevalent than misclassification of obesity [44]. Recently, O'Brien et al. [43] reported that pediatric health care providers diagnosed overweight in only one-half (53%) of overweight children examined for health supervision. Moreover, in children diagnosed as overweight by their physicians, comprehensive treatment programs were not generally prescribed [43]. One study has shown that although plotting BMI enhanced physician recognition of overweight when compared with plotting height and weight for age, survey data in the same report indicatedthat only a minority of pediatricians routinely use BMI [45]. In Chapter 4 of this volume, Gordon provides similar disappointing rates of diagnosis and referral in overweight children in primary care settings [46]. Kiess and colleagues provide a diagnostic algorithm for childhood obesity that primary care providers can use to determine the most appropriate management plan (Figure 7.1) [35].

### MEDICAL HISTORY

Pediatric obesity is a complex condition that is associated, as noted above, with a plethora of medical complications, syndromes, and disorders. An expert panel report [47] suggests that the initial diagnosis should begin with a thorough screening of the patient's medical history. Conditions of primary concern are hypertension, endocrine disorders, orthopedic problems, type 2 diabetes mellitus (or insulin resistance), genetic syndromes, sleep disorders, pseudotumor cerebri, and gastrointestinal disorders.

As part of this medical history, information on the child's current eating and physical activity patterns should be obtained, with a particular focus on behaviors that can be targeted for change.

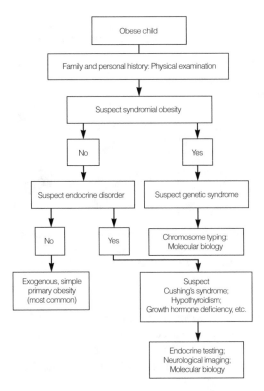

**FIGURE 7.1** Diagnostic algorithm for childhood obesity. Reprinted with permission from Kiess, W., A. Reich, G. Muller, A. Galler, T. Kapellen, K. Raile et al. Obesity in childhood and adolescence: clinical diagnosis and management. *J Pediatr Endocrinol Metabol.* 14(Suppl 6):1431–1440, 2001.

An expert committee has [29] emphasized that both food type and patterns of eating should be assessed to discern origins of excess caloric intake. Likewise, the assessment of physical activity patterns and extent of sedentary behaviors provides information important to increasing energy expenditure [29]. A comprehensive medical history and physical examination form may be found in Appendix A1.6.

## FAMILY HISTORY

Critical to assessment of a child's risk from overweight is the documentation of the family history of disease. The recommended conditions to evaluate when obtaining family history from the patient include overweight, dyslipidemia, hypertension, cardiovascular disease, gallbladder disease, eating disorders in parents, type 2 diabetes mellitus, and other endocrine abnormalities [47]. Emerging research indicates that the health status of the mother immediately before pregnancy, during pregnancy, and during breastfeeding may also be important [48]. Whitaker tracked the weight status of preschool children whose mothers were obese during pregnancy. These youth were twice as likely to be overweight as children whose mothers maintained a healthy weight during pregnancy (Figure 7.2) [49].

## SOCIAL HISTORY

The structure of the family, school and child care arrangements, living situation, parental employment, and history of abuse are examples of information to be obtained in the social history, which will inform the negotiations for health behavior changes.

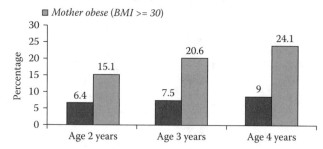

Percentage of newborns obese as preschoolers by
maternal weight in the 1st trimester of pregnancy

■ *Mother normal weight (BMI 18.5 to 24.9)*
□ *Mother obese (BMI >= 30)*

**FIGURE 7.2** Percentage of newborns obese as preschoolers by maternal weight in the first trimester of pregnancy. Reprinted with permission from Whitaker, R. C. Predicting preschooler obesity at birth: the role of maternal obesity in early pregnancy. *Pediatrics*. 114:e29–36, 2004.

## Review of Systems

The review of systems should address symptoms of potential comorbidities of overweight. Examples include asking about the presence of headaches; visual changes; sleep problems such as snoring, restless sleep, inability to lie supine, and daytime somnolence; shortness of breath or wheezing; chest pain; abdominal pain; and joint and skeletal muscle complaints. A brief evaluation of the child's psychological status is also useful.

## Primary Risk Factors

The children who are at the highest risk for becoming obese are those who belong to economically disadvantaged minority populations (Table 7.1). As a result of having a low socioeconomic status, children may have less access to safe places for physical activity and/or less access to healthful food choices such as fruits and vegetables. Recent studies show a consistent rise in the prevalence of obesity among preschool children from low-income families [50]. These children often have low levels of cognitive stimulation, which is associated with a significant increase in the risk for early-onset obesity [51]. Other risk factors that have been linked to an increased risk include unhealthy family and parental dynamics, low or high birth weight, maternal diabetes and obesity, high prevalence of obesity in other family members, and overcontrolling parental behavior (Table 7.1) [2].

## Physical Exam

As for all patients, a patient who is found to be overweight should have a physical examination, in this case with a focus on signs of comorbid conditions that may be present or on any underlying conditions that may contribute to excessive weight gains, such as hypothyroidism, reactive airways disease, tonsillar hypertrophy (contributing to airway obstruction), genu varum (flat feet) or other orthopedic conditions, and genetic or endocrine abnormalities [41]. A patient with insulin resistance may show signs of acanthosis nigricans (darkening of the skin). Hypothyroidism should be suspected with excessive weight gain and plateauing of linear growth; exam findings may include skin and hair changes, enlarged thyroid, and absent deep tendon reflexes. An abdominal exam should assess liver size and tenderness. Postural and gait abnormalities may indicate the presence of orthopedic conditions such as genu varum. Tanner stage should be evaluated and assessed in relation to the child's age. Rare genetic and endocrine abnormalities may manifest themselves through dysmorphic features including abnormal genitalia, developmental delay, poor linear growth, hirsuitism, and striae [41]. Blood pressure measurements should also be obtained using an appropriately sized blood pressure cuff.

## BODY MASS INDEX

### Background

The World Health Organization, the Centers for Disease Control and Prevention, and many national organizations recommend the use of BMI to identify overweight and obesity in youth [2,52,53]. BMI is a convenient measurement for screening for overweight in children. Standard BMI classifications define a BMI between the 85th and 95th percentiles for age and sex as "at risk for overweight," and a BMI greater than the 95th percentile for age as "overweight" (Appendix A1.10). BMI is an accepted screening tool for use by pediatric health care providers as a result of its use of easily accessible data (weight and height) and moderately strong correlation with laboratory measurements of body fatness [2,3,54].

### Calculating Obesity Risk and Status with BMI Percentiles

Pediatric growth charts for the U.S. population now include BMI percentile grids for age and gender and can be used for longitudinal tracking of a patient's BMI from ages 2 through 20 years, and to identify overweight (see Appendix A1.10) [29,53]. BMI is calculated by applying one of the following formulas:

$$\text{weight (kilograms)/height (meters)}^2$$

or

$$[\text{weight (pounds)/height (inches)}^2] \times 703.$$

### Diagnosis

Once BMI is calculated, the physician or health care provider can determine risk and status by plotting on Centers for Disease Control and Prevention growth charts (see Appendix A1.10). This should be done at least annually to facilitate the early recognition of overweight and to monitor weight increases relative to linear growth [2]. If a trend for excessive weight gain is established (e.g., crossing BMI percentile channels or an increase of three to four BMI units in 1 year), contributing factors should be explored and discussed with parents to prevent further progression of excessive weight gain or overweight status. Research, although limited, indicates that early treatment is associated with improved long-term success [29].

## ANTHROPOMETRICS TO ASSESS FAT DISTRIBUTION

### Skinfolds

Subcutaneous fat represents approximately 50% of total body fat, which provides an accessible proxy for assessment of body fatness. The 80th and 95th percentiles of skinfold readings are accepted measures of overweight and obesity in children [6]. Caliper measurement of skinfold thickness requires training and should only be administered by experienced staff. Skinfolds can be measured at a variety of body sites and are used in formulas that predict percent body fat (Appendix A2.3) [6].

### Waist Circumference

An additional method of assessing body composition is the measurement of girth of various body sections. Waist circumference provides an indication of trunk or visceral obesity, which is highly correlated in adults with diabetes and heart disease risk. Similar data are not available for the pediatric population. A metal or fiberglass measuring tape with a metric scale is used to measure the circumference of the waist and hip. The waist circumference is also a useful indicator for determining reduction in fat weight after treatment (Appendix A2.1.3).

### DIRECT MEASUREMENTS OF BODY COMPOSITION

Direct measurements of body fat content can be found using such tools as hydrodensitometry, bioimpedance, or dual-energy x-ray absorptiometry [35]. In Chapter 4 of this text, Gordon discusses the advantages and disadvantages of these various methods, and detailed protocols may be found in Appendix A2.3.

### LABORATORY TESTING — BASIC PANELS

Secondary assessments may include lipid profiles, total cholesterol, insulin, glucose tolerance, glucose, glycohemoglobin, thyroid function, cortisol, and liver enzymes [47].

If the child is diagnosed with a BMI greater than 95th percentile, additional testing may be warranted. Because pediatric overweight (BMI > 95th percentile for age and sex) is associated with many other disease risk factors, practitioners can further define risk by checking a fasting lipid profile (Appendix A2.2) [41]. Other potentially useful biochemical markers of comorbidities include liver profile, and fasting glucose and insulin. It should be recognized that there are not standardized guidelines for biochemical evaluation, especially because identification of biochemical abnormalities will often not change therapeutic interventions.

### MEASUREMENTS OF ENERGY EXPENDITURE

In some cases, measurement of resting energy expenditure may be useful to help caloric intake goals. Resting energy expenditure can be measured through indirect calorimetry. However, it is difficult to obtain an accurate measure because it is affected by diet, exercise, body temperature, growth, and development [55]. In an outpatient setting, it is difficult to optimally control these factors, and thus measurements can at best be viewed as approximations. Therefore, routine assessment of resting energy expenditure is of limited value.

## REFERRALS

Overweight children with more severe medical problems such as obstructive sleep apnea, obesity hypoventilation syndrome, and orthopedic problems may benefit from more aggressive dietary strategies. If a referral is made to an overweight treatment center, it is important to identify a program that is staffed by medical professionals experienced in the management of these serious comorbidities. Massively overweight children without severe comorbidities, but with a history of weight loss failures, may also benefit from consultation with a pediatric obesity center. Ariza and colleagues [41] provide a detailed assessment and action plan for overweight children in the primary care setting (Figure 7.3).

### GENETICS

Genetic syndromes associated with pediatric obesity include Prader–Willi, Turner syndrome, or Laurence–Moon–Bardet–Biedle [41]. Findings such as developmental delay, short stature/delayed growth, dysmorphic features, abnormal or absent genitalia, and digital anomalies should raise suspicion of an underlying genetic etiology and consideration of definitive testing. If any of these conditions is suspected, referral to a geneticist or other relevant subspecialist is recommended [41].

### ENDOCRINOLOGY

There are several endocrine disorders related to pediatric obesity, including primarily hypothyroidism, type 2 diabetes mellitus, and polycystic ovary disease. Although less common, findings

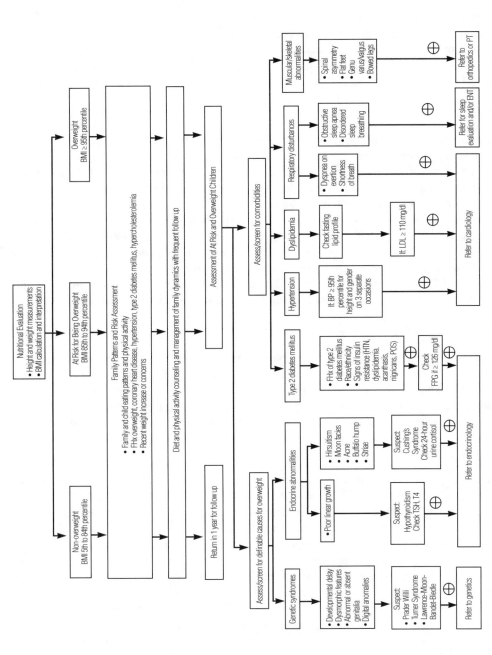

**FIGURE 7.3** Primary care assessment and action plan for overweight children. Reprinted with permission from Ariza, A. J., R. S. Greenberg, and R. Unger. Childhood overweight: management approaches in young children. *Pediatr. Ann.* 33:33–38, 2004.

indicative of Cushing syndrome, including moon facies, short stature, central obesity, and apparent reduced lean body mass should prompt referral to an endocrinologist. If this is the case, then a 24-hour urine cortisol should be ordered [41].

## Thyroid

Symptoms of hypothyroidism include constipation, cold intolerance, fatigue, and lethargy; signs may include poor linear growth, hypotension, bradycardia, anemia, and loss of deep tendon reflexes. If symptoms or signs of hypothyroidism are present, TSH and T4 levels should be checked, and if these levels are diagnostic of hypothyroidism, the child should be referred to a pediatric endocrinologist [41].

## Pancreas

Insulin resistance is common with excess central (or visceral) adiposity. Insulin resistance is associated with hyperinsulinemia, fatty liver, hypertension, and exercise intolerance. Hyperinsulinemia in children can be associated with normal fasting glucose for some time, but with persistence, there is progression to impaired glucose tolerance, and eventually to β-cell failure and elevated fasting glucose and type 2 diabetes. If insulin resistance or type 2 diabetes mellitus is suspected, fasting insulin and blood glucose levels may be obtained. Hyperglycemia is relatively insensitive until there is frank diabetes, but if fasting glucose levels are 126 mg/dL or more, the child should be referred to a pediatric endocrinologist for further examination [41]. The utility of fasting insulin levels is debated, but documentation of elevation is a finding that motivates some families to make changes, especially if there is a strong family history of type 2 diabetes [41]. An elevated fasting insulin is also part of the constellation of findings referred to as metabolic syndrome [56].

## CARDIOLOGY

During the medical examination, if the child's blood pressure is in the 95th (or higher) percentile for height and gender on three separate occasions, then referral to a cardiologist is suggested [41]. Chest pain is another symptom that may require referral. Treatment of hyperlipidemia (LDL ≥ 110 mg/dl) or dyslipidemia (e.g., metabolic syndrome), including initial diet therapy, may also be available through preventive cardiology services, or through nutrition or endocrine subspecialists [41].

## PULMONARY

Pulmonary disorders associated with significant obesity that may require rapid weight loss are obstructive sleep apnea and obesity hypoventilation syndrome [57]. Symptoms indicative of sleep disturbances include snoring, restless sleep, inability to sleep supine, and daytime somnolence. Assessment ideally includes an electrocardiogram to rule out cardiomegaly, sinus dysrhythmias, and right-side heart failure, as well as a sleep study with polysomnography to monitor for hypoxia and cardiac function. Treatment may include supplemental oxygen or positive airway pressure, but at least modest weight loss will also be advantageous. Clinicians should seek guidance from pediatric pulmonologists and obesity treatment specialists [29].

One of the most common pulmonary disorders associated with pediatric obesity is asthma [58]. Asthma is a major cause of chronic pediatric illness and school absenteeism. Moreover, urban minority children with asthma are significantly more overweight than those without asthma [59]. Results of most studies in children do not support a direct causal link between asthma and overweight conditions during childhood [60]. Furthermore, there is insufficient evidence to indicate that asthma precedes overweight conditions in children. Because excess weight exacerbates asthma symptoms, especially during exercise, overweight children with asthma should be monitored closely by a pulmonary specialist.

## ORTHOPEDICS AND PHYSICAL THERAPY

There are several serious orthopedic complications that result from significant obesity during childhood. These include slipped capital femoral epiphysis (manifested as hip or knee pain and limited hip range of motion) and Blount's disease (tibia vara) [29]. Referral should be made to an orthopedic surgeon if radiography confirms either of these conditions [29]. Other related comorbidities include spinal asymmetry, flat feet, genu varus/valgus, Legg–Calve–Perthe disease, and degenerative arthritis. Referral may be made to a physical therapist for an initial evaluation and, in many cases, for therapeutic strategies.

## PSYCHOLOGY

Several psychological disorders are associated with pediatric obesity. Binge-eating disorder should be suspected if the patient reports feeling unable to control food consumption. Depression is commonly found in overweight children, especially in older youth with severe overweight conditions. Jonides and colleagues [61] suggest that the emotional stability of the child and the family will likely determine successful treatment outcomes. If the child displays sadness or reports insomnia, restlessness, or hopelessness, then referral to a psychologist is essential to confirm the diagnosis [29]. In Chapter 9 of this volume, Johnson and von Almen detail appropriate psychological assessment for overweight children.

## SOCIAL SERVICES

The negative effects of food restriction or verbal prompting to consume served food were recently highlighted by the American Academy of Pediatrics [2]. In extreme cases, in which parental behavior results in either food restriction and eating disorders or continued overconsumption and morbid, life-threatening obesity, it may be necessary to refer the patient's family to social services. Likewise, if there is evidence of physical or sexual abuse related to the child's overweight condition, social services should be consulted.

## NUTRITION

Adequate nutrition is vital to growth and development, and both insufficient and imbalanced food consumption can cause nutrient deficiencies, impaired cognitive development, and growth velocity delays [62]. Therefore, if the child's weight condition warrants dietary intervention, referral should be made to a registered dietician. He or she will apply U.S. Department of Agriculture caloric and nutrient guidelines based on the child's age, gender, and medical condition when prescribing a weight-loss plan. A priority for dietary counseling is parent nutrition education so that family-wide changes in food selection and preparation are encouraged [41] (Appendix A3).

## EXERCISE

Pediatric health care professionals should encourage families to engage in regular physical activity to help children achieve and maintain a healthy weight [64]. Local information concerning activity centers, YMCAs, Boys and Girls Clubs, parks, and other recreational areas should be provided to parents [41]. In older children with significant obesity, structured exercise guidelines are useful [64]. Referral to a trained and certified pediatric exercise physiologist will ensure age-appropriate physical activities for the patient.

# EDUCATION

It is now widely accepted that anticipatory guidance on healthy eating habits and physical activity should begin early and for all children (Table 7.2). Readiness for change is essential, and families resistant to lifestyle modification should be referred to a family therapist [34]. Family histories of

**TABLE 7.2**
**Guidelines for Treatment**

Intervention should begin early, with clinicians initiating treatment when children 3 or fewer years of age become overweight. Because the risk of persistent obesity increases with age, it is crucial for the primary care provider to begin treatment as soon as possible [29].

The physician should ensure that the family is ready for change. It is crucial from the outset that physicians, parents, and children have mutually agreeable goals [34]. If the family seems resistant to change, a referral to a therapist who can address the family's readiness may be needed.

The clinician should educate families about the long-term risks and medical complications of obesity. A family history of obesity related disorders will identify children at particular risk [29].

The clinician should involve the family and all caregivers in the treatment program. Doing so will create new family behaviors consistent with the child's new eating and activity goals, which is important for the long-term success of the treatment [29].

Treatment programs should be focused on making permanent changes in physical activity and eating habits. Gradual, long-term changes have higher success rates than multiple, frequent changes [29].

**TABLE 7.3**
**Recommended Steps for Monitoring Patients for Overweight and Obesity**

Identify patients who may be at risk by looking at such factors as family history, birth weight, or socioeconomic, ethnic, cultural, or environmental factors.

Calculate and plot body mass index once a year for all children and adolescent patients to identify those who are obese, overweight, or at risk.

Look for changes in body mass index to identify rates of excessive weight gain relative to linear growth.

Monitor patients for risks of obesity-associated chronic diseases such as hypertension, hyperinsulinemia, impaired glucose tolerance, dyslipidemia, and symptoms of obstructive sleep apnea syndrome [2].

obesity and related disorders increase the child's risk of developing comorbid diseases, and the medical consequences of such diseases should be addressed with the family [29]. Treatment success rates improve with participation by family members and care givers. Gradual, permanent changes to the diet and physical activity patterns of the child are more successful than transient, short-term changes (Table 7.2) [29,34].

The BMI measurements of patients should be evaluated each year, with increased attention paid by the physician to patterns of excessive weight gain relative to linear growth as well as to children identified as at greater risk for overweight and obesity (Table 7.3) [2]. Patients at risk of developing obesity-related comorbidities should be monitored closely for signs of these diseases. Pediatricians and health care providers should routinely encourage parents in the healthy dietary practices of breastfeeding, moderation, and appropriate portion sizes, regular fruit and vegetable consumption, limits on sweetened beverages, and other nutritious food choices (Table 7.4) [2]. Pediatricians should also educate parents and caregivers on their roles in establishing physical activity patterns [2]. Increased physical activity and setting limits on sedentary behaviors should also be promoted. The success of prevention efforts will be more favorable if both dietary and physical activity interventions are emphasized (Table 7.4).

## FOLLOW-UP

### AT RISK FOR OBESITY

Children who are diagnosed with one or more primary risk factors or fall above the 85th percentile on the BMI percentiles may benefit from monitoring more frequently than annually (e.g., every

**TABLE 7.4**
**Preventive Strategies**

Mothers should be encouraged to breastfeed their babies.

Parents and caregivers should be educated in healthy eating patterns as well as on their role in modeling, offering, and regulating food choices.

Families should be educated and given guidance about the effect that they have on their child's development of lifelong physical activity and nutritious eating habits.

Pediatricians should encourage dietary practices that focus on moderation rather than overconsumption, and healthful choices rather than restrictive eating patterns.

Routine physical activity should be consciously promoted by the physician.

Physicians should suggest setting limits for sedentary activities such as watching television or playing video games to less than 2 hours per day.

Steps for optimal prevention should include a combination of dietary and physical activity interventions [2].

6 months) to check for continued upward shifts in BMI [2,36,41]. In addition, anticipatory guidance and brief negotiations for behavior change with parents should be undertaken to change risk eating and physical activity habits.

## OVERWEIGHT

Families of overweight children require consistent feedback from pediatric health care professionals to determine whether nutrition and physical activity recommendations are providing successful outcomes. Height, weight, and BMI should be calculated regularly (e.g., every 3 months).

## SEVERE OVERWEIGHT

Severely overweight youth require intense interventions and regular medical monitoring. This is ideally provided by a multidisciplinary team with experience working with pediatric patients and their families. Patients should be examined at least monthly, especially if they are following a calorie-restricted diet. Monitoring to determine the effect of the weight loss plan on lipid profiles and diabetes risk should be conducted quarterly. An expert committee has provided an algorithm to assist pediatric health care professionals with monitoring [29]. In general, a one-half pound/week weight loss is optimal.

## SUMMARY

For all children, parental education in the medical office setting is strongly recommended regardless of the child's current weight condition, but especially if the parents are obese. Children who are at risk for overweight by virtue of family history or other predisposing factors become increasingly more susceptible as they mature. Thus, age-appropriate, targeted, family-based dietary and physical activity preventive strategies should be consistently promoted, and basic therapeutic interventions should be made available in pediatric clinical settings. The economic burden of obesity-associated illness during childhood in the United States has increased by 43% in the last two decades [66]. Cost-effective individual and group treatment approaches are available and should be both encouraged and financially supported by the pediatric medical community. Academic programs that work simultaneously to conduct research, provide training opportunities for pediatric professionals, and evaluate ongoing interventions to prevent and treat overweight children are also vitally important to reverse this pediatric epidemic.

## REFERENCES

1. Dennison, B. A. and P. S. Boyer. Risk evaluation in pediatric practice aids in prevention of childhood overweight. *Pediatr Ann.* 33:25–30, 2004.
2. Krebs, N., R. Baker, F. Greer, M. Heman, T. Jaksic, F. Lifshitz et al. American Academy of Pediatrics, Committee on Nutrition. Prevention of pediatric overweight and obesity. *Pediatrics.* 112:424–430, 2003.
3. Binns, H. J. and A. J. Ariza. Guidelines help clinicians identify risk factors for overweight in children. *Pediatr Ann.* 33:18–22, 2004.
4. Ogden, C. L., K. M. Flegal, M. D. Carroll, and C. L. Johnson. Prevalence and trends in overweight among US children and adolescents, 1999-2000. *JAMA.* 288:1728–1732, 2002.
5. Flegal, K. M. and R. P. Troiano. Changes in the distribution of body mass index of adults and children in the US population. *Int J Obes Relat Metab Disord.* 24:807–818, 2000.
6. Shephard, R. J. Role of the physician in childhood obesity. *Clin J Sport Med.* 14:161–168, 2004.
6a. Dietz, W. H. and T. N. Robinson. Overweight children and adolescents. *N Engl J Med.* 352:2100–2109, 2005.
7. Fogelholm, M., O. Nuutinen, M. Pasanen, E. Myohanen, and T. Saatela. Parent-child relationship of physical activity patterns and obesity. *Int J Obes Relat Metab Disord.* 23:1262–1268, 1999.
8. Gottlieb, N. H. and M. S. Chen. Sociocultural correlates of childhood sporting activities: their implications for heart health. *Soc Sci Med.* 21:533–539, 1985.
9. Davison, K. and L. Birch. Processes linking weight status and self-concept among girls from ages 5 to 7 years. *Dev Psychol.* 38:735–748, 2002.
10. Jackson, A. A., S. C. Langley-Evans, and H. D. McCarthy. Nutritional influences in early life upon obesity and body proportions. *Ciba Found Symp.* 201:118–129; discussion 129–137, 188–193, 1996.
11. Barker, D. J., C. Osmond, I. Rodin, C. H. Fall, and P. D. Winter. Low weight gain in infancy and suicide in adult life. *BMJ.* 311:1203, 1995.
12. Neel, J. Diabetes mellitus: A "thrifty" genotype rendered detrimental by "progress"? *Am J Hum Gen.* 14:353–362, 1962.
13. Law, C. M., D. J. Barker, C. Osmond, C. H. Fall, and S. J. Simmonds. Early growth and abdominal fatness in adult life. *J Epidemiol Commun Health.* 46:184–186, 1992.
14. Choi, C. S., C. Kim, W. J. Lee, J. Y. Park, S. K. Hong, M. G. Lee et al. Association between birth weight and insulin sensitivity in healthy young men in Korea: role of visceral adiposity. *Diabetes Res Clin Pract.* 49:53–59, 2000.
15. Phillips, D. I., R. McLeish, C. Osmond, and C. N. Hales. Fetal growth and insulin resistance in adult life: role of plasma triglyceride and non-esterified fatty acids. *Diabet Med.* 12:796–801, 1995.
16. Rolland-Cachera, M. F., M. Deheeger, M. Akrout, and F. Bellisle. Influence of macronutrients on adiposity development: a follow up study of nutrition and growth from 10 months to 8 years of age. *Int J Obes Relat Metab Disord.* 19:573–578., 1995.
17. Dietz, W. H. Breastfeeding may help prevent childhood overweight. *JAMA.* 285:2506–2507, 2001.
18. Hediger, M. L., M. D. Overpeck, W. J. Ruan, and J. F. Troendle. Early infant feeding and growth status of US-born infants and children aged 4–71 mo: analyses from the third National Health and Nutrition Examination Survey, 1988-1994. *Am J Clin Nutr.* 72:159–167, 2000.
19. Liese, A. D., T. Hirsch, E. von Mutius, U. Keil, W. Leupold, and S. K. Weiland. Inverse association of overweight and breast feeding in 9 to 10-y-old children in Germany. *Int J Obes Relat Metab Disord.* 25:1644–1650, 2001.
20. Poulton, R. and S. Williams. Breastfeeding and risk of overweight. *JAMA.* 286:1449–1450, 2001.
21. Gillman, M. W., S. L. Rifas-Shiman, C. A. Camargo, Jr., C. S. Berkey, A. L. Frazier, H. R. Rockett et al. Risk of overweight among adolescents who were breastfed as infants. *JAMA.* 285:2461–2467, 2001.
22. Sothern, M. and S. Gordon. Prevention of obesity in young children. *Clin Pediatrics.* 42:101–111, 2003.
23. Lustig, R. H. The neuroendocrinology of childhood obesity. *Pediatr Clin North Am.* 48:909–930., 2001.
24. Strong, J. P., G. T. Malcom, W. P. Newman 3rd, and M. C. Oalmann. Early lesions of atherosclerosis in childhood and youth: natural history and risk factors. *J Am Coll Nutr.* 11(Suppl):51S–54S, 1992.

25. Berenson, G. S., S. R. Srinivasan, W. Bao, W. P. Newman, 3rd, R. E. Tracy, and W. A. Wattigney. Association between multiple cardiovascular risk factors and atherosclerosis in children and young adults. The Bogalusa Heart Study. *N Engl J Med*. 338:1650–1656, 1998.

26. Shulman, G. I. Cellular mechanisms of insulin resistance. *J Clin Invest*. 106:171–176, 2000.

27. Goran, M. I., R. N. Bergman, and B. A. Gower. Influence of total vs. visceral fat on insulin action and secretion in African American and white children. *Obes Res*. 9:423–431, 2001.

28. Teixeira, P. J., L. B. Sardinha, S. B. Going, and T. G. Lohman. Total and regional fat and serum cardiovascular disease risk factors in lean and obese children and adolescents. *Obes Res*. 9:432–442, 2001.

29. Barlow, S. E. and W. H. Dietz. Obesity evaluation and treatment: Expert Committee recommendations. The Maternal and Child Health Bureau, Health Resources and Services Administration and the Department of Health and Human Services. *Pediatrics*. 102:E29, 1998.

30. Edmunds, L., E. Waters, and E. J. Elliott. Evidence based paediatrics: Evidence based management of childhood obesity. *BMJ*. 323:916–919, 2001.

31. Johnson, C. Initial consultation for patients with bulimia and anorexia nervosa: the Diagnostic Survey for Eating Disorders (DSED). In: D. M. Garner, Garfinkel, P.E., Ed. *Handbook of Psychotherapy for Anorexia and Bulimia*. New York: Guilford, 1985, pp. 19–51.

32. Birch, L. Development of food acceptance patterns. *Dev Psychol*. 26:515–519, 1990.

33. Field, A. E., S. B. Austin, C. B. Taylor, S. Malspeis, B. Rosner, H. R. Rockett et al. Relation between dieting and weight change among preadolescents and adolescents. *Pediatrics*. 112:900–906, 2003.

34. Schwimmer, J. B. Managing overweight in older children and adolescents. *Pediatr Ann*. 33:39–44, 2004.

35. Kiess, W., A. Reich, G. Muller, A. Galler, T. Kapellen, K. Raile et al. Obesity in childhood and adolescence: clinical diagnosis and management. *J Pediatr Endocrinol Metabol*. 14(Suppl 6):1431–1440, 2001.

36. Barlow, S. E. and W. H. Dietz. Management of child and adolescent obesity: summary and recommendations based on reports from pediatricians, pediatric nurse practitioners, and registered dietitians. *Pediatrics*. 110:236–238, 2002.

37. Robinson, T. N. Reducing children's television viewing to prevent obesity: a randomized controlled trial. *JAMA*. 282:1561–1567, 1999.

38. Epstein, L. H., A. M. Valoski, L. S. Vara, J. McCurley, L. Wisniewski, M. A. Kalarchian et al. Effects of decreasing sedentary behavior and increasing activity on weight change in obese children. *Health Psychol*. 14:109–115, 1995.

39. Inge, T. H., N. F. Krebs, V. F. Garcia, J. A. Skelton, K. S. Guice, R. S. Strauss et al. Bariatric surgery for severely overweight adolescents: concerns and recommendations. *Pediatrics*. 114:217–223, 2004.

40. Sugerman, H. J., E. L. Sugerman, E. J. DeMaria, J. M. Kellum, C. Kennedy, Y. Mowery, and L. G. Wolfe. Bariatric surgery for severely obese adolescents. *J Gastrointest Surg*. 7:102–107; discussion 107–108, 2003.

41. Ariza, A. J., R. S. Greenberg, and R. Unger. Childhood overweight: management approaches in young children. *Pediatr Ann*. 33:33–38, 2004.

42. Davis, K. and K. K. Christoffel. Obesity in preschool and school-age children. Treatment early and often may be best. *Arch Pediatr Adolesc Med*. 148:1257–1261, 1994.

43. O'Brien, S. H., R. Holubkov, and E. C. Reis. Identification, evaluation, and management of obesity in an academic primary care center. *Pediatrics*. 114:e154–e159, 2004.

44. Robinson, T. N. Defining obesity in children and adolescents: clinical approaches. *Crit Rev Food Sci Nutr*. 33:313–320, 1993.

45. Perrin, E. M., K. B. Flower, and A. S. Ammerman. Body mass index charts: useful yet underused. *J Pediatr*. 144:455–460, 2004.

46. Carlisle, L. K., S. T. Gordon, and M. S. Sothern. Can obesity prevention work for our children? *J La State Med Soc*. 157(Spec No 1):S34–S41, 2005.

47. Barlow, S. E., W. H. Dietz, W. J. Klish, and F. L. Trowbridge. Medical evaluation of overweight children and adolescents: reports from pediatricians, pediatric nurse practitioners, and registered dietitians. *Pediatrics*. 110:222–228, 2002.

48. Sothern, M. S. Obesity prevention in children: physical activity and nutrition. *Nutrition*. 20:704–708, 2004.

49. Whitaker, R. C. Predicting preschooler obesity at birth: the role of maternal obesity in early pregnancy. *Pediatrics*. 114:e29–e36, 2004.

50. O'Loughlin, J., G. Paradis, G. Meshefedjian, and K. Gray-Donald. A five-year trend of increasing obesity among elementary schoolchildren in multiethnic, low-income, inner-city neighborhoods in Montreal, Canada. *Int J Obes Relat Metabol Disord*. 24:1176–1182, 2000.

51. Strauss, R. S. and J. Knight. Influence of the home environment on the development of obesity in children. *Pediatrics*. 103:e85, 1999.

52. Chen, W., C. C. Lin, C. T. Peng, C. I. Li, H. C. Wu, J. Chiang et al. Approaching healthy body mass index norms for children and adolescents from health-related physical fitness. *Obes Rev*. 3:225–232, 2002.

53. Kuczmarski, R. J., C. L. Ogden, L. M. Grummer-Strawn, K. M. Flegal, S. S. Guo, R. Wei et al. CDC growth charts: United States. *Adv Data*. 1–27, 2000.

54. Pietrobelli, A., M. S. Faith, D. B. Allison, D. Gallagher, G. Chiumello, and S. B. Heymsfield. Body mass index as a measure of adiposity among children and adolescents: a validation study. *J Pediatr*. 132:204–210, 1998.

55. Ravussin, E. and J. F. Gautier. [Determinants and control of energy expenditure]. *Ann Endocrinol* (Paris). 63:96–105, 2002.

56. Goran, M. I. *Handbook of Pediatric Obesity: Epidemiology, Etiology, and Prevention*: Boca Raton: Taylor & Francis, 2006.

57. Schechter, M. S. Technical report: diagnosis and management of childhood obstructive sleep apnea syndrome. *Pediatrics*. 109:e69, 2002.

58. Ford, E. S., D. M. Mannino, S. C. Redd, A. H. Mokdad, D. A. Galuska, and M. K. Serdula. Weight-loss practices and asthma: findings from the behavioral risk factor surveillance system. *Obes Res*. 11:81–86, 2003.

59. Gennuso, J., L. H. Epstein, R. A. Paluch, and F. Cerny. The relationship between asthma and obesity in urban minority children and adolescents. *Arch Pediatr Adolesc Med*. 152:1197–1200, 1998.

60. Chinn, S. Obesity and asthma: evidence for and against a causal relation. *J Asthma*. 40:1–16, 2003.

61. Jonides, L., V. Buschbacher, and S. E. Barlow. Management of child and adolescent obesity: psychological, emotional, and behavioral assessment. *Pediatrics*. 110:215–221, 2002.

62. Lee, S., S. Hoerr, and R. Schiffman. Screening for infants' and toddlers' dietary quality through maternal diet. *Amer J Matern/Child Nurs*. 30:60–66, 2005.

63. Rivara, F. P., R. Whitaker, P. M. Sherman, and L. Cuttler. Influencing the childhood behaviors that lead to obesity: role of the pediatrician and health care professional. *Arch Pediatr Adolesc Med*. 157:719–720, 2003.

64. Sothern, M. S. Exercise as a modality in the treatment of childhood obesity. *Pediatr Clin North Am*. 48:995–1015, 2001.

65. Wang, L., Q. Yang, R. Lowry, and H. Wechsler. Economic analysis of a school-based obesity prevention program. *Obes Res*. 11:1313–1324, 2003.

# 8 Nutritional Assessment of the At-Risk for Overweight and Overweight Child and Adolescent

*Nancy Copperman*

## CONTENTS

## INTRODUCTION

In the mid 1900s, pediatric health professionals would screen and treat children and adolescents for issues related to growth and development, but obesity was not a prevalent nutritional concern. Recommending and assessing adequate caloric and nutrient intakes for infants, toddlers, school-aged children, and adolescents in relation to their growth and development was within the routine clinical training and practice of pediatric health professionals. However, in the 21st century, American children and adolescents are plagued with an obesity epidemic. One out of every five children in the United States is classified as overweight [1]. Obesity is now the most prevalent nutritional disease in the pediatric population, and pediatric health professionals are now faced with a disease that has no effective surgical or pharmacological interventions but that, if left untreated, results in signs and symptoms of chronic disease in adolescence [2].

Therefore, health professionals must enhance their clinical skills to become proficient in screening, identifying, and treating at risk for overweight and overweight children and adolescents. They need to be able to identify environmental and genetic promoters of obesity, assess their effect on the child and family, and enable the child and family to make lifestyle changes. The following sections describe various components of the nutritional assessment of children and adolescents that will enable to practitioner to develop a treatment plan that addresses the needs of the child or adolescent and his or her family.

## HOME ENVIRONMENT ASSESSMENT

In the past 40 years, there has been a dramatic increase in dual-income families. More women are working outside the home, with homemaking responsibilities being shared by all family members or outside caretakers. This new dynamic can affect family meal and snack patterns, resulting in more outside dining, prepared convenience foods, or shared meal preparation responsibilities. Children may receive less supervision with after-school food and activity selections. Older siblings may be responsible for child care of younger siblings and for food preparation for the family. Extended family members such as grandparents or other relatives may assume the roles of caretaker and food preparer. Child care may be provided in a commercial daycare or after-school care setting in which younger children consume two meals and daily snacks up to 5 days per week and school-age children receive afternoon snacks. Therefore, understanding which family member or caretaker plays significant roles in food selection and preparation is key to helping the family develop nutrition strategies to foster healthful eating. Specific queries as to who is responsible for purchasing, preparing, and serving food must be included in a comprehensive nutrition assessment.

As family schedules become more hectic, family meals occur less frequently in households. Often, families rely on outside dining or frozen convenience meals between or after activities. Meals may be consumed in cars in transit to or from an activity. Eating may be rushed or hurried to conform to the family schedule. Data from the U.S. Department of Agriculture indicates that from 1977 to 1996, energy consumed outside the home increased from 17% to almost 35% of the daily energy intake, with the percentage of energy contributed from fast food almost tripling [3]. In addition, several studies have shown the relationship between fast food consumption and total energy intake and body weight in adolescents [4,5]. Children have been shown to consume more energy when dining outside the home than when eating in the home [6]. Conversely, in-home, family meals have been shown to increase nutrient quality of the meal by decreasing nutrient-sparse foods and increasing fruit and vegetable consumption [7]. Assessing the frequency of outside or "on the run" dining verses in-home family meals may provide the practitioner with an insight into problematic family eating behaviors.

Family composition can be an important influence on dietary intake and feeding practices in families. Children of divorced parents with various custody arrangements and visitation rights can live in separate households, consuming significantly different foods and beverages in each setting. The divorced spouses' awareness and priority in addressing the issue of overweight may be similar or markedly different. The children may use family discord to manipulate family dining practices causing inconsistencies in applying nutrition interventions between households. Inquiring about these issues in divorced families can aid the practitioner in identifying supportive family members, in communicating with the different households, and in assessing the educational needs of each household to support recommended lifestyle changes. The relationship between the parents may dictate scheduling joint or separate consultation sessions with the parents, child, and practitioner.

An inventory of the variety and amounts of foods and beverages available to the child or adolescent and his or her family in the home may reveal the degree to which the home food environment is nutritious or toxic. A pantry full of high-calorie, nutrient-sparse foods and beverages provides stiff competition to the bowl of fruits and a bottle of water on the kitchen table. Grimm et al. demonstrated that parental soda consumption was correlated with increased soda consumption of children, especially when the beverage was stocked in the home [8]. Inquiring about the food habits and preferences of individual family members may identify barriers to the successful weight management of the child or adolescent. Some examples may be parental concerns about weight gain for thin siblings conflicting with concerns about weight loss for overweight siblings. Parental ambivalence about eating habits and their effect on weight management may lead to the presence of nonnutritious family food selections in the home. It is important to address the presence of calorically dense but nutrient-sparse foods and beverages in the home, their role in family eating patterns, and the effect these items have on the nutritional status of the family. This focus will enable the family to modify their home feeding environment to foster healthy food choices for the entire family.

## SCHOOL ENVIRONMENT ASSESSMENT

According to data from the USDA Economic Research Council, school meals account for approximately 10% of foods eaten outside the home [3]. Participation in school meals can include school breakfast, snack, and lunch programs. Some children and adolescents are eligible for free or reduced school meals, whereas others are required to self pay at a nominal cost. Other sources of food and beverages provided in schools include *à la carte* snack programs, vending machines, special events, and fundraising drives. Recent advocacy by parents, community groups, health professionals, government agencies, and legislators has led to reforms in school food and beverage nutrient standards that affect meals, snacks and vending machines, and fundraising food selections in some school districts. However, the reforms have not reached the majority of the schools in the United States.

The degree of participation in these programs varies, as do the food selections offered by the schools and chosen by the children and adolescents. The practitioner can assess the effect of school dining on weight management interventions by gathering information on the extent of participation (how many meals/snacks per week including after-school programs), reason for participation (economic, food preference, peer pressure, religious dietary restrictions), and the food choices available for the student. All these factors influence the food selections made by the child or adolescent, and ultimately the nutritional quality of his or her diet.

## COMMUNITY ENVIRONMENT ASSESSMENT

Food availability is a major factor in the food purchasing habits of a family that can determine the nutrient quality of the family's diet. Food availability includes economic resources, food purchasing options, and transportation. Families that have limited financial resources may qualify for federal food programs such as WIC and food stamps. Participation in these programs can provide nutrition education and the financial support to help stretch food dollars, thereby enabling the family to purchase and consume healthier foods. Community food banks may provide sources for foods that can supplement household food inventories during periods of financial hardship that might occur for a short time between household paychecks. Some families opt to shop at food warehouses to reduce food costs. These outlets provide bulk foods at a lower per unit cost than at traditional supermarkets. However, although some bulk foods may be attractive in cost, they may contain significant amounts of energy, saturated fats, and sugar.

The type of store accessible to the family determines food-purchasing options. If the family has transportation and the ability to carry quantities of foodstuffs home from the store, many options such as food warehouses, supermarkets, or food cooperatives may be available to the family. However, if transportation and delivery of foodstuffs are limited, then food-purchasing options are limited. Depending on the neighborhood, small grocery stores or bodegas that stock limited inventories at high cost may be the only option for some households. Assessing the family's food availability as well as the family's understanding of food consumerism principles, such as menu planning, food preparation, and food purchasing practices, can identify hurdles to the implementation of healthy lifestyle changes.

## PHYSICAL ACTIVITY ASSESSMENT

Recent data have shown that children and adolescents in the United States have become more sedentary, with significant declines in physical activity as children, especially females, become adolescents [9]. Increased body mass index (BMI) has been correlated to increased hours spent television viewing as well as increased time playing video games [10,11]. The American Academy of Pediatrics recommends less than 2 hours of television time per day and 1 hour or more of physical activity per day [12,13]. Making parents aware of these guidelines can help frame the discussion about appropriate activity patterns. Several questions may provide an insight into the child's/adolescent's and family's physical activity patterns. How often do you (the child/adolescent/ parent/family) participate in physical activity each day or week? How much time do you spend participating in sedentary activities such as television viewing and playing video games? Is it safe to play outside in your neighborhood? (Safety issues can include crime rate, sidewalks, supervision, safe parks or fields, and the amount of daylight hours.) Are there any opportunities to engage in physical activity inside the home or apartment? (The opportunities can include lighted safe stairs, exercise machines, a play area such as a basement or den, and audio players.) The answers to these questions can identify barriers and opportunities to increasing physical activity.

## PSYCHOSOCIAL ASSESSMENT

An assessment of the child's/adolescent's and family's readiness to make lifestyle changes is an important barometer of whether weight-management interventions will be effective. Several studies in adults and adolescents have shown that stage of change can influence behavioral change [14,15]. An adolescent who is ambivalent about modifying his or her lifestyle may exhibit opposition and poor adherence to weight-management interventions, leading to subsequent program failure and weight gain. A family who is not ready to make lifestyle changes will not provide a supportive environment for their child. By identifying the older child's/adolescent's and family's readiness to change, the practitioner can integrate specific counseling strategies related to their stage of change into the weight management intervention. A tool for addressing these stages of change and developing appropriate intervention strategies can be found in the tool section of *Bright Futures in Practice: Physical Activity* [16].

Overweight children and adolescents can present psychological manifestations that include low self-esteem, poor peer socialization, and depression. Overweight children and adolescents may also have eating disorders such as bulimia and binge-eating disorders. Screening children and adolescents for psychological issues and eating disorders is an important component of the nutritional assessment. Several screening tools are available [17–19]. If any of these psychological disorders is suspected, referral for a comprehensive psychological evaluation is warranted. In the case of a suspected eating disorder, an evaluation by a multidisciplinary team that specializes in pediatric eating disorders is recommended.

## DIETARY INTAKE ASSESSMENT

The self-report of dietary intake by overweight children and adults has been shown to be inaccurate. Researchers have shown that food records from overweight pediatric patients tend to underestimate caloric intake when compared with actual energy expenditure [20]. The assessment of the dietary intake of overweight children and adolescents can be performed using a global assessment that is composed of self-administered 3-day food records, nutrition questionnaires, and a dietary interview performed by a registered dietitian [21] or other health professional. By using self-report coupled with a dietary interview, the resulting nutritional intake data can be more reliable for the practitioner. The use of either the global assessment or an individual component will depend on personnel, time constraints, technology, and clinical care needs.

The global assessment requires the child or adolescent and family to be trained in the recording of a 3-day food record (2 weekdays and 1 weekend day). The training includes educating the child and family on how to list (including times and places the foods were consumed) and describe (portion size, brand, food preparation) all foods and beverages consumed over the 3-day period. The recorders need to know how to record accurate portion sizes or amounts of all food consumed inside and outside of the home. A packet containing contact information for a person of whom the family can ask questions related to the food records, food recording sheets, written instructions, and pictorial methods of describing foods will improve the quality of the records. For younger children in daycare centers or at babysitters' homes, the caretaker needs to be involved in this food recording process. Adding questions to the end of each day's recording that prompt for missing items, assessment of daily intake (less, more, or typical), and completeness of record (complete, incomplete) can improve accuracy and analysis. The practitioner can explain to the family that the purpose of the record is to accurately represent what the child or adolescent is eating rather than judge whether his or her diet is "good or bad." Adolescents may prefer to complete their records on their own with the understanding that the analysis will be kept confidential and not shared with their parents. If the child or adolescent spends time in two households, two sets of food records may be warranted.

The food records offer the child or adolescent and family the opportunity to actually reflect on what types and amounts of foods are eaten, as well as where they are consuming these foods. This simple form of self-monitoring can be very enlightening for the child or adolescent, family, and practitioner. In research settings, a 24-hour multiple-day food record pass may be used. In this case, the child, adolescent, and family receive similar training to that above, but the dietary intake data is collected by means of a 24-hour food recall and 24-hour food record, reviewed by a dietitian either in person or via telephone. This method was found to be more reliable for group intakes than for individual intakes [22].

The food records can be returned before the counseling session and analyzed with computer software. Several nutrient analysis programs are available, and their features vary according to their cost. The practitioner must determine the needs of the practice such as client education, clinical care, research, or a combination of these. If the records are to be used for research, then the accuracy and scope of the database; the flexibility of analysis of meals, snacks, foods, and food components; and the ease of export of nutritional data for statistical analysis using commercial software would be of concern to the researcher. In clinical care situations, the accuracy of the database, ease of data entry, cost, and client education reports would be of greater importance. Some practitioners may choose not to formally analyze the food records but, rather, to clinically review them to assess for overall dietary quality.

Nutritional questionnaires include food frequency questionnaires that inquire how many times in a specified time period a person consumes certain foods, beverages, or food groups. The format of the questionnaire can require the respondent to provide a written answer to a question or circle a response on a scale. The answers to the questions can be used in conjunction with a Likert Scale, which can be used to score the questionnaire. The score can then be used to evaluate the quality of the diet. Limitations of this method include the validity of the measurement or questionnaire and the scope of the nutrient information obtained. The advantage of nutritional questionnaires is that they are easy to administer, require minimal patient training, are inexpensive, and can be designed to address specific eating patterns and food consumption. Health professionals, other than registered dietitians, may find this measure easier to interpret than a formal food record nutrient analysis.

The third component of nutrient intake assessment is a dietary interview. The dietary interview is usually conducted by a registered dietitian or other health professional with nutrition training. The interview comprises a nutrition history of allergies, supplements, medications, and past feeding practices; recent changes to child or adolescent or family diets; typical intake for meals and snacks for weekdays and weekends, including foods and beverages eaten inside and outside the home; schedule of meals/snacks; current feeding practices; and child or adolescent and family nutritional concerns or conflicts. If the child or adolescent spends time in multiple households or has multiple caretakers, all parents or caretakers should be interviewed either in person or by phone when possible.

Feeding practices that have been related to overweight in children and adolescents have been identified. They include parental restriction of childhood eating [23], speed of eating [24–26], increased portion size [27], increased consumption of soda [28], and frequency of fast food meals [5]. Children ages 6 to 11 years consume on average only 2.5 servings of fruit and vegetables per day, which is only half of their recommended 5 servings per day. Data from the National Health and Nutrition Examination Survey (NHANES) III survey indicate that adolescents consume less than one third of their recommended fruit and vegetable intakes [3]. Data from the 1994–1996 and 1998 U.S. Department of Agriculture Continuing Survey of Food Intakes by Individuals for youth, ages 6 to 17 years, indicate that individuals with increased consumption of sugar-sweetened beverages, sugars and sweets, and sweetened grains had a decreased likelihood of meeting the dietary reference intakes for calcium, folate, and iron [29].

The information from the dietary intake assessment should identify overly consumed, high-calorie, nutrient-sparse foods and beverages; locations and times that these foods are consumed; feeding practices that promote the overconsumption of these foods; and child or adolescent and family awareness of these eating behaviors. In addition, nutrient intake deficiencies such as inadequate intakes of calcium, fiber, iron, folic acid, and fat-soluble and water-soluble vitamins should become apparent. Identifying obesegenic feeding practices and nutrient intake deficiencies can aid the practitioner, child or adolescent, and family to develop strategies to modify these eating behaviors.

## PHYSICAL AND LABORATORY ASSESSMENTS

In the context of nutritional assessment of the at risk for overweight or overweight child or adolescent, physical findings obtained by a medical exam, coupled with anthropometrics, blood pressure measurements, and laboratory assessments obtained by a health professional, are important in the formulation of weight management goals and evaluation of treatment outcomes. Initial assessment of anthropometrics including accurate height and weight measurements, calculation of BMI, and correct plotting of data points on age- and sex-appropriate growth charts enables the practitioner to assess the weight status of the child or adolescent. This assessment along with the absence or presence of any comorbidity allows the practitioner to determine weight management goals (see Figures 8.1 and 8.2) [30].

Anthropometrics are the most widely used clinical tool in the evaluation of pediatric growth and development. In assessing the overweight status of a child or adolescent, accurate and reliable weight and height measurements are essential because they will be used to calculate the BMI

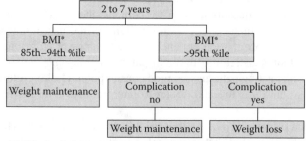

**FIGURE 8.1** Obesity evaluation and treatment: expert committee recommendations for ages 2–7 years. Reprinted with permission from Barlow E and Deitz WH. Obesity evaluation and treatment: Expert Committee recommendations. *Pediatrics.* 102(3):1–11, 1998.

**Recommendations for Weight Goals**

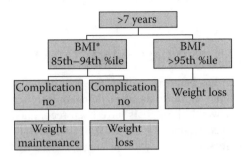

- ° Children and adolescents in this group should be encouraged to reduce their weight by 1 pound per month to eventually achieve a BMI less than the 85th %ile
- Medical complications include mild hypertension, dyslipidemias, insulin resistance, sleep apnea, genu varum, and cutaneous candidiasis

**FIGURE 8.2** Obesity evaluation and treatment: expert committee recommendations for ages >7 years. Reprinted with permission from Barlow E and Deitz WH. Obesity evaluation and treatment: Expert Committee recommendations. *Pediatrics.* 102(3):1–11, 1998.

(weight [kg]/height [m²]). Weights can be recorded on a digital or triple-beam balance scale, and heights can be measured by a wall-mounted stadiometer. Children and adolescents should be gowned and in bare feet. Some pediatric patients refuse to wear gowns; therefore, they should be instructed to bring the same lightweight clothing to every visit for anthropometric measurements. The practitioner should also stock large adult gowns suitable for adolescents weighing over 200 lbs in addition to pediatric gowns. Heights should be measured on a wall-mounted stadiometer with the child or adolescent in bare feet; he or she should be standing comfortably erect against a perpendicular measuring unit with a sliding headboard (wall-mounted stadiometer). The feet should be as close together as possible, and the heels, buttocks, and shoulders should touch the measuring unit. The headboard should be lowered against the top of the head with the head upright and the chin parallel to the floor. The height, weight, and calculated BMI can be plotted on appropriate Centers for Disease Control and Prevention age and gender growth charts. More information on calculating BMI and plotting anthropometrics is available at http://www.cdc.gov/nchs. Serial laboratory assessments, height and weight measurements, and BMI calculations provide a method of formulating initial treatment goals and evaluating treatment outcomes as long as the measurements are consistent and accurate.

Other physical findings are important components in nutritional assessment. Tanner Staging, which assigns a stage of sexual development to the child or adolescent, can be used to assess the growth potential of a child or adolescent. Menstrual history for females is also important for assessment of growth potential, as the female adolescent's growth spurt generally occurs in the year before the onset of menses. By monitoring weight fluctuations during the menstrual cycle, the practitioner can track weight status according to the effect of fluid retention before menses (wet weight) and diuresis postmenses (dry weight) to assess overall anthropometric response to lifestyle changes. The presence of acanthosis nigricans is significant in that it is a cutaneous marker of insulin resistance. All of these physical and laboratory findings highlight the importance of a multidisciplinary team approach to the evaluation of the overweight child or adolescent.

Educating the child or adolescent and family about the significance of abnormal physical findings and laboratory assays, BMI, and the BMI percentiles can be a useful counseling tool in pediatric weight management. Using the changes in laboratory parameters and physical findings as outcome measures for evaluating the progress of the child or adolescent can help the family reduce the emphasis on weight as the only outcome. Reduction of cardiac risk factors coupled with a stable weight or BMI will positively affect health outcomes for the child or adolescent. Understanding the importance of multiple outcomes as a measure of progress toward weight management can enable the child or adolescent and family to realize that healthy eating and exercise are lifelong commitments.

## NUTRITIONAL CARE PLAN AND CASE MANAGEMENT

Once the nutritional assessment has been completed, the practitioner can refer to the recommendations of Barlow and Dietz for weight goals. Depending on the age, BMI, and comorbidities present, weight-maintenance or weight-loss goals have been recommended for children ages 2 to 7 years and 7 years and older (see Figures 8.1 and 8.2). It is important to note that a weight loss goal of 1 pound per month is recommended with an appropriate weight goal below the 85% for BMI for age and sex. Before their pubertal growth spurt, children usually grow 2 inches per year. Each inch in growth without subsequent weight gain represents approximately a 5-pound weight loss, as demonstrated by a reduction in BMI. A child who loses 1 pound per month for a year and gains 2 inches in height during that year, even though he or she only loses 12 lb, actually exhibits almost a 22-lb weight loss, resulting in a significant reduction in BMI and BMI percentile. Explaining the rationale of the recommended weight goals to children, adolescents, and their families can help clarify unrealistic weight loss expectations and lead to more attainable weight goals.

The practitioner can adapt the intensity of lifestyle interventions to the severity of the overweight condition, the findings of nutritional assessment, the readiness of the child or adolescent and family to make lifestyle modifications, and the clinical resources available in the community. In other chapters of this book, several nutrition, physical activity, and behavioral interventions and their appropriateness will be discussed. A common aspect of all these interventions/programs is frequent visits with the staff, such as weekly, biweekly, or monthly for an extended period of time greater than 1 year. Each practitioner should communicate with other disciplines (medical, nutrition, psychology, exercise) involved in the care of the child or adolescent to coordinate and provide optimum care. Weight management for the at risk for overweight or the overweight pediatric patient and his or her family should include an interdisciplinary approach to modify the families' nutritional and physical activity patterns to enable them to attain the needed skills for a lifetime of weight management.

## REFERENCES

1.  Hedley A, Ogden C, Johnson C, Carroll M, Curtin L, Flegal K. Prevalence of overweight and obesity among US children, adolescents, and adults, 1999–2002. *JAMA*. 2004;291:2847–2850.
2.  Bao W, Srinivasan SR, Wattigniey WA, Berenson GS. Persistance of multiple cardiovascular risk clustering related to syndrome X from childhood to adulthood. The Bogalusa Heart Study. *Arch Intern Med*. 1994;1954:1842–1847.
3.  Economic Research Service, UDSA. *Food Rev*. 2002;25(3).
4.  French SA, Story M, Newmark-Szainer D, Fulkerson JA, Hannan P. Fast food restaurant use among adolescents: associations with nutrient intake, food choices and behavioral and psychosocial variables. *Intl J Obes*. 2001;25:1823–1833.
5.  Bowman SA, Gortmaker SL, Ebbeling CB, Pereira MA, Ludwig DS. Effects of fast-food consumption on energy intake and diet quality among children in a national household survey. *Pediatrics*. 2004;113:112–118.
6.  Zoumas-Morse C, Rock CL, Sobo EJ, Neuhouser ML. Children's pattern of macronutrient intake and associations with restaurant and home eating. *J Amer Diet Assoc*. 2001;101:923–925.
7.  Gillman MW, Rifas-Shiman SL, Fraiser AL. Family dinner and diet quality among older children and adolescents. *Arch Family Med*. 2000;9:235–240.
8.  Grimm GC, Harnack L, Story M. Factors associated with soft drink consumption in school-aged children. *J Amer Diet Assoc*. 2004;104:1244–1249.

9. Kimm SY, Glynn NW, Kriska AM, Barton BA, Kronsberg SS, Daniels SR et al. Decline in physical activity in black girls and white girls during adolescence. *New Engl J Med.* 2002;5;347:709–715.

10. McMurray RG, Harrell JS, Deng S, Bradley CB, Cox LM, Bangdiwala. The influence of physical activity, socioeconomic status, and ethnicity on weight status of adolescents. *Obes Res.* 2000;8:130–139.

11. Anderson RE, Crespo CJ, Bartlett SJ, Cheskin LJ, Pratt M. Relationship of physical activity and television watching with body weight and level of fatness among children. *JAMA.* 1998;279(12):938–942.

12. American Academy of Pediatrics. Committee on Communications. Children adolescents, and television. *Pediatrics.* 1995;96:786–787.

13. American Academy of Pediatrics. Committee on Nutrition. Prevention of pediatric overweight and obesity. *Pediatrics.* 2003;112(2):424–430.

14. Watt RG. Stages of change for sugar and fat reduction in an adolescent sample. *Commun Dental Health.* 1996;14:102–107.

15. Curry SJ, Kristal AR, Bowen DJ. An application of the stage of change model of behavior change to dietary fat restriction. *Health Educ Res.* 1992;7:97–105.

16. Patrick K, Spear B, Holt K, Sofka D. Eds. *Bright Futures in Practice: Physical Activity.* Arlington, VA: National Center for Education in Maternal and Child Health, 2002.

17. Story M, Holt K, Sofka D. Eds. *Bright Futures in Practice: Nutrition.* Arlington, VA: National Center for Education in Maternal and Child Health, 2002.

18. American Dietetic Association. Position of the American Dietetic Association: Nutrition intervention in the treatment of anorexia nervosa, bulimia nervosa, and eating disorders not otherwise specified (EDNOS). *J Amer Diet Assoc.* 2001;101:810–819.

19. Garner DM, Garfinkel PE. Eds. *Handbook of Treatment for Eating Disorders.* New York: Guilford Press, 1997.

20. Bandini LG, Schoeller DA, Cyr HN, Dietz WH. Validity of reported energy intakes in obese and non-obese adolescents. *Amer J Clin Nutr.* 1990;52:421–425.

21. Copperman N, Jacobson MS. Medical nutritional therapy for the treatment of adolescent overweight. In: Fisher M, Golden N, Eds. *Adolescent Medicine: State of the Art Reviews: Spectrum of Disordered Eating: Anorexia Nervosa, Bulimia Nervosa and Obesity.* Chicago: American Academy of Pediatrics, 2003: pp. 11–22.

22. Johnson RK, Driscoll P, Goran MI. Comparison of multiple-pass 24-hour recall estimates of energy intake with total energy expenditure determined by the doubly labeled water method in young children. *J Amer Diet Assoc.* 1996;96:1140–1144.

23. Johnson SL, Birch LL. Parents' and children's adiposity and eating style. *Pediatrics.* 1994;94:653–661.

24. Drabman RS, Cordura GD, Hammer D, Jarvie GJ, Horton W. Developmental trends in eating rates of normal and overweight preschool children. *Child Devel.* 1979;50:211–216.

25. Marston AR, London P, Cooper LM. A note on the eating behavior of children varying in weight. *J Child Psychol Psych.* 1976;17:221–225.

26. Barkling B, Ekman S, Rossner S. Eating behaviour in obese and normal weight 11-year-old children. *Intl J Obes.* 1992;16:355–360.

27. Fisher JO, Rolls BJ, Birch LL. Children's bite size and intake of an entrée are greater with large portions than with age-appropriate or self-selected portions. *Amer J Clin Nutr.* 2003;77:1164–1170.

28. Ludwig DS, Peterson KE, Gortmaker SL. Relationship between consumption of sugar sweetened drinks and childhood obesity: a prospective, observational analysis. *Lancet.* 2001;357:505–508.

29. Frary CD, Johnson RK, Wang MQ. Children and adolescents' choices of foods and beverages high in added sugars are associated with intakes of key nutrients and food groups. *J Adolesc Health.* 2004;34:56–63.

30. Barlow E, Deitz, WH. Obesity evaluation and treatment: Expert Committee recommendations. *Pediatrics.* 1998;102(3):1–11.

# 9 Behavioral and Psychosocial Assessment Tools

*T. Kristian von Almen*

## CONTENTS

Some cross-sectional, population-based studies of children and adolescents report little to no differences on standardized psychosocial or behavioral assessment measures in obese and nonobese subjects, whereas many reports have documented significant differences between these groups. The same is true when examining longitudinal, population-based studies of obese versus nonobese children and adolescents. Some researchers have reported significant differences, particularly in adolescent females, whereas others have failed to observe significant differences between groups. There are also discrepancies in data collected from clinic-referred samples of obese children and adolescents. Some researchers report little to no differences, yet most researchers have reported significant differences. The discrepancies found in these studies have been postulated to relate to differences in the study group's social status, age, sex, ethnicity, geographic region, and parental factors, and even recent trends toward a heavier population of children and adolescents. This controversy is compounded by the fact that many of the reviewed studies have failed to use standardized or psychometrically sound psychosocial or behavioral measures. In addition, in some cases, the standardized assessment used across studies has been abbreviated, dissimilar, or a newer version of the original measure.

This chapter summarizes standardized behavioral and psychosocial instruments that have been widely used in baseline and follow-up assessment of overweight children and adolescents in both population-based and clinic-referred samples. This is not meant to be a comprehensive listing of behavioral or psychosocial assessment instruments available to clinicians but, instead, details those assessments that have been most widely used to date. Though standardized, psychometrically sound assessments take 10 to 15 minutes to complete, future research should attempt to use these measures, when possible, to allow for more accurate comparisons within and between study groups.

## BEHAVIORAL ASSESSMENTS

### ACHENBACH CHILD BEHAVIOR CHECKLIST

The Achenbach Child Behavior Checklist (CBCL) [1,2], parent form, is likely to be the most widely used standardized behavior problem assessment tool of obese children and adolescents, aged 6 to 18 years. The scale takes about 15 minutes to complete and consists of 118 items or statements that describe specific behavioral and emotional problems, with two open-ended items for reporting additional problems. Parents rate their child for how true each item is now or within the last 6 months, using the following scale: 0 = not true; 1 = somewhat or sometimes true; 2 = very true. The CBCL can be hand or computer scored. A total behavior problem (T) score is obtained, as are T scores for two broad categories: internalizing (e.g., withdrawn, depressed) and externalizing (e.g., acting out, aggression). The CBCL is further divided into T scores for eight subcategories of problematic behavior: aggressive behavior, anxious/depressed, attention problems, rule-breaking behavior, social problems, somatic complaints, thought problems, and withdrawn/depressed. There are also six DSM -oriented scales: affective problems, anxiety problems, somatic problems, attention deficit/hyperactivity problems, oppositional defiant problems, and conduct problems. In general, a T score greater than 67 indicates significant behavior problems in that category. There is also a social competence scale that yields a total T score, as well as T scores for involvement in activities, social interactions, and school performance. A T score less than 33 on the social competence scale indicates problems.

The CBCL has been well standardized, and norms exist for both clinic-referred and normative populations. The items of the CBCL were factor analyzed to empirically identify the forms of psychopathology that actually occur in children. Further, the scales are based on new factor analyses of parents' ratings of 4994 clinically referred children and were normed on 1753 children aged 6 to 18 years. The normative sample was reportedly representative of the 48 contiguous states across socioeconomic status, ethnicity, region, and urban–suburban–rural residence. Children were excluded from the normative sample if they had been referred for mental health or special education services within the last year. The CBCL is also available in a newly revised Spanish version. A teacher version and youth self-report version are also available, but they have been used much less frequently.

### SOCIAL SKILLS RATING SYSTEM

The Social Skills Rating System [3] has been used much less frequently and allows professionals to screen and classify children and adolescents suspected of having significant social behavior problems. A teacher, parent, and self-report form are available and take about 15 minutes to complete. The respondent is asked to report how often the child or teen engages in 39 to 49 statements as 0 = never, 1 = sometimes true, or 2 = very often true. The Social Skills Rating System can be scored by hand or computer. A score is generated for social skills (cooperation, assertion, responsibility, empathy, and self-control), problem behaviors (externalizing problems, internalizing problems, and hyperactivity), and academic competence.

The test–retest reliability of the Social Skills Rating System ranges from .65 to .93, whereas coefficient alpha reliability ranges from .81 to .85. The subscale reliabilities range from .48 to .88.

## PSYCHOSOCIAL ASSESSMENTS

### CHILDREN'S DEPRESSION INVENTORY

The Children's Depression Inventory [4] is a 27-item, self-report measure and takes about 10 minutes to complete. It is the most often used measure for child depression and is appropriate for use in children and adolescents 7 to 17 years old. The individual is asked to select the statement that best describes his or her feelings during the last 2 weeks. For each item, the child has three possible answers: 0 = absence of symptoms, 1 = mild symptoms, and 2 = definite symptoms. A total score and five scaled scores are generated for negative mood, interpersonal problems, ineffectiveness, anhedonia, and negative self-esteem. A clinical cutoff score has been established to facilitate referral to a mental health professional when necessary. Hand and computer scoring are available.

The normative sample included 1266 public school students (592 boys, 674 girls). Twenty-three percent of the participants were African-American, American Indian, or Hispanic in origin. Twenty percent of the children came from single-parent homes. In addition, the normative sample used for scoring the Children's Depression Inventory was divided into groups based on age (ages 6 to 11, 12 to 17) and gender. The internal consistency coefficients of the Children's Depression Inventory range from .71 to .89. Test–retest reliability coefficients (2 to 3-week time interval) range from .74 to .83.

### REYNOLDS ADOLESCENT DEPRESSION SCALE 2

The Reynolds Adolescent Depression Scale 2 (RADS-2) [5,6] is a less frequently used adolescent self-report measure that consists of 30 items, rated on a 4-point scale, which takes 5 to 10 minutes to complete. The RADS-2 yields five scores: overall depression, demoralization, worry and despondency, somatic, and anhedonia. The RADS-2 is hand scored using a single scoring template. Internal consistency coefficients for grades 7 to 12 range from .91 to .94. The RADS-2 has a total sample alpha reliability of .92 and a split half reliability of .91. Test–retest coefficients of .80 and .79 are reported.

## SELF-ESTEEM

### PIERS–HARRIS CHILDREN'S SELF CONCEPT SCALE, SECOND EDITION

The Piers–Harris Children's Self Concept Scale 2 [7–9] is the most widely used measure to date of children and adolescent self-esteem. It is a revised version of the 80-item scale developed in 1969. It is appropriate for use with 7 to 18 year olds, and consists of 60 yes or no items. The measure is designed to evaluate the child's psychological health on the basis of their perceptions and takes 10 to 15 minutes to complete. A total score and six subscale scores for physical appearance and attributes, freedom from anxiety, intellectual and school status, behavior adjustment, happiness and satisfaction, and popularity are generated.

The Piers-Harris-2 has new, nationally representative norms, which are based on a sample of 1387 students, ages 7 to 18 years, from across the United States. Because the revised scales remain psychometrically equivalent to the original scales, results from the Piers–Harris 2 can be compared with those obtained using the original test. Computer scoring and interpretation are available, as is a Spanish version of the scale.

### SELF-PERCEPTION PROFILE FOR CHILDREN

The Self-Perception Profile for Children [10] is a less frequently used, 36-item self-report scale. A global self-worth score and five domain scores — scholastic competence, social acceptance, athletic competence, physical appearance, and behavioral conduct — are generated. The manual on the Self-Perception Profile for Children is a revised version of the Perceived Competence Scale for Children. The reported internal reliability of subscales is ($r = .73$ to $.86$), and 9-month test–retest reliability is $r = .8$.

## ANXIETY

### STATE-TRAIT ANXIETY INVENTORY FOR CHILDREN

The State-Trait Anxiety Inventory for Children (STAIC) [11] is composed of separate, self-report scales for measuring two distinct anxiety concepts: state anxiety (S-Anxiety) and trait anxiety (T-Anxiety). It is designed for use by 9 to 12 year olds. The STAIC requires about 10 minutes to complete each scale, and children respond to items on a 3-point rating scale. The STAIC S-Anxiety scale consists of 20 statements that ask children how they feel at a *particular moment in time.* The S-Anxiety scale is designed to measure transitory anxiety; that is, subjective feelings of apprehension, tension, and worry that vary in intensity and fluctuate over time. The STAIC T-Anxiety scale also consists of 20 items, but children respond to these items by indicating how they *generally* feel. The T-Anxiety scale measures more stable individual differences in anxiety proneness.

The normative group consisted of two large samples of fourth-, fifth-, and sixth-grade elementary school children from six different schools.

## MEASURES OF EATING DISORDERS

### THE KIDS' EATING DISORDER SURVEY

The Kids' Eating Disorder Survey [12] is a 14-item self-report inventory of eating disorder attitudes and behaviors. The instrument has been shown to have a 4-month test–retest reliability of $r = 0.83$ and an internal consistency of Cronbach's $\alpha = 0.73$ in a sample of 1883 fifth- through eighth-grade students. Children are asked to respond "yes", "no", or "I don't know" to questions concerning five attitudes and behaviors: desire to lose weight (Do you want to lose weight now?), feeling fat (Have you ever thought that you looked fat to other people?), fear of gaining weight (Have you ever been afraid to eat because you thought you would gain weight?), dieting to lose weight (Have you ever tried to lose weight by dieting?), and fasting to lose weight (Have you ever tried to lose weight by fasting?).

### THE EATING DISORDER INVENTORY

The Eating Disorder Inventory [13,14] is a commonly used, standardized, self-report screening instrument for the assessment of specific eating attitudes and behavior commonly associated with anorexia nervosa and bulimia nervosa. It is a revised version of the original measure published in 1984. The original 64 items were retained and are grouped into eight scales (drive for thinness, bulimia, body dissatisfaction, ineffectiveness, perfectionism, interpersonal distrust, interoceptive awareness, and maturity fears). Twenty-seven new items were added into three provisional scales of asceticism, impulse regulation, and social insecurity.

Internal consistency reliability of the Eating Disorder Inventory 2 scales range between .44 and .93, and test–retest reliability at 1-week ranges from .79 to .95 (for all subscales except interoceptive awareness). Reliability and construct, convergent, and discriminant validity have been demonstrated for the Eating Disorder Inventory, which has included use with adolescent populations.

### THE EATING ATTITUDES TEST

The Eating Attitudes Test (EAT-26) [15,16] is a widely used, standardized, self-report, 20-item screening measure adapted from the original 40-item test developed in 1979. The EAT-26 assesses a broad range of symptoms and provides a total score for disturbed eating attitudes and behavior in adolescents. The EAT-26 has acceptable criterion-related validity by significantly predicting group membership. The reliability (internal consistency) of the EAT-26 was reportedly high ($\alpha = 0.90$) for an anorexia nervosa group. Total scores on the EAT-26 are derived as a sum of all items, ranging from 0 to 78. Scores that are greater than or equal to 20 on the EAT-26 are frequently associated with abnormal eating attitudes and behavior and may identify those with an eating disorder. The EAT-26 manual clarifies that although a score of 20 or higher is a cause of concern, it does not necessarily mean that a life-threatening condition exists. As such, individuals scoring 20 or higher on this test are encouraged to seek the advice of a qualified mental health professional who has experience with treating eating disorders.

## THE DIAGNOSTIC SURVEY FOR EATING DISORDERS

The Diagnostic Survey for Eating Disorders (DSED) [17] is a self-report questionnaire that allows for the quantification of the frequency of disturbed eating behaviors. The DSED was not developed as a standardized, scaled instrument but, instead, provides a format for the collection of information about eating and purging behaviors. Despite having been widely used, the reliability of the DSED has not been reported, mainly because the self-reported eating and purging behaviors that are assessed appear to be somewhat changeable over time.

# FAMILY MEASURES

## FAMILY ADAPTABILITY AND COHESION EVALUATION SCALES

Family Adaptability and Cohesion Evaluation Scales III (FACES III) [18] is a self-report questionnaire composed of 20 statements that asks family members to circle, on a 5-point Likert-type scale, the degree to which their family possesses certain qualities. A separate rating scale measures what the family member would like in the ideal situation. It is intended for use with all family types and can be administered to any family member over 12 years of age. It has been used to measure the degree of family functioning after intervention and treatment and to compare differences with control group families.

The reliability of the subscales of FACES III has been fairly well established. Internal consistency reliability estimates of .62 for adaptability and .77 for cohesion, with a test–retest (4 to 5 weeks) estimate of .80 for adaptability and .83 for cohesion reported in the manual. FACES III is the third of a series of scales developed to assess two major dimensions of the circumplex model: adaptation and cohesion of the family. Further, the circumplex model is based on the assumption that the difference between functional and dysfunctional families is determined by the two interrelated dimensions of cohesion and adaptability.

Cohesion refers to the level of attachment and emotional bonding between family members. There are four graded levels to the cohesion dimension: disengaged, separated, connected, and enmeshed. Families that are disengaged lack closeness or loyalty and are characterized as highly independent. At the other end of the cohesion scale are enmeshed families. These families are characterized by a high level of closeness, loyalty, or dependence.

Adaptability is defined as the ability of the family to change in power structure, roles, and relationships to adjust to varied stressors. There are four graded levels: rigid, structured, flexible, and chaotic. Families with low levels of adaptability are classified as rigid. Rigid families are characterized by authoritarian leadership, strict negotiation, and lack of change or role modification. Families with high levels of adaptability are classified as chaotic. Chaotic family types are characterized by a lack of leadership, dramatic role shifts, erratic negotiation, and a high degree of change.

A score is obtained for adaptability and cohesion, and then a specific family type is determined. There are three distinct family types, based on the interaction of adaptability and cohesion. Balanced families (assumed to be ideal) are those with a moderate level of both adaptability and cohesion. Midrange family types are extreme on one dimension and moderate on the other. Finally, extreme family types are those who are extreme on both adaptability and cohesion measures.

## FAMILY ENVIRONMENT SCALE

The Family Environment Scale (FES) [19] is a self-report inventory designed to measure social and environmental aspects of the family; it takes about 10 minutes to complete. The FES consists of 90 true or false questions and is divided into 10 subscales. Three of the FES subscales focus on the internal aspects of the family's interpersonal relationship: cohesion, expressions, and conflict. Five of the FES subscales are concerned with goal orientation and personal growth. They are independence, achievement orientation, intellectual–cultural orientation, active–recreational orientation, and moral religious emphasis. The last two subscales (organization and control) measure aspects of family structure wuch as planning family activities or the rules and regulations used to run the family.

The FES subscales have internal consistencies ranging from .61 to .79. The item-to-subscale correlation coefficients range from .45 to .58, and the test–retest reliability for a 2-month interval ranges from .68 to .86. In addition, a low to moderate interscale correlation has been reported for the 10 subscales ($n = .25$), indicating that the FES subscales may measure distinct but moderately related aspects of families. No significant gender difference was reported for the scale.

Three separate forms of the FES are available. The Real Form (Form R) measures an individual's perception of the actual family environment. The Ideal Form (Form I) assesses an individual's perceptions of his or her ideal family environment. The Expectations Form (Form E) measures what an individual expects his or her family environment would be like with anticipated family changes.

## CONCLUSION

This chapter details standardized, psychometrically sound, behavioral and psychosocial instruments available to clinicians, which have been used in population and treatment studies of overweight children and adolescents. Although there has been a recent emphasis to screen children and adolescents on psychological, behavioral, activity and dietary parameters [20,21], few studies have used standardized assessments to measure these variables. It is no wonder, then, that there is a lack of consensus among studies related to the effects of being overweight on children's and adolescents' psychological and behavioral characteristics when compared with normative samples. Standardized behavioral and psychosocial measures are often criticized because they take too long to complete. Yet each measure takes an average of only 10 to 15 minutes to complete. As such, future research must attempt to use one or more of these measures, depending on time constraints, to allow for a more accurate understanding and comparison within and between overweight and normal-weight children and adolescents. A clear delineation of variables such as social status, age, sex, ethnicity, and geographic region is also essential to gain a fuller understanding of the effects of overweight on children and teens.

## REFERENCES

1. Achenbach, T. M. Manual for the Child Behavior Checklist/ 4-18 and 1991 Profile. Burlington, VT, 1991.
2. Achenbach, T. M. Integrative Guide to the 1991 CBCL/ 4-18, YSR and TRF Profiles. Burlington, VT, 1991.
3. Gresham, F., Elliot, S. *Social Skills Rating System*. Circle Pines, MN, 1990.
4. Kovacs, M. *Children's Depression Inventory*. San Antonio, TX: Multi-Health Systems, 1981.
5. Reynolds, W. M. *Reynolds Adolescent Depression Scale: Professional Manual*. Odessa, FL: Psychological Assessment Resources, Inc., 1987.
6. Reynolds, W. M. Reynolds Adolescent Depression Scale. In: A. B. M. Hersen. Ed. *Dictionary of Behavioral Assessment Techniques*. New York: Pergamon, 1988, pp. 381–383.
7. Piers, E., Harris, D. *The Piers-Harris Children's Self-Concept Scale*. Los Angeles, CA: Western Psychological Services, 1969.
8. Piers, E. V. *Piers-Harris Children's Self-Concept Scale: Revised Manual*. Los Angeles, CA: Western Psychological Services, 1984.

9. Piers, E., Harris, D., Herzberg, D. *The Piers-Harris Children's Self Concept Scale*. 2nd ed. Los Angeles: Western Psychological Services, 2002.
10. Harter, S. *Manual for Self-Perception Profile for Children*. Denver, CO, 1985.
11. Speilberger, C. D. *Manual for the State-Trait Anxiety Inventory for Children*. Palo Alto, CA: Consulting Psychologists Press, 1973.
12. Childress, A. C., Brewerton, T. D., Hodges, E. L., Jarrell, M. P. The Kids' Eating Disorder Survey (KEDS): a study of middle school students. *J Am Acad Child Adolesc Psychiatry*. 32:843–850, 1993.
13. Garner, D. M., Olmsted, M. P. *Eating Disorder Inventory (EDI Manual)*. Odessa, FL: Psychological Assessment Resources, 1984.
14. Garner, D. M. *The Eating Disorder Inventory-2 Professional Manual*. Odessa, FL: Psychological Assessment Resources, 1991.
15. Garner, D. M., Olmsted, M. P., Bohr, Y., Garfinkel, P. E. The Eating Attitudes Test: psychometric features and clinical correlates. *Psychol Med*. 12:871–878, 1982.
16. Garner, D. M., Garfinkel, P. E. The Eating Attitudes Test: an index of symptoms of anorexia nervosa. *Psychol Med*. 9:273–279, 1979.
17. Johnson, C. Initial consultation for patients with bulimia and anorexia nervosa: The Diagnostic Survey for Eating Disorders (DSED). In: D. M. Garner, P. E. Garfinkel. Eds. *Handbook of Psychotherapy for Anorexia and Bulimia*. New York: Guilford Press, 1985, pp. 19–51.
18. Olson, D. H., Porner, J., Lavee, Y. Family Adaptability and Cohesion Evaluation Scales (FACES III). In: F. S. Science. Ed. *Handbook of Measurements for Marriage and Family Therapy*. New York: Brunner Mazel, 1985, pp. 180–185.
19. Moos, R. H., Moos, B. S. *Family Environment Scale Manual*. Palo Alto, CA: Consulting Psychologists Press, 1981.
20. Barlow, S. E., Dietz, W. H. Obesity evaluation and treatment: Expert Committee recommendations. The Maternal and Child Health Bureau, Health Resources and Services Administration and the Department of Health and Human Services. *Pediatrics*. 102:E29, 1998.
21. Jonides, L., Buschbacher, V., Barlow, S. E. Management of child and adolescent obesity: psychological, emotional, and behavioral assessment. *Pediatrics*. 110:215-221, 2002.

# 10 Exercise Testing

*Thomas Rowland and Mark Loftin*

## CONTENTS

## PHYSIOLOGICAL CONSIDERATIONS

The exercising obese subject demonstrates a number of physiologic characteristics that distinguish him or her from the nonobese individual. In general, these findings reflect the amount of excessive body fat; that is, the quantitative changes in these physiologic variables during exercise are exhibited in direct proportion to level of obesity. Such effects of adiposity need to be appreciated when interpreting physiologic findings during exercise testing of overweight individuals.

## CARDIOVASCULAR FITNESS

Excessive body fat can profoundly affect cardiovascular fitness (considered in this discussion to be synonymous with aerobic fitness). The nature of this influence, however, depends on the definition of "cardiovascular fitness" being considered.

### ENDURANCE PERFORMANCE

The ability to perform in a distance exercise event, either time over distance or distance covered in a given time, is indirectly related to body fat content. This effect of obesity is more obvious in weight-supported activities (running, walking) and will therefore be more evident during treadmill compared with cycle exercise in the testing laboratory [1].

The effect of obesity on endurance performance is not minimal. For example, Rowland et al. found that body fat content accounted for 28% of the variance in mile run times in preadolescent boys [2], an influence similar to that of maximal oxygen uptake ($VO_2$ max). Watson demonstrated that a 46-yard decrement in distance covered in a 12-minute walk/run occurred for every 1% increase in body fat in adolescent boys [3].

It has generally been considered that this negative effect on endurance performance reflects the inert load created by excessive fat that must be transported in weight-bearing events. Still, the potential roles of depressed fitness from a sedentary lifestyle as well as depression of "true" cardiovascular fitness (see below) need to be considered.

## MAXIMAL OXYGEN UPTAKE (VO₂ MAX)

The highest rate of oxygen use by the body during a progressive exercise test ($VO_2$ max) is a physiologic marker of cardiovascular fitness. When expressed relative to body mass, $VO_2$ max is inversely related to body fat — obesity depresses mass-relative aerobic fitness. Correlation coefficients between level of obesity and $VO_2$ max per kilogram body mass have generally been approximately $r = 0.50$ [4].

The depression of $VO_2$ max per kilogram in obese youth is largely the effect of an inflated denominator, as "per kilogram" includes their inert body fat burden. Obesity does not appear to affect the numerator, as absolute values of $VO_2$ max in overweight youth are equal or greater than those of lean subjects [4–6]. Allometric scaling of $VO_2$ peak has been found to have less bias than the traditional ratio method. In this procedure, stature and mass are raised to a particular power function on the basis of the association of $VO_2$ peak (L/min) and stature and mass. Loftin et al. found that adjusting $VO_2$ peak for stature and mass reduced the difference from 50%, found in the ratio method, to 10% (allometric method) when obese were compared with normal-weight youth [7].

## "TRUE" CARDIOVASCULAR FITNESS

When cardiovascular fitness is defined as the greatest level of cardiac output that can be achieved in an exhaustive exercise test (so-called "true" cardiovascular fitness), obese subjects possess a superior level of fitness compared with the nonobese. Combining data from a series of three cycle studies of height-matched nonobese [5], moderately obese [5], and morbidly obese (unpublished data) adolescent girls, Rowland et al. found a direct correlation between body mass index and absolute maximal cardiac output ($r = .77$) [5]. The increased maximal cardiac output in obese subjects appears to parallel their greater lean body mass rather than body fat per se [6–8]. When the maximal cardiac values in the studies by Rowland et al. [5] were related to body surface area, the positive relationship with body mass index was eliminated.

These findings indicate that the reduced endurance performance and lower $VO_2$ max per kilogram observed in obese subjects are not indicators of depressed cardiac functional reserve. As a consequence, exercise interventions for obese youth do not need to be designed with a frequency, intensity, and duration that would be required to improve true cardiovascular fitness. Instead, lower-intensity exercise (certainly more palatable to the obese child) is more appropriate as a means of increasing caloric expenditure and reducing fat burden.

## AUTONOMIC FUNCTION

The autonomic nervous system responds to alterations in body energy balance, and cardiac autonomic dysfunction has been identified frequently in adult subjects. The reported patterns of this response, however, have been variable and sometimes conflicting, with descriptions of decreases in both sympathetic and parasympathetic activity [9,10], increased sympathetic tone [11,12], and depressed parasympathetic influence alone [13].

Limited information is available in children. Using measures of heart rate variability, Gutin et al. found that resting vagal (parasympathetic) activity was inversely related to fat mass in 7- to 11-year-old children [14]. Supporting this, Yakinci et al. found evidence of depressed parasympathetic activity but normal sympathetic tone in obese boys and girls (mean age, 9.5 years) [15]. These observations would explain the direct correlation between body mass index and resting heart rate ($r = .53$) in the three studies of nonobese and obese subjects described by Rowland et al., cited above [5].

How autonomic changes might influence cardiovascular variables during exercise in youth remains to be clarified. Most studies have indicated no differences in maximal heart rate between obese and nonobese youth [6,16]. However, Loftin et al. [17] observed significant differences in HR peak when obese were compared with normal-weight female youth. Some investigators have found a lower HR max in obese as compared with normal-weight adults [18,19]. Salvadori and colleagues also found a reduced catecholamine response in the obese adults [19]. Other researchers have also observed this response [20]. The reduced catecholamine response may have led to a lower heart rate maximum. Further research is needed to more fully explore this phenomenon.

## BLOOD PRESSURE

Obese children and adolescents often demonstrate systemic hypertension, and level of resting blood pressure relates to degree of adiposity [21]. As systolic blood pressure at maximal exercise typically correlates with resting values [16], greater levels of systolic pressure can be expected during exercise testing of obese subjects. Gutin et al. [22] for instance, found that maximal systolic blood pressure correlated directly with percentage body fat ($r = .35$) during treadmill exercise in 9- to 11-year-old children. As observed by Owens and Gutin [23], however, even in obese subjects systolic pressure at high exercise intensities is unlikely to reach levels that would interfere with completion of a treadmill or cycle testing.

Tulio et al. [16] measured blood pressure responses to maximal treadmill exercise in 30 lean normotensive, 30 obese hypertensive, and 10 obese normotensive males ages 13 to 18 years. In the obese hypertensive subjects, mean systolic blood pressure rose from 148 ± 11 mm Hg at rest to 212 ± 21 mm Hg at maximal exercise, compared with respective values of 117 ± 15 to 166 ± 20 mm Hg in the lean normotensives and 107 ± 16 to 168 ± 16 mm Hg in the normotensive obese subjects. At maximal exercise systolic blood pressure was significantly related to body mass index ($r = .44$) [16].

## VENTILATORY ANAEROBIC THRESHOLD

Ventilatory anaerobic threshold (VAT) is the exercise intensity or oxygen uptake at which the rise in minute ventilation diverges upward from $VO_2$ in a progressive exercise test. This submaximal marker of aerobic fitness may be particularly useful in assessing subjects with significant obesity, who may be less prone to provide an exhaustive effort during exercise testing. Values are typically expressed as $VO_2$ per kilogram or as a percentage of $VO_2$ max.

Studies of VAT in obese subjects have generally indicated parallel findings to the other indicators of aerobic fitness outlined above [24,25]. That is, VAT expressed as $VO_2$ per kg is typically lower in overweight children and adolescents, reflecting the influence of body fat on "kilogram body mass" in the denominator. However, VAT as percentage of $VO_2$ max is no different from that in nonobese youth. These findings support the concept that expressions of aerobic fitness in obese subjects are depressed by the effect of fat as an inert load rather than as an indication of negative influence of excessive body fat on cardiovascular function.

## RUNNING/WALKING ECONOMY

The energy cost of moving body mass in weight-bearing activities is defined by exercise economy, or the $VO_2$ per kilogram at a given treadmill speed or elevation. Determinants of economy are multifold, including muscular efficiency (work accomplished relative to energetic expenditure of muscle contraction), stride length and frequency, and gait coordination.

Most studies have indicated little or no difference in exercise economy in obese compared with nonobese subjects [4,26,27]. For instance, when comparing submaximal treadmill energy expenditure at 67 m/min (2.5 mph) 0% grade in 7- to 10-year-old obese and nonobese girls, Treuth et al. [26]

found values of $16.6 \pm 2.5$ and $14.7 \pm 2.6$ ml kg[1] min[1], respectively. These findings indicate that any differences in gait kinematics or muscular efficiency that might occur in obese subjects are not of sufficient magnitude to significantly alter the energy cost of submaximal treadmill exercise.

## EXERCISE TESTING

In a recent review, Owens and Gutin [23] indicated that limited information is available regarding peak exercise test protocols for obese children and youth. Investigators have typically employed exercise protocols at less strenuous treadmill speeds/inclines or cycle power outputs than protocols implemented for apparently healthy, normal-weight youth [6,7,28]. The excess adiposity presents added burden to movement, in particular, movement where the individual supports his or her own mass, such as walking or running. Loftin et al. [7] employed a walking treadmill test for the obese participants, as they were not able to tolerate a running test. Treadmill speed ranged from 67 m/min to 94 m/min (2.5 to 3.5 mph), with elevation increased by 2% every 2 minutes until volitional termination [7]. During cycle ergometry, Sothern et al. [28] employed a protocol that set the initial power output at 29 W and increased by 29 W every 2 minutes until 118 W. Power output was increased by 15 W for each additional workload. Maffeis [6] employed a similar protocol (25 W initial power output), with 15-W increments every 6 minutes.

Typically, protocols for normal-weight youth have been more strenuous. For example, treadmill protocols have been either walking or running at various inclines. Boileau et al. [29] used a walking protocol at 94 m/min (3.5 mph) that began at 10% incline. Each 3 minutes thereafter, the incline was increased by 2.5% until volitional termination. Turley et al. [30] used a protocol that included both walking and running (80 m/min to 134 m/min) with incline increased from level walking to 5% while running. Boileau et al. [29] used a peak cycle ergometer protocol that had the youth exercising at an initial workload of 88W with increases of 29W every three minutes until volitional termination. Turley et al. [30] used a protocol that began at zero resistance (65 rpm) and increased by 16 W every minute until volitional termination.

In comparing treadmill with cycle peak $VO_2$ values, Loftin et al. [31] found no significant differences for either absolute $VO_2$ (L/min) or $VO_2$ peak relative to mass. The authors speculated that the excess adiposity in the severely obese participants may have limited their performance during the treadmill peak test as they had to support their mass during this test. Typically, treadmill $VO_2$ peak has yielded higher values than peak cycle ergometry in normal-weight youth. In summary, less strenuous peak treadmill and cycle ergometry protocols are typically used for obese youth when compared with apparently healthy, normal-weight youth. Either ergometer yields peak responses.

## REFERENCES

1. Cumming, G. R., D. Everatt, and L. Hastman. Bruce treadmill test in children: normal values in a clinic population. *Am J Cardiol.* 41:69–75, 1978.
2. Rowland, T., G. Kline, D. Goff, L. Martel, and L. Ferrone. One-mile run performance and cardiovascular fitness in children. *Arch Pediatr Adolesc Med.* 153:845–849, 1999.
3. Watson, A. W. Quantification of the influence of body fat content on selected physical performance variables in adolescent boys. *Ir J Med Sci.* 157:383–384, 1988.
4. Rowland, T. W. Effects of obesity on aerobic fitness in adolescent females. *Am J Dis Child.* 145:764–768, 1991.
5. Rowland, T., R. Bhargava, D. Parslow, and R. A. Heptulla. Cardiac response to progressive cycle exercise in moderately obese adolescent females. *J Adolesc Health.* 32:422–427, 2003.
6. Maffeis, C., F. Schena, M. Zaffanello, L. Zoccante, Y. Schutz, and L. Pinelli. Maximal aerobic power during running and cycling in obese and non-obese children. *Acta Paediatr.* 83:113–116, 1994.

7.  Loftin, M., M. Sothern, L. Trosclair, A. O'Hanlon, J. Miller, and J. Udall. Scaling VO(2) peak in obese and non-obese girls. *Obes Res.* 9:290–296, 2001.

8.  Daniels, S. R., T. R. Kimball, J. A. Morrison, P. Khoury, S. Witt, and R. A. Meyer. Effect of lean body mass, fat mass, blood pressure, and sexual maturation on left ventricular mass in children and adolescents. Statistical, biological, and clinical significance. *Circulation.* 92:3249–3254, 1995.

9.  Peterson, H. R., M. Rothschild, C. R. Weinberg, R. D. Fell, K. R. McLeish, and M. A. Pfeifer. Body fat and the activity of the autonomic nervous system. *N Engl J Med.* 318:1077–1083, 1988.

10. Laederach-Hofmann, K., L. Mussgay, and H. Ruddel. Autonomic cardiovascular regulation in obesity. *J Endocrinol.* 164:59–66, 2000.

11. Arone, L. J., R. Mackintosh, M. Rosenbaum, R. L. Leibel, and J. Hirsch. Autonomic nervous system activity in weight gain and weight loss. *Am J Physiol.* 269:R222–R225, 1995.

12. Zahorska-Markiewicz, B., E. Kuagowska, C. Kucio, and M. Klin. Heart rate variability in obesity. *Int J Obes Relat Metab Disord.* 17:21–23, 1993.

13. Valensi, P., B. N. Thi, B. Lormeau, J. Paries, and J. R. Attali. Cardiac autonomic function in obese patients. *Int J Obes Relat Metab Disord.* 19:113–118, 1995.

14. Gutin, B., P. Barbeau, M. S. Litaker, M. Ferguson, and S. Owens. Heart rate variability in obese children: relations to total body and visceral adiposity, and changes with physical training and detraining. *Obes Res.* 8:12–19, 2000.

15. Yakinci, C., B. Mungen, H. Karabiber, M. Tayfun, and C. Evereklioglu. Autonomic nervous system functions in obese children. *Brain Dev.* 22:151–153, 2000.

16. Tulio, S., S. Egle, and B. Greily. Blood pressure response to exercise of obese and lean hypertensive and normotensive male adolescents. *J Hum Hypertens.* 9:953–958, 1995.

17. Loftin, M., M. Sothern, C. VanVrancken, A. O'Hanlon, and J. Udall. Effect of obesity status on heart rate peak in female youth. *Clin Pediatr* (Phila). 42:505–510, 2003.

18. Salvadori, A., P. Fanari, P. Mazza, S. Baudo, A. Brunani, M. De Martin et al. Metabolic aspects and sympathetic effects in the obese subject undergoing exercise testing. *Minerva Med.* 84:171–177, 1993.

19. Salvadori, A., M. Arreghini, G. Bolla, P. Fanari, E. Giacomotti, E. Longhini et al. Cardiovascular and adrenergic response to exercise in obese subjects. *J Clin Basic Cardiol.* 2:229–236, 1999.

20. Gustafson, A. B., P. A. Farrell, and R. K. Kalkhoff. Impaired plasma catecholamine response to submaximal treadmill exercise in obese women. *Metabolism.* 39:410–417, 1990.

21. Lauer, R. M., W. E. Connor, P. E. Leaverton, M. A. Reiter, and W. R. Clarke. Coronary heart disease risk factors in school children: the Muscatine Study. *J Pediatr.* 86:697–706, 1975.

22. Gutin, B., S. Islam, F. Treiber, C. Smith, and T. Manos. Fasting insulin concentration is related to cardiovascular reactivity to exercise in children. *Pediatrics.* 96:1123–1125, 1995.

23. Owens, S. and B. Gutin. Exercise testing of the child with obesity. *Pediatr Cardiol.* 20:79–83, 1999; discussion 84.

24. Reybrouck, T., M. Weymans, J. Vinckx, H. Stijns, and M. Vanderschueren-Lodeweyckx. Cardiorespiratory function during exercise in obese children. *Acta Paediatr Scand.* 76:342–348, 1987.

25. Zanconato, S., E. Baraldi, P. Santuz, F. Rigon, L. Vido, L. Da Dalt, and F. Zacchello. Gas exchange during exercise in obese children. *Eur J Pediatr.* 148:614–617, 1989.

26. Treuth, M. S., R. Figueroa-Colon, G. R. Hunter, R. L. Weinsier, N. F. Butte, and M. I. Goran. Energy expenditure and physical fitness in overweight vs non-overweight prepubertal girls. *Int J Obes Relat Metab Disord.* 22:440–447, 1998.

27. Katch, V., M. D. Becque, C. Marks, C. Moorehead, and A. Rocchini. Oxygen uptake and energy output during walking of obese male and female adolescents. *Am J Clin Nutr.* 47:26–32, 1988.

28. Sothern, M. S., M. Loftin, U. Blecker, and J. N. Udall, Jr. Impact of significant weight loss on maximal oxygen uptake in obese children and adolescents. *J Investig Med.* 48:411–416, 2000.

29. Boileau, R. A., A. Bonen, V. H. Heyward, and B. H. Massey. Maximal aerobic capacity on the treadmill and bicycle ergometer of boys 11-14 years of age. *J Sports Med Phys Fitness.* 17:153–162, 1977.

30. Turley, K. R., Rogers, D.M., Harper, K.M., Kujawa, K.I., Wilmore, J.H. Maximal treadmill versus cycle ergometry testing in children: differences, reliability, and variability of responses. *Pediatr Exerc Sci.* 7:49–60, 1995.

31. Loftin, M., Sothern, M., Warren, B., Udall, J. Comparison of VO$_2$ peak during treadmill and cycle ergometry in severely overweight youth. *J Sports Sci Med.* 3:254–260, 2004.

# Section 5

## Dietary Approaches

# 11 Pediatric Obesity Dietary Approaches in Clinical Settings: A Survey of the Options and Recommendations

*Melinda S. Sothern, Connie VanVrancken-Tompkins, and Lauren Keely Carlisle*

## CONTENTS

## INTRODUCTION

The clinical management of pediatric obesity requires the application of scientifically sound and medically relevant dietary approaches. The most successful approaches are implemented in conjunction with behavioral counseling, including the promotion of physical activity and medical supervision [1]. The child's medical history and current weight condition during critical periods of obesity development may help to define the appropriate dietary approach and optimal weight loss schedule or maintenance plan (Table 11.1). These critical periods include birth, 4 to 6 years of age, and adolescence [2].

Although successful weight loss is rare in overweight adults, research indicates that weight loss during childhood can be maintained into adulthood [3]. However, few studies have reported success in treating more severe conditions of childhood and adolescent obesity.

The most successful dietary approaches are those that the patient will most likely follow with a high level of compliance. Dietary plans should include a combination of nutrients and daily calorie levels that best promotes the optimal schedule of weight loss or maintenance associated with the patient's medical history, current weight condition, and age. Younger, less overweight children

**TABLE 11.1**
**Critical Opportunities for Dietary Intervention**

Normal and overweight children ≤6 years of age, with parental obesity
At risk for overweight (>85th percentile BMI) children and adolescents, 7–18 years
Overweight (>95th percentile BMI) children and adolescents, 7–18 years
Severely overweight (>97th percentile BMI) children and adolescents, 7–18 years

probably require less structure and more family education. Older, more severely overweight children may need comprehensive, aggressive therapy that promotes significant weight loss. Furthermore, increasing levels of obesity decrease exercise performance in some children [4]. This decreased ability makes it more difficult to encourage increased physical activity [5]. Increasing physical activity especially during caloric restriction is absolutely necessary to prevent adult obesity and promote normal muscle and bone development. Therefore, in children with more severe overweight conditions, aggressive dietary therapy may be required initially. In all cases, a pediatrician or family physician must supervise the dietary plan and monitor the child's growth and development.

In this chapter, we review studies of pediatric overweight treatment over the last two decades and then present varied dietary approaches to the management of pediatric obesity in clinical settings. Finally, we provide recommendations with consideration for medical history, age, and level of obesity.

## INDIVIDUAL- AND FAMILY-BASED DIETARY INTERVENTIONS IN CLINICAL SETTINGS

The Committee on Nutrition of the American Academy of Pediatrics recommends family-based therapies including diet, psychosocial therapy, and exercise [6]. However, the presence of medical complications, age, and obesity level should be considered when developing prevention and treatment plans. The clinical management of pediatric obesity includes dietary strategies to prevent excessive weight gain, especially in children at high risk, and treatment diets to reduce adiposity in overweight children. Several different types of diets have been suggested for treating clinically relevant pediatric obesity. These include portion-controlled diets, with a primary focus on reducing sugar and saturated fat while increasing fruits and vegetables; low-fat, moderately low calorie diets; low-glycemic load diets; low-carbohydrate diets; very low calorie diets (VLCDs); and other, including liquid diets (Table 11.2). Research to support any one individual approach to the clinical management of pediatric obesity is limited. With few exceptions, the results of research studies

**TABLE 11.2**
**Dietary Approaches for the Clinical Management of Pediatric Obesity**

Nutrition education (prevention)
Portion controlled, with a focus on reducing sugar and saturated fat, while increasing fruits and
  vegetables
Low-fat, moderately low-calorie diet
Low-glycemic diet
Low-carbohydrate diet
Very low calorie diets:
    Protein sparing modified fast
    Protein modified fast
Other: meal replacement plans

employing these varied types of diets are confounded. The majority were conducted in family-based, multidisciplinary settings, in which diets were examined in conjunction with other therapies such as behavioral counseling and exercise. Thus, studies that examine specific dietary approaches independently in overweight children and adolescents are urgently needed. Until such studies are conducted, pediatric health care professionals must refer to studies that use dietary approaches in conjunction with behavioral counseling and exercise to determine appropriate dietary interventions for their overweight patients.

Recently, Crawford and others conducted a systematic, evidence-based review of the pediatric overweight treatment literature over the last two decades [7]. Studies were included if they were conducted after 1980 and before 2002. Over 100 studies were evaluated, and in this chapter we focus on studies that include nutrition education or dietary therapy based on the following criteria: targeted subjects were greater than the 85th percentile body mass index (BMI), study was conducted in a clinical setting, study included at least 15 subjects per group (if randomized controlled trials (RCT), a total of 15 subjects was acceptable), the intervention duration was greater than 8 weeks, the study included a dietary intervention, and the study included a measure of weight loss or adiposity.

Interventions reviewed included 42 family-based interventions, one individual-based intervention [8], and one individual- versus family-based intervention [9–11]. Individual-based interventions were defined as those that involved one-on-one counseling only, and family-based interventions involved group counseling, with family participation within at least one intervention group. All individual- and family-based interventions involved treatment of overweight youth rather than prevention of excessive weight gain in nonoverweight individuals. Of the 44 studies evaluated, 29 were RCTs, and 15 were studies of other designs. One study by Epstein [12] duplicated a later report [13], and therefore the two reports were combined and treated as one intervention. One metaanalysis, by LeMura and Maziekas [14], was reviewed but was not included in the final report because of differing study exclusion criteria.

No studies examined dietary counseling exclusively, and only one study examined nutrition education without dietary counseling. Thirty-eight studies examined dietary counseling in conjunction with behavior modification and counseling or physical activity and exercise that resulted in significant reductions in weight status and adiposity. Of these, 24 studies were randomized controlled trials, and 14 were studies of other design [15–20]. In the majority of these studies, both short- and long-term reductions in weight status/adiposity in children and adolescents were significant.

Most of the studies used techniques such as portion control and recommendations to reduce access to higher-density foods. Many studies used the U.S. Food and Drug Administration's Food Guide Pyramid for prescribing a low-fat diet. The pyramid conveys messages about eating a variety of grains, fruits, and vegetables and limiting fat intake to 30% or less of total calories. Although the pyramid has been widely recommended for promoting healthful eating among children in general [21–24], there are no randomized and controlled studies comparing its direct use as an intervention with other dietary approaches in children and adolescents. Furthermore, the educational benefits of the food guide pyramid remain understudied and inconclusive [25]. A recent study concluded that promoting a diet with a variety of foods, such as the food guide pyramid does, increases the probability of nutrient adequacy in adults [26]. However, no such studies have been conducted in children.

Eight studies [5,27–33] prescribed balanced hypocaloric diets with a 300- to 500-calorie-per-day reduction based on current American Diabetes Association (ADA) age-appropriate standards. Two studies examined dietary counseling alone versus dietary counseling and nutrition education combined with physical activity (lifestyle exercise) or structured exercise with mixed findings. Epstein et al. [34] examined the effect of diet plus lifestyle exercise versus diet only and waiting list control over 6 months. Both treatment groups had significant reductions in weight status and adiposity compared with controls. However, there were no significant differences in the reduction of weight status and adiposity between diet only and diet plus exercise groups at 6 months or at 12-month follow up. In contrast, in a subsequent study, Epstein et al. [35] showed that interventions with diet plus structured exercise resulted in a significantly greater reduction in weight status/adiposity than those with diet alone at 6 months and at 1-year follow up.

Two randomized controlled studies [18,19] and seven nonrandomized, clinical observational studies [5,20,28–33] evaluated reduced-calorie diets with different nutrient compositions (alternative approaches). In all of the studies, significant reductions were observed in weight status/adiposity from baseline. When alternative approaches were compared with standard diets in two randomized controlled trials [18,19], a significantly greater change in weight status was seen in the subjects receiving the alternative diet. However, none of the studies was greater than 1 year in duration. Thus, the long-term effect of such diets is not known. More RCTs, are needed to confirm these results.

Research over the last 2 decades indicates that there is sufficient evidence to support family-based, group dietary counseling in conjunction with exercise or physical activity and behavior modification in children 12 year of age and under. Individual- and family-based studies contain several common elements. Most studies use a combination of dietary counseling, nutrition education, exercise/physical activity, and behavioral counseling. Because dietary recommendations vary from one study to another, it is not possible at this time to conclude that any one particular type of diet is more effective for the treatment of pediatric obesity.

Long-term interventions designed for diverse populations are lacking; most of the long-term studies were conducted in white, middle-upper class youth. Long-term studies in older children are also lacking. At present, there is little information concerning the optimal overweight treatment program for adolescents 13 years or older in clinical settings. There is a need for tailored, developmentally appropriate overweight treatment programs for adolescents. With regard to this age group, there is little consensus as to what constitutes an effective approach.

## DIETARY PREVENTION AND TREATMENT RECOMMENDATIONS FOR CHILDREN AND ADOLESCENTS

### NORMAL AND OVERWEIGHT CHILDREN 6 OR FEWER YEARS OF AGE WITH PARENTAL OBESITY

Because both normal and overweight children who are 6 or fewer years of age, with obese parents, are at increased risk for adult obesity, researchers recommend programs that combine nutrition education and parent training. Parents are encouraged to create a healthy home food environment [36]. They are advised to limit the quantities of high-calorie snacks, especially those with excessive sugar and saturated fat, in the home and to promote fruit and vegetable consumption. Parents are also encouraged to observe their child's behavior for important cues such as excessive hunger, inability to become satiated, or excessive shyness or isolation, and to report this behavior to their child's pediatrician or family physician [37].

Clinical management of these at-risk children has not been systemic. Moreover, there are no studies in the literature that specifically target young, healthy-weight children with primary risk factors for developing obesity in a clinical setting [38,39]. A recent publication of the American Academy of Pediatrics offers pediatric obesity prevention guidelines for medical professionals, which include increased monitoring of at-risk children and parent education [6]. Parents are advised to implement strategies such as avoiding snacking, replacing high-sugar beverages with water, and regulating meal times, which are examples of simple measures to reduce the risk of obesity in young children [37,40–42] The potential role of prevention through primary care is currently underrated by the medical community [43]. In one study, it was concluded that frequent medical clinic visits in preschool-aged children might reduce the degree of obesity in the patients [44]. Furthermore, targeting families of susceptible children with nutrition and lifestyle behavior education may create an added benefit to the other family members [43]. By the time children enter kindergarten, their food preferences and the social context with which they associate foods are already established [45]. Infants whose parents were instructed in health education emphasizing

**TABLE 11.3**

**Proposed Initial Dietary Strategies by Medical History, Age, and Level of Obesity**

| Level | Medical History, Age and Weight Condition (BMI %) | Dietary Approach |
|---|---|---|
| I | ≤6 years, normal or overweight with one or more obese parents | Family nutrition education and parent training emphasizing appropriate food portions, reduced sugar and saturated fat, increased fruits and vegetables, and recommended dairy and fiber intake |
| II | 7–18 years, at risk for overweight (>85th percentile BMI) | Family nutrition education and parent training in combination with portion control methods or balanced calorie meal plans emphasizing appropriate food portions, reduced sugar and saturated fat, increased fruits and vegetables, and recommended dairy and fiber intake |
| III | 7–18 years, overweight (>95th percentile BMI) | Family nutrition education and parent training in combination with balanced hypocaloric diets emphasizing appropriate food portions, reduced sugar and saturated fat, increased fruits and vegetables, recommended dairy and fiber intake, and Low Glycemic Index Diet |
| IV | 7–18 years, severely overweight (>97th percentile BMI) | Family nutrition education and parent training in combination with dietary approaches as follows: Low Glycemic Index Diet, Atkins Diet, protein modified fast diet followed by balanced hypocaloric diet |

diets low in saturated fat and sugar were less likely to be obese at 3 years of age than were age-matched controls [46]. Therefore, educating the families of young children about nutrition may have a powerful, positive effect on the obesity risk of those children, and especially on those with obese parents (Table 11.3) [36,37].

Recently Passehl and others [47] implemented a clinical pediatric obesity prevention program called "Take Charge," an on-site training program for primary health care providers (Appendix A3.1.2). Six health care provider sites pilot tested the curriculum. Results indicated that over one-third of providers used the materials with their patients daily or weekly. However, individual patient results were not available. Although it is generally recommended as a method of preventing pediatric obesity, the effects of including a nutrition curriculum to prevent pediatric obesity in at-risk preschool youth in the clinical setting remain unclear.

## AT RISK FOR OVERWEIGHT CHILDREN AND ADOLESCENTS, 7 TO 18 YEARS OF AGE

Children, 7 years or older, who are classified as at risk for overweight are more likely to become overweight adults [48]. The risk is higher in adolescents [49]. Several dietary approaches based on portion control or balanced-calorie healthy meal plans low in saturated fat and sugar and higher in fiber have been shown to be successful [9,50,51]. The Traffic Light Diet [52] (Appendix A3.2) uses a color-coded system to promote increased consumption of healthy foods that are less nutrient dense and, therefore, lower in saturated fat and sugar and higher in fiber, and decreased intake of those foods that are less nutritious and higher in calories. In our review, we found 12 studies that prescribed the Traffic Light Diet [52]. In all cases, studies using the Traffic Light Diet demonstrated significant reductions in weight status. The dietary pattern consisted of green (go foods — unlimited), yellow (eat with caution foods — limit), and red (stop foods — avoid) (Appendix A3.2).

Several studies [16,17,20,53–56] specify diets with daily caloric recommendations based on current ADA age-appropriate standards. As stated earlier, it is difficult to assess the direct effect of ADA standard diets, but when they are used in combination with behavioral counseling and exercise, weight loss results are generally significant. In addition, several of these studies use portion control techniques to reduce calorie intake by limiting the amount of food (portions) consumed by the child [32,33,55,56]. Because portion control may help to reteach the body to normalize food intake over a period of time, it can be routinely used in clinical settings as a method to prevent the onset of significant obesity in children.

## OVERWEIGHT CHILDREN AND ADOLESCENTS, 7 TO 18 YEARS OF AGE

The overweight child presents the greatest challenge to the health care professional. Excess weight limits exercise tolerance and promotes sedentary behaviors [57]. Thus, it may be necessary to limit the daily calorie intake of an obese child to promote a noticeable weight loss. In addition, caloric restriction may be necessary if previous attempts to promote reduced fat/healthy food choices were unsuccessful. In our review, eight studies [5,27–33] prescribed hypocaloric diets with a 300 to 500 calorie per day reduction based on current ADA age-appropriate standards. All of these studies showed significant reductions in weight status or adiposity after 8 to 10 weeks. In one clinical observation [9], growth velocity delays were observed in some of the participants. However, none of the randomized and controlled trials using hypocaloric diets showed growth abnormalities. Because the risk of growth delays is possible, caloric reduction requires close medical monitoring. Therefore, reduced-calorie diets should only be prescribed and monitored by registered dietitians in conjunction with physician supervision and long-term follow-up.

## SEVERELY OVERWEIGHT CHILDREN AND ADOLESCENTS, 7 TO 18 YEARS OF AGE

Research consistently supports the concept that traditional dietary approaches may not promote successful weight management in severely overweight children [58,59]. In older overweight children with a history of dietary failures, it may be necessary initially to prescribe a more restrictive diet for a short period. Typically, these children have other emotional concerns that must be addressed during dietary treatment [13,60–62]. Several alternative dietary approaches have been proposed and scientifically tested in short-term, clinical settings (Table 11.2).

## LOW-GLYCEMIC INDEX DIET

Changing patterns of macronutrient consumption have arguably contributed to the epidemic of obesity [63]. With an estimated 302 million adults worldwide classified as obese by the World Health Organization, high-fat diets have been viewed by many as a leading cause of this energy excess [63]. In the United States, however, there has been a substantial decline in the percentage of total energy obtained from fat [64]. Therefore, it is important to consider the effects of other dietary changes on body weight — in particular, high-glycemic index (GI) carbohydrates.

Traditionally, carbohydrates were classified according to saccharide chain length, as "simple sugars" or "complex carbohydrates" [65]. In 1981, Jenkins and colleagues introduced an alternative system for characterizing carbohydrate-containing foods according to how they affect postgrandial glycemia [66]. Thus, the GI is determined by comparing the blood glucose response to ingestion of 50 g of available carbohydrate from a test food with that of a reference food (either glucose or white bread), as follows:

$$GI = \frac{\text{Incremental area under the glucose response curve to 50 g carbohydrate from test food}}{\text{Incremental area under the glucose response curve to 50 g carbohydrate standard}} \times 100$$

A related term, *glycemic load*, has been proposed to take into account differences in carbohydrate content among foods, meals, or diets [67]:

Glycemic load = GI of food (meal, diet) × carbohydrate content of food (meal, diet).

Thus, glycemic load facilitates application of GI to the clinical setting, where macronutrient composition differs among individuals.

Weight loss on energy-restricted, reduced-fat diets may be increased when such diets are modified to lower GI. In an outcomes assessment study of 107 patients attending a pediatric obesity clinic, Spieth et al. [68] prescribed either an ad libitum low-glycemic load diet (45 to 50% carbohydrate, 30 to 35% fat, 20 to 25% protein) emphasizing low-GI carbohydrate sources or an energy-restricted low-fat diet (55 to 60% carbohydrate, 25 to 30% fat, 15 to 20% protein). Children in the low-glycemic load group were specifically instructed to eat to satiety and snack when hungry. Patients on the low-glycemic load diet lost more weight, resulting in a group difference of 1.5 kg/m$^2$ for change in BMI over a mean of 4 months. Ebbeling et al. conducted a randomized and controlled study, which indicated that low-glycemic diets promote significantly greater improvements in the weight status/adiposity and metabolic profiles of sedentary, overweight adolescents when compared with a low-fat diet [18]. By 12 months, BMI had decreased more in the low-glycemic load group compared with the low-fat group (1.3 vs. +0.7 kg/m$^2$). This ad libitum reduced-glycemic load diet, without strict limitation on carbohydrate intake, may be a promising alternative to conventional dietary therapy.

The metabolic profile associated with consumption of low-GI diets may foster satiety and reduce food intake [69,70]. The decreased availability of metabolic fuels in the late postprandial period after consumption of a high-GI diet would be expected to stimulate hunger and promote food intake in an environment of food abundance [65]. Single-meal studies show GI to be directly related to postprandial hunger and subsequent voluntary food intake [69–71]. Studies have also shown that this satiety effect is likely to extend beyond the short term (one meal). In addition, soluble fiber has been shown to lower hunger ratings [72,73] and the desire to eat for as long as 13 hours after the meal [72] and to promote longer-term negative energy balance [74].

According to low-fat dietary guidelines set by the American Heart Association to prevent and treat cardiovascular disease, total fat intake should be less than 30% of the diet, with saturated fat less than 10%. Independent of weight loss and physical activity, the effectiveness of this diet on cardiovascular disease remains unclear [75–78]. It is possible that low-GI diets may modify the unfavorable risk factors caused by obesity by decreasing postprandial hyperinsulinemia [79]. Studies have demonstrated decreased blood glucose profiles and lower levels of C-peptide (a marker of insulin secretion) on nutrient-controlled low-, compared with high-, GI diets [80–83]. It was also reported that glucose tolerance improved after consuming low- versus high-GI test meals [84–87]. In addition, two of three observational studies found significant associations after controlling for body weight and other potentially confounding factors to further support a role of GI or glycemic load in diabetes risk [88,89].

There is concern that the GI concept is too complex to be practical in the clinical setting; however, several studies have reported clinically significant improvement in relevant endpoints among subjects consuming self-selected low-GI diets. In addition, in newly diagnosed diabetic adults and children, the low-GI diets facilitated better glycemic control and were perceived as "simple and practical" [90,91]. The benefits of low-GI diets in the treatment and prevention of obesity and type 2 diabetes should be considered by the clinician for dietary counsel. Ebbeling and Ludwig provide a detailed overview of the ad libitum low-glycemic load approach in Volume 1 of the *Handbook of Pediatric Obesity*, including lesson plans, student handouts, and study results [92].

## VERY LOW CALORIE DIETS IN THE CLINICAL SETTING

There have been few randomized and controlled trials using very low calorie diets (VLCDs) in children and adolescents. In a short-term study, Sondike et al. [93] reported greater reductions in weight status/adiposity (9.9 vs. 4.1 kg) in adolescents who were instructed to follow an ad libitum VLCD versus an ad libitum low-fat diet for 12 weeks. In this study, two diets were compared on their effects on weight loss and serum lipid profiles in 30 obese adolescents (BMI > 95th percentile for age) in a controlled 12-week trial. The low-carbohydrate and low-fat diets were chosen because of previous research showing that they are well-tolerated and effective treatments for short-term weight loss in both children and adults. The low-carbohydrate diet consisted of <20 g/day of carbohydrates for the first 2 weeks and <40 g/day for the remaining 10 weeks. The low-fat diet (control) consisted of consumption of <30% of energy from fat per day. Any additional calorie consumption was self-selected. Diet composition and weight were monitored every 2 weeks throughout the trial. Serum lipid profiles were obtained at the beginning and end of the 12-week trial period.

The low-carbohydrate group lost more weight (9.9 ± 9.3 kg) compared with the low-fat diet group (4.1 ± 4.9 kg) and showed significantly better average BMI improvements (3.3 ± 3.0 kg/m²) than the low-fat group (1.5 ± 1.7 kg/m²). The low-carbohydrate group also showed improvements in non-high-density-lipoprotein cholesterol levels, as well as greater decreases in serum triglyceride values, than the low-fat group. Improvements in low-density lipoprotein cholesterol levels were seen only in the low-fat group. Neither group showed adverse effects on serum lipid profiles.

Total caloric intake estimates show that on average, the low-carbohydrate group consumed more energy than the low-fat group and reported higher fat and cholesterol intakes and lower carbohydrate intakes than the low-fat group. Greater weight loss despite higher caloric, fat, and cholesterol intakes in the low-carbohydrate group indicates that a low-carbohydrate diet may be more effective than a low-fat diet in promoting short-term weight loss in obese adolescents. However, the long-term effect of such approaches is unknown.

Brown et al. [28] demonstrated improvements in the lipid profiles and weight status/adiposity of 53 children, 7 to 17 years of age, after a VLCD, nutrition education, structured exercise, increased physical activity, and behavior modification. In a series of three clinical observations, [29,31,33] Sothern and colleagues examined the change in weight status/adiposity in children and adolescents, 7 to 17 years of age, after participation in behavior modification, nutrition education, structured exercise, increased physical activity, and a VLCD or balanced hypocaloric diet (based on initial weight status). The multidisciplinary program included a VLCD called a protein-sparing modified fast that provided 600 to 800 kcal/day and 1.5 to 2.0 gm/kg of ideal body weight in severely obese children (BMI = 34.1 ± 4.8 and >97th percentile BMI). Subjects reduced weight approximately 30% after 10 weeks and maintained the weight loss at 1 year. In one study, however, two males and four females exhibited growth velocities below the 3rd percentile for their chronological age. In females, but not males, heights at the end of the study were normal for an adult North American individual. Regardless, in some patients this severe caloric restriction may negatively affect growth velocity, even in the presence of exercise and close medical supervision. Recently, a modified version of the protein-sparing modified fast called the protein modified fast has been suggested and observed in clinical settings [94]. It is a nonketogenic VLCD of approximately 1000 calories per day, 50 to 75 g/day of carbohydrates, and 2.5 gm/kg ideal body weight (average 90 to 140 g/day) of protein. Because this diet emphasizes the intake of low-starch vegetables, includes dairy and fruit up to 45 to 50 grams, and reduces saturated fat, it is less like a VLCD and, in concept, is a structured reduced-calorie diet that includes low-glycemic recommendations. In Chapter 12 of this text, Schumacher and colleagues detail this approach and provide preliminary findings in children 7 to 17 years of age.

## SUMMARY

The goal for preventing and treating childhood obesity is regulating body weight and fat with adequate nutrition for growth and development. Clinical pediatric obesity dietary interventions should be delivered by a team of health care experts in a medically supervised, nurturing, and nonintimidating environment. In children, from birth to 6 years of age, parental nutrition education is strongly recommended regardless of the child's current weight condition, especially if the parents are obese (Table 11.3). Children and adolescents 7 years or older at risk for overweight become increasingly more susceptible as they mature. Therefore, appropriate, targeted, family-based dietary interventions are recommended to prevent the onset of a clinically significant overweight condition (Table 11.3). Children, 7 years of age or older with clinically relevant overweight conditions require more comprehensive, structured, and in severe cases, aggressive dietary approaches (Table 11.3). Low-GI diets have been safely and effectively used to promote weight loss in adolescents in a 1-year randomized and controlled study. The results of VLCDs in youth are limited to one short-term randomized and controlled trial and several 1-year clinical observations. Strict medical supervision is absolutely necessary when developing children are prescribed diets low in calories. Research is needed to determine the safest and most effective dietary strategy for children and, especially, adolescents with more severe conditions of obesity under randomized and controlled conditions over long-term periods.

## REFERENCES

1. Batch, J. A. and L. A. Baur. Management and prevention of obesity and its complications in children and adolescents. *Med J Aust*. 182:130–135, 2005.
2. Dietz, W. H. Critical periods in childhood for the development of obesity. *Am J Clin Nutr*. 59:955–959, 1994.
3. Epstein, L. H., A. Valoski, R. R. Wing, and J. McCurley. Ten-year follow-up of behavioral, family-based treatment for obese children. *JAMA*. 264:2519–2523, 1990.
4. Bar-Or, O., J. Foreyt, C. Bouchard et al. Physical activity, genetic and nutritional considerations in childhood weight management. *Med Sci Sports Exerc*. 30:2–10, 1998.
5. Sothern, M. S., S. Hunter, R. M. Suskind, R. Brown, J. N. Udall, Jr., and U. Blecker. Motivating the obese child to move: the role of structured exercise in pediatric weight management. *South Med J*. 92:577–584, 1999.
6. Krebs, N. F. and M. S. Jacobson. Prevention of pediatric overweight and obesity. *Pediatrics*. 112:424–430, 2003.
7. Crawford, P., M. S. Sothern, D. Hoest, and L. Ritchie. Pediatric overweight: Position statement and evidence-based analysis of interventions. *J Am Dietetic Assoc*. in press.
8. Saelens, B. E., E. Jelalian, and D. M. Kukene. Physician weight counseling for adolescents. *Clin Pediatr* (Phila). 41:575–585, 2002.
9. Nuutinen, O. and M. Knip. Long-term weight control in obese children: persistence of treatment outcome and metabolic changes. *Int J Obes Relat Metabol Disord*. 16:279–287, 1992.
10. Nuutinen, O. and M. Knip. Predictors of weight reduction in obese children. *Eur J Clin Nutr*. 46:785–794, 1992.
11. Nuutinen, O. and M. Knip. Weight loss, body composition and risk factors for cardiovascular disease in obese children: long-term effects of two treatment strategies. *J Am Coll Nutr*. 11:707–714, 1992.
12. Epstein, L. H. Methodological issues and ten-year outcomes for obese children. *Ann N Y Acad Sci*. 699:237–249, 1993.
13. Epstein, L. H., K. R. Klein, and L. Wisniewski. Child and parent factors that influence psychological problems in obese children. *Int J Eat Disord*. 15:151–158, 1994.
14. LeMura, L. M. and M. T. Maziekas. Factors that alter body fat, body mass, and fat-free mass in pediatric obesity. *Med Sci Sports Exerc*. 34:487–496, 2002.
15. Van Horn, L., E. Obarzanek, B. A. Barton, V. J. Stevens, P. O. Kwiterovich Jr., N. L. Lasser et al. A summary of results of the Dietary Intervention Study in Children (DISC): lessons learned. *Prog Cardiovasc Nurs*. 18:28–41, 2003.
16. Obarzanek, E., F. M. Sacks, W. M. Vollmer, G. A. Bray, E. R. Miller 3rd, P. H. Lin et al. Effects on blood lipids of a blood pressure-lowering diet: the Dietary Approaches to Stop Hypertension (DASH) Trial. *Am J Clin Nutr*. 74:80–89, 2001.
17. Obarzanek, E., S. Y. Kimm, B. A. Barton, L. L. Van Horn, P. O. Kwiterovich, Jr., D. G. Simons-Morton et al. Long-term safety and efficacy of a cholesterol-lowering diet in children with elevated low-density lipoprotein cholesterol: seven-year results of the Dietary Intervention Study in Children (DISC). *Pediatrics*. 107:256–264, 2001.
18. Ebbeling, C. B., M. M. Leidig, K. B. Sinclair, J. P. Hangen, and D. S. Ludwig. A reduced-glycemic load diet in the treatment of adolescent obesity. *Arch Pediatr Adolesc Med*. 157:773–779, 2003.
19. Sondike, S. B., N. Copperman, and M. S. Jacobson. Effects of a low-carbohydrate diet on weight loss and cardiovascular risk factor in overweight adolescents. *J Pediatr*. 142:253–258, 2003.

20. Spieth, L. E., J. D. Harnish, C. M. Lenders, L. B. Raezer, M. A. Pereira, S. J. Hangen, and D. S. Ludwig. A low-glycemic index diet in the treatment of pediatric obesity. *Arch Pediatr Adolesc Med.* 154:947–951, 2000.

21. U.S. Department of Agriculture, Department of Health and Human Services. Dietary guidelines for Americans, 2000. Accessed from: http:www.health.gov/dietaryguidelines/

22. Barlow, S. E. and W. H. Dietz. Obesity evaluation and treatment: expert committee recommendations. *Pediatrics.* 102:e29, 1998.

23. Nicklas, T., R. Johnson, and American Dietetic Association. Position of the American Dietetic Association: dietary guidance for healthy children ages 2 to 11 years. *J Am Diet Assoc.* 104:660–677, 2004.

24. Goldberg, J. P., M. A. Belury, P. Elam, S. C. Finn, D. Hayes, R. Lyle et al. The obesity crisis: don't blame it on the pyramid. *J Am Diet Assoc.* 104:1141–1147, 2004.

25. Kinney, J. M. Challenges to rebuilding the US food pyramid. *Curr Opin Clin Nutr Metabol Care.* 8:1–7, 2005.

26. Foote, J. A., S. P. Murphy, L. R. Wilkens, P. P. Basiotis, and A. Carlson. Dietary variety increases the probability of nutrient adequacy among adults. *J Nutr.* 134:1779–1785, 2004.

27. Chen, W., S. C. Chen, H. S. Hsu, and C. Lee. Counseling clinic for pediatric weight reduction: program formulation and follow-up. *J Formos Med Assoc.* 96:59–62, 1997.

28. Brown, R., M. Sothern, R. Suskind, J. Udall, and U. Blecker. Racial differences in the lipid profiles of obese children and adolescents before and after significant weight loss. *Clin Pediatr* (Phila). 39:427–431, 2000.

29. Sothern, M. S., M. Loftin, U. Blecker, and J. N. Udall, Jr. Impact of significant weight loss on maximal oxygen uptake in obese children and adolescents. *J Investig Med.* 48:411–416, 2000.

30. Sothern, M. S., J. M. Loftin, J. N. Udall, R. M. Suskind, T. L. Ewing, S. C. Tang, and U. Blecker. Safety, feasibility, and efficacy of a resistance training program in preadolescent obese children. *Am J Med Sci.* 319:370–375, 2000.

31. Sothern, M. S., B. Despinasse, R. Brown, R. M. Suskind, J. N. Udall, Jr., and U. Blecker. Lipid profiles of obese children and adolescents before and after significant weight loss: differences according to sex. *South Med J.* 93:278–282, 2000.

32. Sothern, M. S., H. Schumacher, T. K. von Almen, L. K. Carlisle, and J. N. Udall. Committed to kids: an integrated, 4-level team approach to weight management in adolescents. *J Am Diet Assoc.* 102:S81–S85, 2002.

33. Sothern, M., J. Udall, R. Suskind, A. Vargas, and U. Blecker. Weight loss and growth velocity in obese children after very low calorie diet, exercise and behavior modification. *Acta Paediatrica.* 89:1036–1043, 2000.

34. Epstein, L., Woodall, K., Goreczny, A. et al. The modification of activity patterns and energy expenditure in obese young girls. *Behav Ther.* 15:101–108, 1984.

35. Epstein, L. H., R. R. Wing, B. C. Penner, and M. J. Kress. Effect of diet and controlled exercise on weight loss in obese children. *J Pediatr.* 107:358–361, 1985.

36. Sothern, M. S. Obesity prevention in children: physical activity and nutrition. *Nutrition.* 20:704–708, 2004.

37. Sothern, M. S. and S. T. Gordon. Prevention of obesity in young children: a critical challenge for medical professionals. *Clin Pediatr* (Phila). 42:101–111, 2003.

38. Bautista-Castano, I., J. Doreste, and L. Serra-Majem. Effectiveness of interventions in the prevention of childhood obesity. *Eur J Epidemiol.* 19:617–622, 2004.

39. Campbell, K., E. Waters, S. O'Meara, S. Kelly, and C. Summerbell. Interventions for preventing obesity in children. *Cochrane Database Syst Rev.* CD001871, 2002.

40. Bouchard, C. Can obesity be prevented? *Nutr Rev.* 54:S125–S130, 1996.

41. Kranz, S., D. C. Mitchell, A. M. Siega-Riz, and H. Smiciklas-Wright. Dietary fiber intake by American preschoolers is associated with more nutrient-dense diets. *J Am Diet Assoc.* 105:221–225, 2005.

42. Frary, C. D., R. K. Johnson, and M. Q. Wang. Children and adolescents' choices of foods and beverages high in added sugars are associated with intakes of key nutrients and food groups. *J Adolesc Health.* 34:56–63, 2004.

43. Gill, T. P. Key issues in the prevention of obesity. *Br Med Bull.* 53:359–388, 1997.

44. Davis, K. and K. K. Christoffel. Obesity in preschool and school-age children. Treatment early and often may be best. *Arch Pediatr Adolesc Med.* 148:1257–1261, 1994.

45. Birch, L. Development of food acceptance patterns. *Dev Psychol.* 26:515–519, 1990.

46. Schonfeld-Warden, N. and C. H. Warden. Pediatric obesity. An overview of etiology and treatment. *Pediatr Clin North Am.* 44:339–361, 1997.

47. Passehl, B., C. McCarroll, J. Buechner, C. Gearring, A. E. Smith, and F. Trowbridge. Preventing childhood obesity: establishing healthy lifestyle habits in the preschool years. *J Pediatr Health Care.* 18:315–319, 2004.

48. Krebs, N., R. Baker, F. Greer, M. Heyman, T. Jaksic, F. Lifshitz et al. American Academy of Pediatrics, Committee on Nutrition. Prevention of pediatric overweight and obesity. *Pediatrics.* 112:424–430, 2003.

49. Ogden, C. L., K. M. Flegal, M. D. Carroll, and C. L. Johnson. Prevalence and trends in overweight among US children and adolescents, 1999-2000. *JAMA.* 288:1728–1732, 2002.

50. Epstein, L. H., A. Valoski, R. R. Wing, and J. McCurley. Ten-year outcomes of behavioral family-based treatment for childhood obesity. *Health Psychol.* 13:373–383, 1994.

51. Schwimmer, J. B. Managing overweight in older children and adolescents. *Pediatr Ann.* 33:39–44, 2004.

52. Epstein, L. H., S. J. McKenzie, A. Valoski, K. R. Klein, and R. R. Wing. Effects of mastery criteria and contingent reinforcement for family-based child weight control. *Addict Behav.* 19:135–145, 1994.

53. Epstein, L. H., R. Koeske, R. R. Wing, and A. Valoski. The effect of family variables on child weight change. *Health Psychol.* 5:1–11, 1986.

54. Epstein, L. H., A. Valoski, R. Koeske, and R. R. Wing. Family-based behavioral weight control in obese young children. *J Am Diet Assoc.* 86:481–484, 1986.

55. Flodmark, C. E., T. Ohlsson, O. Ryden, and T. Sveger. Prevention of progression to severe obesity in a group of obese schoolchildren treated with family therapy. *Pediatrics.* 91:880–884, 1993.

56. Eliakim, A., G. Kaven, I. Berger, O. Friedland, B. Wolach, and D. Nemet. The effect of a combined intervention on body mass index and fitness in obese children and adolescents — a clinical experience. *Eur J Pediatr.* 161:449–454, 2002.

57. Sothern, M. S. Exercise as a modality in the treatment of childhood obesity. *Pediatr Clin North Am.* 48:995–1015, 2001.

58. Kiess, W., A. Galler, A. Reich, G. Muller, T. Kapellen, J. Deutscher et al. Clinical aspects of obesity in childhood and adolescence. *Obes Rev.* 2:29–36, 2001.

59. Yanovski, J. A. and S. Z. Yanovski. Treatment of pediatric and adolescent obesity. *JAMA.* 289:1851–1853, 2003.

60. Eisenberg, M. E., D. Neumark-Sztainer, and M. Story. Associations of weight-based teasing and emotional well-being among adolescents. *Arch Pediatr Adolesc Med.* 157:733–738, 2003.

61. Schwimmer, J. B., T. M. Burwinkle, and J. W. Varni. Health-related quality of life of severely obese children and adolescents. *JAMA.* 289:1813–1819, 2003.

62. Erermis, S., N. Cetin, M. Tamar, N. Bukusoglu, F. Akdeniz, and D. Goksen. Is obesity a risk factor for psychopathology among adolescents? *Pediatr Int.* 46:296–301, 2004.

63. Bray, G. A. and B. M. Popkin. Dietary fat intake does affect obesity! *Am J Clin Nutr.* 68:1157–1173, 1998.

64. Putnam, J., Allshouse, JA. *Food Consumption, Prices, and Expenditures, 1970–97.* Washington, DC: U.S. Department of Agriculture, 1999.

65. Ludwig, D. S. The glycemic index: physiological mechanisms relating to obesity, diabetes, and cardiovascular disease. *JAMA.* 287:2414–2423, 2002.

66. Jenkins, D. J., T. M. Wolever, R. H. Taylor, H. Barker, H. Fielden, J. M. Baldwin et al. Glycemic index of foods: a physiological basis for carbohydrate exchange. *Am J Clin Nutr.* 34:362–366, 1981.

67. Liu, S. *Dietary Glycemic Load, Carbohydrate and Whole Grain Intakes in Relation to Risk of Coronary Heart Disease.* Boston: Harvard University, 1998, pp. 1–121.

68. Spieth, L. E., J. D. Harnish, C. M. Lenders, L. B. Raezer, M. A. Pereira, S. J. Hangen, and D. S. Ludwig. A low glycemic index diet in the treatment of pediatric obesity. *Arch Pediatr Adolesc Med,* 154:947–951, 2000.

69. Roberts, S. B. High-glycemic index foods, hunger, and obesity: is there a connection? *Nutr Rev.* 58:163–169, 2000.

70. Ludwig, D. S. Dietary glycemic index and obesity. *J Nutr.* 130:280S–283S, 2000.

71. Ebbeling, C. B. and D. S. Ludwig. Treating obesity in youth: should dietary glycemic load be a consideration? *Adv Pediatr.* 48:179–212, 2001.

72. Krotkiewski, M. Effect of guar gum on body-weight, hunger ratings and metabolism in obese subjects. *Br J Nutr.* 52:97–105, 1984.

73. Rigaud, D., F. Paycha, A. Meulemans, M. Merrouche, and M. Mignon. Effect of psyllium on gastric emptying, hunger feeling and food intake in normal volunteers: a double blind study. *Eur J Clin Nutr.* 52:239–245, 1998.

74. Delargy, H. J., V. J. Burley, K. R. O'Sullivan, R. J. Fletcher, and J. E. Blundell. Effects of different soluble: insoluble fibre ratios at breakfast on 24-h pattern of dietary intake and satiety. *Eur J Clin Nutr.* 49:754–766, 1995.

75. Parks, E. J. and M. K. Hellerstein. Carbohydrate-induced hypertriacylglycerolemia: historical perspective and review of biological mechanisms. *Am J Clin Nutr.* 71:412–433, 2000.

76. Reaven, G. M. Do high carbohydrate diets prevent the development or attenuate the manifestations (or both) of syndrome X? A viewpoint strongly against. *Curr Opin Lipidol.* 8:23–27, 1997.

77. Yu-Poth, S., G. Zhao, T. Etherton, M. Naglak, S. Jonnalagadda, and P. M. Kris-Etherton. Effects of the National Cholesterol Education Program's Step I and Step II dietary intervention programs on cardiovascular disease risk factors: a meta-analysis. *Am J Clin Nutr.* 69:632–646, 1999.

78. Program, U.S. Department of Health and Human Services, *Report of the Expert Panel on Detection, Evaluation and Treatment of High Blood Cholesterol in Adults (ATP II).* Washington, DC: U.S. Department of Health and Human Services, 1993.

79. Lamarche, B., A. Tchernof, P. Mauriege, B. Cantin, G. R. Dagenais, P. J. Lupien, and J. P. Despres. Fasting insulin and apolipoprotein B levels and low-density lipoprotein particle size as risk factors for ischemic heart disease. *JAMA.* 279:1955–1961, 1998.

80. Wolever, T. M., D. J. Jenkins, V. Vuksan, A. L. Jenkins, G. S. Wong, and R. G. Josse. Beneficial effect of low-glycemic index diet in overweight NIDDM subjects. *Diabetes Care.* 15:562–564, 1992.

81. Miller, J. C. Importance of glycemic index in diabetes. *Am J Clin Nutr.* 59:747S–752S, 1994.

82. Jenkins, D. J., T. M. Wolever, G. Buckley et al. Low-glycemic-index starchy foods in the diabetic diet. *Am J Clin Nutr.* 48:248–254, 1988.

83. Jenkins, D. J., T. M. Wolever, G. R. Collier, A. Ocana, A. V. Rao, G. Buckley, Y et al. Metabolic effects of a low-glycemic-index diet. *Am J Clin Nutr.* 46:968–975, 1987.

84. Liljeberg, H. G., A. K. Akerberg, and I. M. Bjorck. Effect of the glycemic index and content of indigestible carbohydrates of cereal-based breakfast meals on glucose tolerance at lunch in healthy subjects. *Am J Clin Nutr.* 69:647–655, 1999.

85. Jenkins, D. J., T. M. Wolever, R. H. Taylor, C. Griffiths, K. Krzeminska, J. A. Lawrie et al. Slow release dietary carbohydrate improves second meal tolerance. *Am J Clin Nutr.* 35:1339–1346, 1982.

86. Jenkins, D. J., T. M. Wolever, R. Nineham, D. L. Sarson, S. R. Bloom, J. Ahern et al. Improved glucose tolerance four hours after taking guar with glucose. *Diabetologia.* 19:21–24, 1980.

87. Wolever, T. M., D. J. Jenkins, A. M. Ocana, V. A. Rao, and G. R. Collier. Second-meal effect: low-glycemic-index foods eaten at dinner improve subsequent breakfast glycemic response. *Am J Clin Nutr.* 48:1041–1047, 1988.

88. Salmeron, J., A. Ascherio, E. B. Rimm, G. A. Colditz, D. Spiegelman, D. J. Jenkins et al. Dietary fiber, glycemic load, and risk of NIDDM in men. *Diabetes Care.* 20:545–550, 1997.

89. Salmeron, J., J. E. Manson, M. J. Stampfer, G. A. Colditz, A. L. Wing, and W. C. Willett. Dietary fiber, glycemic load, and risk of non-insulin-dependent diabetes mellitus in women. *JAMA.* 277:472–477, 1997.

90. Frost, G., J. Wilding, and J. Beecham. Dietary advice based on the glycaemic index improves dietary profile and metabolic control in type 2 diabetic patients. *Diabet Med.* 11:397–401, 1994.

91. Gilbertson, H. R., J. C. Brand-Miller, A. W. Thorburn, S. Evans, P. Chondros, and G. A. Werther. The effect of flexible low glycemic index dietary advice versus measured carbohydrate exchange diets on glycemic control in children with type 1 diabetes. *Diabetes Care.* 24:1137–1143, 2001.

92. Ebbeling, C. B. and D L. Ludwig. Dietary approaches for obesity treatment and prevention in children and adolescents. In: M. Goran MI and V. L. Sothern. Eds. *Handbook of Pediatric Obesity: Epidemiology, Etiology and Prevention.* New York: Taylor & Francis, 2006.

93. Sondike, S. B., N. Copperman, and M. S. Jacobson. Effects of a low-carbohydrate diet on weight loss and cardiovascular risk factors in overweight adolescents. *J Pediatr.* 142:253–258, 2003.

94. Sothern, M., C. VanVrancken, H. Schumacher, L. Carlisle, S. Gordon, J. Reed et al. A controlled comparison of high protein, low carbohydrate diets with different daily calories levels in severely obese children. *Obesity Res.* 9:204S, 2001.

# 12 Nutrition Education

*Heidi Schumacher, Connie VanVrancken-Tompkins, and Melinda S. Sothern*

## CONTENTS

## INTRODUCTION

Nutrition education is the cornerstone of the management of several chronic diseases in children, including diabetes mellitus and hyperlipidemia. However, its application in the clinical management of pediatric obesity is unclear. Moreover, systematic evaluation of the effect of including nutrition education in pediatric obesity prevention and treatment is unavailable.

## NUTRITION EDUCATION AND INDIVIDUAL COUNSELING

Over the last two decades only one study has been published that evaluated individual nutrition education counseling alone. Saelens et al. [1] implemented a weight management program in 44 overweight 12 to 16 year olds that included nutrition education based on the Traffic Light Diet [2]. The subjects participated in an intervention called Healthy Habits, which included use of a computer program designed for normal and overweight adolescents. The computer program provided individualized plans after assessing each subjects' eating, physical activity, and sedentary behavior. Action plans were then printed for each individual that identified strategies for increasing fruit and vegetable intake and decreasing overeating and snacking. The subjects then reviewed the action plan with a pediatrician to discuss and finalize their programs. After this visit, the subjects met with the pediatrician to discuss food self-monitoring and the upcoming mail and phone contact obligations. Subjects were counseled weekly by phone for the first 8 weeks and then biweekly for the last three or four calls, for a total of 14 to 16 weeks. Subjects received nutritional and behavioral counseling over the phone in addition to a participant manual designed to help them acquire various behavioral skills for weight control. They were instructed by the food counselors to reduce food quantity while being encouraged to eat healthier. The subjects were also given self-monitoring booklets and encouraged to monitor all food and beverage intake. The foods were then categorized as a green, red, or no-color food similar to the Traffic Light Diet [2]. Green foods included foods with less than 1 gram of fat per serving, with fewer than 150 calories per serving, and that provided a good source of one or more dietary components such as calcium, fiber, or protein. The red foods consisted of foods having 5 g or more of fat per serving. The goal of the diet was to consume 40 green food servings and fewer than 15 red food servings per week. Parents were provided with information sheets that directed them on ways to help promote and encourage their child's behavior changes. At the end of the intervention period, a significant decrease was observed in the subjects' body mass index (BMI) z-score.

## NUTRITION EDUCATION AND GROUP COUNSELING

There has been only one study in the last 20 years that examined nutrition education alone without dietary counseling [3]. Kirschenbaum and Rosenberg [3] recruited overweight children along with one overweight parent for a weight-reduction program. The children ranged in age from 9 to 13 years and were at least 20% overweight relative to norms for height, age, and sex. Parents were at least 10% overweight relative to ideal weights. The program participants were randomly assigned to one of three groups. The first group included a cognitive behavioral program and was comprised of the parent plus the child. The second group included the cognitive behavioral program as well but consisted of the child only. The third group was a waiting list control group in which the children agreed to participate in the assessments with the guarantee that they would be placed in the next treatment program. The cognitive behavioral sessions consisted of nine weekly, 90-minute sessions at which the subjects were provided detailed written lessons and homework assignments. The homework and lessons consisted of self-monitoring food intake, documenting exercise, stimulus control, self-reward, and decelerated eating. In the parent-plus-child group, both attended these sessions together. In the child-only group, the child was alone at the sessions and was responsible for submitting his or her parent's homework assignments. Significant weight decreases were observed at 3 months in both of the treatment groups, and significant weight increases were observed in the control group.

## NUTRITION EDUCATION IN MULTIDISCIPLINARY SETTINGS

Twenty-nine studies evaluated an intervention of nutrition education in conjunction with dietary counseling, exercise or physical activity, and behavioral counseling. Twenty of these 29 studies were randomized and controlled trials, and all but five studies [2,4–7] provided evidence-based results.

In the Dietary Intervention Study in Children (DISC) study [8] and a study by Obarzanek et al. [9], researchers implemented a diet intervention that was similar to the National Cholesterol Education Program Step 2 diet. Both studies included over six hundred 7 to 9 year olds. The DISC diet consisted of 28% of energy from total fat, less than 8% from saturated fat, up to 9% from polyunsaturated fat, and less than 75 mg/4200 kJ (1000 kcal) per day of cholesterol (not to exceed 150 mg/day). Although overall dietary total fat, saturated fat, and cholesterol decreased significantly in the subjects, there were no significant changes in the subject's BMI at the end of the study.

Epstein et al. implemented the Traffic Light Diet in both children and their families in 11 studies over the course of 16 years [10–18]. The Traffic Light Diet developed by Epstein et al. is a diet that classifies foods in the Food Guide Pyramid according to their fat and sugar contents. The foods are labeled as green, "go," yellow, "caution," and red, "stop." Foods with 0 to 1.9 g fat per serving are categorized as green, 2.0 to 4.9 g fat as yellow, and 5 g fat or more as red. The focus of the diet is to reduce calorie consumption by promoting the green foods and decreasing the intake of the red foods. The energy target ranged from 4200 to 6300 kJ per day and was adjusted according to the subjects weight change. The subjects were provided targets not to exceed a certain number of red foods per week. Typically, students reduced weight status significantly in these studies.

Mellin et al. [19] implemented the SHAPEDOWN program in 66 subjects aged 12 to 18 years. The SHAPEDOWN program consists of a variety of cognitive and behavioral techniques, including a self-directed change format. The program encourages adolescents to make sustainable, small diet modifications, while the parents are instructed on strategies to help facilitate their child's weight loss efforts. At 3 and 15 months, the subjects displayed a significant decrease in relative body weight (actual weight divided by expected weight, multiplied by 100).

Rescinow et al. [20] implemented a nutrition and activity intervention in 11- to 17-year-old inner-city female adolescents biweekly for 4 months, and then weekly for the last 2 months of the program, for a total of 6 months. The goal of the nutrition education was to increase fruit and vegetable intake and decrease fat and fast food intake. The subjects were instructed in satiety awareness, portion control, reading food labels, and healthy grocery shopping. The subjects also participated in hands-on cooking sessions and easy-to-prepare food sessions and were given new foods to taste. Subjects completed food frequency and 24-hour dietary food recall questionnaires and from there developed a list of target foods on which they focused their behavior change efforts. Subjects were asked to complete a take-home assignment involving the nutrition education just learned or involving food or physical activity goals. Although a decrease in total kilocalories was observed in high-attending subjects (attended at least 50% of the sessions), there was no significant difference in body weight or BMI.

Eliakim et al. [21] implemented a dietary–behavioral–exercise intervention in 177 obese youth, ages 6 to 16 years. The primary intervention was for 3 months; however, 65 of the 177 subjects continued in the multidisciplinary program for an additional 3 months, for a total of 6 months. Each subject met with a dietician on a monthly basis to receive various nutrition education (food labels, food preparation, eating habits) in addition to receiving handouts with other diet and nutrition information. Subjects received either a balanced diet that consisted of 1200 to 2000 kcal per day, depending on the individual's age and weight, or a caloric deficit of approximately 30% of the reported intake, or 15% less of the estimated daily required intake. Following both the 3- and 6-month interventions, there was a significant decrease in both weight and BMI.

The purpose of a study by Nuutinen and Knip [22] was to examine the characteristics of successful and unsuccessful weight losers in obese children ages 6 to 15 years. Forty-eight children participated in a 2-year weight reduction program. The children received treatment the first year and were observed for the second. Sixteen received individual counseling, sixteen received group therapy, and the other sixteen were treated in a school heath care setting. The individual treatment consisted of physician check-ups once per month for the first year in addition to five meetings with a nutritionist for dietary counseling. Dietary counseling entailed reducing fat and sugar intake, increasing fruit and vegetable intake, and individual meal plans. The children in the group setting received monthly check-ups as well with the physician for the first year and participated in a group behavior modification session with a psychiatrist seven times in the first year. The nutritionist participated in the group sessions with the psychiatrist every other time. The nutritionist provided similar dietary counseling to the group as the individual dietary counseling. The children who were treated in the school health care setting met with the school nurse once per month for approximately 20 to 40 minutes during the first year. The nurse tried to encourage the child to identify his or her dietary problems and provide a solution for those problems. Only half of the children kept food records, and only a quarter received a meal plan. The school nurse provided a treatment program tailored to what each child felt that he or she could handle. Of the 45 children who completed the study, 21 were found to be successful weight losers (1.5 standard deviation score at 1 year and 1.7 standard deviation score at 2 years). Twenty-four children were unsuccessful weight losers, with a 0.2 standard deviation score decrease after year 1 and a return to baseline at the end of the 2 years. Of the 21 successful weight losers, 11 subjects were in the individual treatment group, 6 were in the group behavior-modification group, and 4 were in the school health care treatment.

The Committed to Kids program uses portion control techniques to reduce calorie intake by limiting the amount of food (portions) consumed by the child. Portion guidelines for each nutrient, which are provided by the American Dietetic Association, are used to reteach the children to normalize food intake over a period of time (Table 12.1). Once a desired calorie level for weight

**TABLE 12.1**
**Nutrition Plan Portion Control Chart**

| Daily Weight Loss, Calorie Level (Approx.)[a] | Carbohydrate Food Units (OK to mix and match) | | | Total (Starch/Fruit/Milk) Daily Carbohydrate Units | Total Daily Meat and Protein-Substitute Units | Total Daily Fat Units | Vegetable Group — Lower-Carbohydrate Units |
|---|---|---|---|---|---|---|---|
| | Starch | Fruit | Milk/Dairy | | | | |
| 1200 | 3-4 | 2 | 3 | 8 | 4–5 | 4 | Unlimited |
| 1500 | 5-6 | 2-3 | 3 | 10 | 6 | 5 | Unlimited |
| 1800 | 7-8 | 2-3 | 3 | 12 | 6 | 6 | Unlimited |
| 2000 | 9 | 2-3 | 3 | 14 | 6–8 | 7 | Unlimited |

[a] Try to include at least 2 to 3 servings of vegetables per day.

*Source:* Sothern et al. *Trim Kids*, New York: Harper Collins, 2001.

**TABLE 12.2**
**Daily Energy Needs and Average Calorie Requirements**

| Age, years | Average Daily Calorie Needs | Average Calories Needed to Reduce Weight |
|---|---|---|
| 7–10 (male and female) | 1600–2200 | 1200–1600 |
| 11–14 (male) | 2200–2800 | 1500–2000 |
| 11–14 (female) | 1600–2400 | 1200–1800 |
| 15–18 (male) | 2400–3400 | 1800–2400 |
| 15–18 (female) | 1800–2400 | 1200–1800 |

*Source:* Sothern et al. *Trim Kids*, New York: Harper Collins, 2001.

management is established, these guidelines can be used to assist with prescribing appropriate nutrient portions (see Appendix A3.6 for full meal plans). The average calories recommended to normalize intake through the use of portion control strategies are listed in Table 12.2. The recommended calorie reductions for children who are already overweight are also provided in Table 12.2.

## NUTRITION EDUCATION AND ALTERNATIVE DIETARY APPROACHES

Two randomized controlled studies [23,24] and seven non-randomized, clinical observational studies [4–6,25–28] evaluated reduced-calorie diets with different nutrient compositions (alternative approaches). In all of the studies, significant reductions were observed in weight status/adiposity from baseline. Spieth et al. [6] examined the effects of a low-glycemic diet in 107 children (mean age about 10 years) attending the Optimal Weight for Life Program. Subjects were instructed on either a low-glycemic diet or a standard reduced-fat diet. The standard reduced-fat diet followed U.S. Department of Agriculture recommendations as depicted by the Food Guide Pyramid. A special emphasis was placed on limiting intake of high-fat, high-sugar, and energy-dense foods and promoting the intake of grain products, vegetables, and fruit. Recommendations were customized for the subject to incorporate an energy restriction of approximately 1042 to 2084 kJ (250 to 500 kcal) per day compared with usual energy intake. Specific macronutrient goals included 55 to 60% carbohydrate, 15 to 20% protein, and 25 to 30% fat. The goal of the low-glycemic diet was to obtain the lowest glycemic response possible while providing adequate dietary carbohydrates and satisfying all nutritional recommendations for children. The researchers employed a "Low-GI Pyramid" modeled after the Food Guide Pyramid. The Low-GI pyramid placed a primary emphasis on vegetables, legumes, and fruits; a secondary emphasis on lean proteins and dairy products; a third on whole-grain products; and limited the refined-grain products, potatoes, and concentrated sugars. The low-glycemic diet recommendations included macronutrient goals of 45 to 50% carbohydrate, 20 to 25% protein, and 30 to 35% fat. The results demonstrated a significant difference in BMI in the low-GI group compared with that of the reduced-fat group. Details of the Optimal Weigh for Life Program are provided in a chapter by Ebbeling and Ludwig [29].

Ebbeling et al. [23] examined the effect of a reduced glycemic-load (GL) diet compared with an energy-restricted, reduced-fat diet in obese adolescents aged 13 to 21 years. Fourteen subjects completed the study, with seven subjects assigned to each diet. The reduced-GL diet emphasized selection of carbohydrate-containing foods that are characterized by a low to moderate glycemic index (GI). The macronutrient goals of this diet included 45 to 50% of energy from carbohydrates, 30 to 35% from fat, and the remaining proportion from protein. The subjects were instructed to consume the carbohydrates along with protein and fat at every meal and snack. The reduced-fat diet emphasized limiting fat intake and increasing the consumption of grains, vegetables, and fruits. Tailored individual meal prescriptions were developed to elicit a negative energy balance of 250 to 500 kcal per day. The macronutrient goals of the reduced-fat diet were 55 to 60% of energy intake from carbohydrates, 25 to 30% from fat, and the remainder from protein. At the end of 12 months, the subjects in the low-GI group displayed a significant decrease in fat mass and BMI compared with the reduced-fat diet subjects.

In the Committed to Kids weight management program, Brown and others [25] demonstrated improvements in the lipid profiles and weight status/adiposity of 53 children, 7 to 17 years of age, after a very low calorie diet, nutrition education, structured exercise, increased physical activity, and behavior modification. In a series of three studies, Sothern and colleagues [5,25,27,30] examined the change in weight status/adiposity in children and adolescents, 7 to 17 years of age, after participation in behavior modification, nutrition education, structured exercise, increased physical activity, and a very low calorie diet or balanced hypocaloric diet (based on initial weight status). The multidisciplinary program included a very low calorie diet that provided 600 to 800 kcal/day and 1.5 to 2.0 gm/kg of ideal body weight in severely obese children (BMI = 34.1 ± 4.8 and greater than 97th percentile BMI). The protein-sparing modified fast (PSMF) restricted carbohydrate intake to 20 to 25 g/day to induce ketosis. The diet was supplemented with additional calorie-free liquids (2 L/day), a multivitamin with minerals, 800 mg/day of calcium, and 25 meq/day KCl. Subjects reduced weight approximately 30% after 10 weeks and maintained the weight loss at 1 year. Resting energy expenditure and lean body mass were maintained, relative $VO_2$ max (but not absolute) was improved, and relative fat (percentage), total cholesterol, and low-density lipoproteins were reduced after 10 weeks. In one study, however, two males and four females exhibited growth velocities below the third percentile for their chronological age. However, the females' heights at the end of the study were normal for the height of an adult North American female. Regardless, in some patients this severe caloric restriction may negatively affect growth velocity even in the presence of exercise and close medical supervision.

Clinical trials conducted in adults using very low calorie diets illustrate that it may be unnecessary to reduce the daily calorie level below 800 kcal/day. Sothern and colleagues conducted clinical outcome trials using an alternative high-protein dietary approach called the Protein Modified Fast (PMF) diet (Table 12.3). The PMF diet is higher in total calories, protein, and carbohydrate than the PSMF diet and is a nonketogenic approach. Subjects receiving the PMF diet plus exercise and behavioral counseling were compared with subjects who were prescribed the traditional PSMF diet plus exercise and behavioral counseling. Both groups had significant reductions in BMI percentile at 10 weeks that were maintained at 1 year. In addition, although the PMF was higher in calories, the change in BMI did not differ significantly between the groups [32]. Although preliminary, these results indicate that it may be unnecessary to reduce calories below 800 kcal/day. Because PSMF may

---

**TABLE 12.3**
**Protein Modified Fast Diet**

800–1000 calories (depending on the protein prescription)
High protein: 2–2.5 g/kg ideal body weight (average 90–140 g/day)
Reduced carbohydrate: 50–75 g/day
Reduced fat: 30–45 g/day
Lean meat and substitutes: 13–20 oz/day
Vegetables (reduced carbohydrate)
Bread/Starch/Fruit/Milk: 2–3 units/day combined (45–50 g carbohydrates)
Free foods such as tea, mustard, bouillon, pickles, spices
Fluid: 64–96 oz minimum per day
Supplements: Daily multivitamin with minerals; elemental calcium: 1200–1400 mg/day; additional potassium
  may be necessary
Duration: 10–20 weeks

*Note:* For full description of the Protein Modified Fast diet, refer to Appendix A3.8.

---

negatively affect growth velocity in some children, PMF may provide a useful alternative in severely obese children. However, this warrants further investigation under randomized, controlled conditions.

The remainder of this chapter provides a sample nutrition education curriculum that can be implemented in a group, family-based, multidisciplinary setting.

## A SAMPLE NUTRITION EDUCATION CURRICULUM IN THE CLINICAL SETTING

Nutrition education centers on identifying high-calorie and low-calorie foods in each food group. Nutrition sessions are conducted in a group with patients, parents, siblings, and extended family and friends in attendance. Patient participation is encouraged during the cooking demonstrations, calorie-counting, and food-measuring activities. During the early lessons of the program, nutrition information is delivered in a simple, knowledge-based format. As the groups progress through the different levels, the activities require more advanced levels of comprehension and problem-solving skills. The long-term goal of education is to enable patients and their families to adequately identify, select, and prepare foods that are appropriate to continued weight maintenance and good health. Sample lesson plans follow.

### DIET INSTRUCTION

Participants will need to have a copy of Table 12.1, Nutrition Plan Portion Control Chart, the Table of Food Portions and Units located in Appendix A3.4, a notepad and a pen, and the program book [31].

First, review what calories are and how they relate to a weight-loss diet: Calories are the energy produced in our body from the foods that we eat. When we eat more food (calories) than our bodies need, the extra calories are stored in our bodies as fat (weight gain). When we eat fewer calories than we need, our bodies will break down fat (weight loss) to get the energy they need. It takes about 3500 extra calories to make 1 pound of body fat. For example, if you eat 500 calories per day fewer than what your body needs, you will lose one pound of body fat per week. You can also burn off extra calories by increasing your activity. For example, if you eat 500 fewer calories per day than what you need and you burn an additional 250 calories per day by exercising, you will lose about 1.5 pounds of body fat per week.

Second, review where calories in foods come from: There are three major kinds of nutrients in food that give us calories: carbohydrate, protein, and fat. Protein helps to build and maintain your muscle tissue. Carbohydrate helps to give us energy. Small amounts of fat are necessary to maintain certain body functions. Carbohydrate and protein produce 4 calories per gram. Fat produces 9 calories per gram. Because the same amount of fat has more than twice the calories as carbohydrate or protein, choosing foods that are low in fat will help reduce the amount of calories you consume. Because carbohydrate and protein still produce calories, eating too much of even low-fat foods can give you too many calories. Choosing low-fat foods and watching portion sizes should be used as part of a weight-loss diet.

Third, review the rationale of the food unit system: Foods can be grouped into food groups or food units based on their nutrient content. There are six basic food units: meat and meat substitutes, vegetables, starches and breads, fruit, milk and dairy, and fat groups. You will be allowed a certain number of servings or "units" from each food group to meet your calorie requirements (see Appendix A3.4).

Fourth, review Table 12.1, the Nutrition Plan Portion Control Chart. Next, review Table 12.2, Daily Energy Needs and Average Calorie Requirements. Last, review the Table of Food Portions and Units in Appendix A3.4.

## FOOD LABS: THE MEAT AND PROTEIN GROUP

The instructor will need the following items for this lesson: food scale; cooked meat, fish, and poultry (e.g., large steak, chicken breast, filet of fish); tuna (canned in water); mayonnaise (regular); packaged cheese; and the program book [31].

First, review the specific meat and substitute group and fat grams. Second, have participants volunteer to weigh and measure items. Calculate the calories and fat grams and weigh meats to demonstrate portion sizes. Have group guess the weights before weighing. After weighing the meat, calculate the calories and fat grams based on exchange values. Emphasize caloric and fat difference. Specifically emphasize caloric density.

Third, measure one cup of tuna and calculate the calories (1/2 cup of water-packed tuna = 100 calories and 4 g fat). Add 1 tablespoon of mayonnaise (1 tablespoon of mayonnaise = 100 calories and 11 g fat) at a time, calculating the calories and fat grams until the tuna salad is made. Emphasize caloric difference between plain tuna and tuna salad.

Fourth, weigh the cheese. Have the group estimate the caloric and fat gram value before weighing. Emphasize the caloric density of cheese.

## COOKING DEMONSTRATIONS: FUN IN THE KITCHEN — LOW-CALORIE PIZZA

The instructor will need the following items for this lesson: baking sheet, nonstick cooking spray, "lite" bread, tomato sauce, Italian seasoning, low-fat mozzarella cheese, vegetable toppings (sliced tomatoes, mushrooms, bell peppers, onions, artichokes, etc.), oven/broiler, and program book [31].

First, in a group setting, have participants help prepare low-calorie pizza (see Appendix A3.6.1 for full recipe). Second, review ingredients during preparation, including "lite" bread calories (one-half the calories of regular bread), tomato sauce, low-fat cheese, and vegetable toppings. Third, review the low-fat cheese label; compare with regular cheese. Emphasize the importance of measuring cheese — have participants measure and review one-quarter cup volume. Fourth, review and emphasize the low-calorie vegetable topping options. Fifth, review and emphasize the use of nonstick cooking spray versus oil. Finally, review the importance of serving appropriate portion sizes as you serve the participants.

## NUTRITION GAMES: SNACK-FOOD JEOPARDY

The instructor will need the following materials for this lesson: assorted snack samples (Table 12.4) and small incentive prizes for participants, such as stickers, pencils, balls, coloring books [31], and so on.

**TABLE 12.4**
**Snack-Food Jeopardy Instructor List**

| Item | Calories | Fat, grams |
|---|---|---|
| Raisins | 60 | 0 |
| Cake (medium slice) | 600 | 30 |
| Nachos and cheese (medium serving) | 800 | 40 |
| Fresh fruit (1 medium) | 60 | 0 |
| Low-fat, sugar-free yogurt (4 oz) | 40 | 0 |
| Candy bar, jumbo | a | a |
| Potato chips (3 oz) | 450 | 30 |
| Graham crackers (3 squares) | 80 | 0 |
| Hot cocoa, sugar-free (1 packet) | 50 | 0 |
| Life Savers™ (1 packet) | 120 | 0 |
| Popcorn, air-popped (6 cups) | 140 | 0 |
| Peanuts (1 cup) | 930 | 35 |
| Carrot or celery sticks (3 cups) | 40 | 0 |

a Check calories and fat grams on the package label.

Instruct the participants to gather around the table. Place various snack foods on the table with small cards (placed face down) indicating the calorie and fat grams contained in each. Call out a calorie or fat value and ask participants to identify the snack that contains those values. Turn the card over and compare answers. Provide a small incentive prize to the participant who first correctly identifies the correct snack. You may also want to include sugar grams when you call out a value. Refer to package labeling or the program book [31] for the specific sugar grams contained in each snack.

## CLASS DISCUSSION: CALCIUM: THE BONE-BUILDER

The participants will need the hand-out "Calcium: The Bone-Builder," located in Appendix A3.7, and the program book [31].

First, review and discuss the importance of adequate calcium intake. Children should consume 800 to 1200 mg calcium per day, depending on age. Adult women should consume 800 to 1000 mg calcium per day, and those at higher risk should consume 1000 to 1500 mg per day.

Second, review calcium content of various foods and daily requirements (Table 12.5). Although a number of foods contain calcium, dairy products are the chief source of calcium in the diet. Recommended daily intake of the milk/dairy group is two to four servings per day to meet the minimum calcium requirements.

Third, discuss the risk of developing bone disorders such as osteoporosis. Osteoporosis is a gradual loss of structural minerals or decalcification of bones that begins at adulthood and progresses with increasing age. It is a crippling bone disease that affects one of every four Caucasian women over the age of 65 years. Women at highest risk for developing osteoporiosis include Caucasian and Asian women; small-framed, thin women; women who do not exercise; women who do not drink milk; chronic dieters; postmenopausal women; and smokers. Inadequate calcium intake is a major contributing factor to osteoporosis, because a low calcium intake accelerates bone loss.

**TABLE 12.5**
**Calcium Content of Common Foods**

| Milk and Dairy Products | (milligrams of calcium) |
|---|---|
| Low-fat or skim milk, 1 cup | 300 |
| Low-fat yogurt (plain), 1 cup | 415 |
| Low-fat yogurt (fruit-flavored), 1 cup | 345 |
| American cheese, 1 oz | 174 |
| Swiss cheese, 1 oz | 272 |
| Cheddar cheese, 1 oz | 204 |
| Mozzarella cheese, 1 oz | 207 |
| Cottage cheese, 1 cup | 145 |
| Ice milk, 1/2 cup | 88 |
| Sherbet, 1/2 cup | 52 |
| Pudding, 1/2 cup | 133 |
| Custard, 1/2 cup | 149 |

| Other Sources | (milligrams of calcium) |
|---|---|
| Beans, 1 cup | 90 |
| Broccoli, 1/2 cup | 47 |
| Cheese pizza, 1 slice | 220 |
| Collard greens, 1/2 cup | 179 |
| Macaroni and cheese, 1/2 cup | 181 |
| Salmon (with bones), 3 oz | 167 |
| Sardines (with bones) 3 oz | 371 |
| Shrimp, 3 oz | 98 |
| Soups made with milk, 1 cup | 165 |

## SUMMARY

Typically, children begin gaining unnecessary weight between the ages of 3 and 7 years. By then, they are spending a good deal of time sitting behind a desk at school. After school, they might play video or computer games or watch several hours of television. Meanwhile, they may be eating fast food three to six times per week (the national average). Once they become overweight, other children may tease them relentlessly, and they may turn to food for comfort, which causes more weight gain. Pediatric health care providers can help parents to stop the vicious cycle on all fronts by guiding the children to make changes in the home environment that will promote healthy eating. In fact, the family environment has the greatest effect of all on children's weight gain. The flip side of this fact is that the family environment also has the greatest effect on the child's ability to achieve a healthy weight and build a lifetime of healthy habits — but it doesn't happen overnight. Change must come gradually for parents to experience success. Establishing just one nutrition goal per pediatric office visit can go a long way to creating a nutritious, physically active home environment (Table 12.6). Providing brief information on strategies to help achieve these goals takes only a few minutes. The rewards to the patient's health far exceed the extra time and attention.

## TABLE 12.6
## Nutrition Education: Goals and Strategies for Parents

| Nutrition Goals | Strategies |
|---|---|
| Replace unhealthy snacks with fruits, vegetables, and other healthy offerings. | 1. Allow infrequent consumption of nonnutritious foods away from the home.<br>2. Keep within reach nutritious foods naturally low in saturated fat and sugar and high in fiber.<br>3. Gradually reduce fast food consumption to less than one time per week.<br>4. Take children along when shopping.<br>5. Have them select one fruit and one vegetable to try for the week and skip the candy, cookie, and soft drink aisle.<br>6. Purchase bottled water instead of soda, which is high in sugar.<br>7. Give your children water when they are thirsty, not high-sugar beverages. |
| Decrease eating in front of the TV/computer. | 1. Establish family dinners on the weekend.<br>2. Include children in meal preparation.<br>3. Use the china and make it special.<br>4. Gradually include weekdays.<br>5. Eventually restrict all eating and drinking (except water) to the kitchen counter, table, or dining room.<br>6. Serve children an appropriate portion size (usually about 1/2 cup) of each food prepared. Children will eat more if you serve them more.<br>7. Encourage at least three bites of each food on the plate.<br>8. Grade the foods, A, B, C, or F. High-scoring veggies are served again and often. |
| Promote regular consumption of healthy breakfasts. | 1. Discourage snacking after dinner. (If children are not hungry when they awake, they may be eating too late at night.)<br>2. Plan breakfast the night before and make it attractive.<br>3. Select high-fiber cereals, breads, and other baked goods.<br>4. Serve reduced-fat turkey bacon, turkey sausage, or veggie substitutes<br>5. Try a low-fat cheese omelet made with scrambled egg substitute.<br>6. Serve low-fat milk rather than fruit drinks.<br>7. Serve fruits instead of concentrated juice.<br>8. Try a fruit juice "spritzer": 3 oz fruit juice mixed with 5 oz club soda or sparkling water. |
| Establish a healthy relationship with food. | 1. Help your child to understand that there are no "bad" or "good" foods.<br>2. Encourage your child to select more of the healthy variety, and NEVER give food as a reward.<br>3. Teach children that it is okay to leave food on their plate. This teaches them to self-regulate and not to overeat.<br>4. Stop the nagging. Do not draw attention to negative behaviors.<br>5. Rather, spend your energy praising your child when she chooses healthy foods or physical activity.<br>6. When your child selects an unhealthy snack or heads for the television, try to redirect and give choices: "Do you want strawberries, carrots, or melon for your snack?" He can't choose what is not offered. |

*Source:* Sothern et al. *Trim Kids*, New York: Harper Collins, 2001.

## REFERENCES

1. Saelens, B. E., J. F. Sallis, D. E. Wilfley, K. Patrick, J. A. Cella, and R. Buchta. Behavioral weight control for overweight adolescents initiated in primary care. *Obes Res.* 10:22–32, 2002.
2. Epstein, L. H., R. R. Wing, and A. Valoski. Childhood obesity. *Pediatr Clin North Am.* 32:363–379, 1985.
3. Kirschenbaum, H. L. and J. M. Rosenberg. Educational programs offered by colleges of pharmacy and drug information centers within the United States. *Am J Pharm Educ.* 48:155–157, 1984.
4. Sothern, M. S., S. Hunter, R. M. Suskind, R. Brown, J. N. Udall, Jr., and U. Blecker. Motivating the obese child to move: the role of structured exercise in pediatric weight management. *South Med J.* 92:577–584, 1999.
5. Sothern, M. S., H. Schumacher, T. K. von Almen, L. K. Carlisle, and J. N. Udall. Committed to kids: an integrated, 4-level team approach to weight management in adolescents. *J Am Diet Assoc.* 102:S81–S85, 2002.
6. Spieth, L. E., J. D. Harnish, C. M. Lenders, L. B. Raezer, M. A. Pereira, S. J. Hangen, and D. S. Ludwig. A low-glycemic index diet in the treatment of pediatric obesity. *Arch Pediatr Adolesc Med.* 154:947–951, 2000.
7. Schwingshandl, J., K. Sudi, B. Eibl, S. Wallner, and M. Borkenstein. Effect of an individualised training programme during weight reduction on body composition: a randomised trial. *Arch Dis Child.* 81:426–428, 1999.
8. The Writing Group for the DISC Collaborative Research Group. Efficacy and safety of lowering dietary intake of fat and cholesterol in children with elevated low-density lipoprotein cholesterol: The Dietary Intervention Study in Children (DISC). *JAMA.* 273:1429–1435, 1995.
9. Obarzanek, E., S. Y. Kimm, B. A. Barton, L. L. Van Horn, P. O. Kwiterovich, Jr., D. G. Simons-Morton et al. Long-term safety and efficacy of a cholesterol-lowering diet in children with elevated low-density lipoprotein cholesterol: seven-year results of the Dietary Intervention Study in Children (DISC). *Pediatrics.* 107:256–264, 2001.
10. Epstein, L., Woodall, K., Goreczny, A. et al. The modification of activity patterns and energy expenditure in obese young girls. *Behav Ther.* 15:101–108, 1984.
11. Epstein, L. H., R. R. Wing, B. C. Penner, and M. J. Kress. Effect of diet and controlled exercise on weight loss in obese children. *J Pediatr.* 107:358–361, 1985.
12. Epstein, L. H. Methodological issues and ten-year outcomes for obese children. *Ann N Y Acad Sci.* 699:237–249, 1993.
13. Epstein, L. H., S. J. McKenzie, A. Valoski, K. R. Klein, and R. R. Wing. Effects of mastery criteria and contingent reinforcement for family-based child weight control. *Addict Behav.* 19:135–145, 1994.
14. Epstein, L. H., A. Valoski, R. Koeske, and R. R. Wing. Family-based behavioral weight control in obese young children. *J Am Diet Assoc.* 86:481–484, 1986.
15. Epstein, L. H., A. Valoski, and J. McCurley. Effect of weight loss by obese children on long-term growth. *Am J Dis Child.* 147:1076–1080, 1993.
16. Epstein, L. H., A. Valoski, R. R. Wing, and J. McCurley. Ten-year follow-up of behavioral, family-based treatment for obese children. *JAMA.* 264:2519–2523, 1990.
17. Epstein, L. H., A. Valoski, R. R. Wing, and J. McCurley. Ten-year outcomes of behavioral family-based treatment for childhood obesity. *Health Psychol.* 13:373–383, 1994.
18. Epstein, L. H., R. R. Wing, R. Koeske, and A. Valoski. Effect of parent weight on weight loss in obese children. *J Consult Clin Psychol.* 54:400–401, 1986.
19. Mellin, L. M., L. A. Slinkard, and C. E. Irwin, Jr. Adolescent obesity intervention: validation of the SHAPEDOWN program. *J Am Diet Assoc.* 87:333–338, 1987.
20. Resnicow, K., A. L. Yaroch, A. Davis, D. T. Wang, S. Carter, L. Slaughter et al. GO GIRLS! Results from a nutrition and physical activity program for low-income, overweight African American adolescent females. *Health Educ Behav.* 27:616–631, 2000.
21. Eliakim, A., G. Kaven, I. Berger, O. Friedland, B. Wolach, and D. Nemet. The effect of a combined intervention on body mass index and fitness in obese children and adolescents — a clinical experience. *Eur J Pediatr.* 161:449–454, 2002.
22. Nuutinen, O. and M. Knip. Predictors of weight reduction in obese children. *Eur J Clin Nutr.* 46:785–794, 1992.

23. Ebbeling, C. B., M. M. Leidig, K. B. Sinclair, J. P. Hangen, and D. S. Ludwig. A reduced-glycemic load diet in the treatment of adolescent obesity. *Arch Pediatr Adolesc Med.* 157:773–779, 2003.

24. Sondike, S. B., N. Copperman, and M. S. Jacobson. Effects of a low-carbohydrate diet on weight loss and cardiovascular risk factor in overweight adolescents. *J Pediatr.* 142:253–258, 2003.

25. Brown, R., M. Sothern, R. Suskind, J. Udall, and U. Blecker. Racial differences in the lipid profiles of obese children and adolescents before and after significant weight loss. *Clin Pediatr* (Phila). 39:427–431, 2000.

26. Sothern, M. S., B. Despinasse, R. Brown, R. M. Suskind, J. N. Udall, Jr., and U. Blecker. Lipid profiles of obese children and adolescents before and after significant weight loss: differences according to sex. *South Med J.* 93:278–282, 2000.

27. Sothern, M., J. Udall, R. Suskind, A. Vargas, and U. Blecker. Weight loss and growth velocity in obese children after very low calorie diet, exercise and behavior modification. *Acta Paediat.* 89:1036–1043, 2000.

28. Sothern, M. S., J. M. Loftin, J. N. Udall, R. M. Suskind, T. L. Ewing, S. C. Tang, and U. Blecker. Safety, feasibility, and efficacy of a resistance training program in preadolescent obese children. *Am J Med Sci.* 319:370–375, 2000.

29. Ebbeling, C. B. and D. L. Ludwig. Dietary approaches for obesity treatment and prevention in children and adolescents. In: M. Goran and M.I Sothern. Ed. *Handbook of Pediatric Obesity: Epidemiology, Etiology and Prevention.* Boca Raton, FL: Taylor & Francis, 2006.

30. Sothern, M. S., M. Loftin, U. Blecker, and J. N. Udall, Jr. Impact of significant weight loss on maximal oxygen uptake in obese children and adolescents. *J Investig Med.* 48:411–416, 2000.

31. Sothern, M., T. K. Von Almen, and H. Schumacher. *Trim Kids: The Proven Plan That Has Helped Thousands of Children Achieve a Healthier Weight.* New York: Harper Collins Publishers, 2001.

32. Sothern, M., C. vanVrancken, H. Schumacher, L. Carlisle, S. Gordon, J. Reed et al. A controlled comparison of high protein, low carbohydrate diets with different daily calorie levels in severely obese children. *Obes Res.* 9:204S, 2001.

# Section 6

---

*Behavioral Counseling*

# 13 Behavioral Counseling: Family-Based Behavioral Counseling in Clinical Settings

*Valerie H. Myers and Pamela Davis Martin*

## CONTENTS

Childhood obesity is a worldwide health concern of epidemic proportions. The prevalence of obesity in children and adolescents has risen over the last 20 years among all ethnicities, ages, and genders [1–3]. According to the U.S. Surgeon General, 13% of children aged 6 to 11 years and 14% of adolescents aged 12 to 19 years in the United States are overweight. Overweight adolescents have a 70% chance of becoming overweight or obese adults. This risk increases to 80% if one or more parents are overweight or obese.

There are a significant number of medical sequelae and risk factors associated with pediatric obesity, many of which are commonly believed to occur only in the adult population. Specifically, hypertension, hypercholesterolemia, type II diabetes, glucose intolerance, some forms of cancer, musculoskeletal injuries [4], premature pubarche [5,6], and future cardiovascular disease [7] are associated with childhood obesity. Research indicates that the psychosocial consequences of over-weight/obesity among children and adolescents are serious and highly prevalent [2]. Obese children may experience higher levels of depression and lower self-esteem [2,8]. In addition, overweight and obese children can be targets of social discrimination by peers, family members, and teachers [9,10].

Research suggests that familial factors impact the development of childhood obesity. However, it is unclear the impact that environment and genetics play on these familial factors [11]. Estimates suggest that only 7% of children will become obese when born to parents of normal weight [12,13]. However, if one parent is obese, the risk of childhood obesity increases to 40%, and the lifetime risk factor for developing obesity doubles; to 80% for that child if both parents are obese [12,13]. Behavior is influenced by numerous factors, making behavior change a complex process. Healthy dietary intake and physical activity are important aspects in reducing obesity in children and adolescents and are both behavioral and modifiable in nature [2]. Family behavioral counseling and parent training sessions are effective methods for preventing and treating childhood obesity [14–19] and are considered a vital component of the majority of published studies that show efficacious results. There are several types of effective behavioral treatment strategies in the management of overweight, and many of the family-based behavioral counseling interventions used are based on well-estab-lished theories such as social learning theory, social cognitive theory, and social action theory [20]. In more than 100 controlled studies (mostly adult), behavioral weight loss treatments have dem-onstrated efficacy over placebo, traditional diet, insight therapy, nutritional information, and control groups [21,22]. Weight loss has been shown to be positively correlated with a number of behavioral therapy techniques [23]. The importance of behavior therapy in the pediatric obesity program has also been demonstrated, making this a standard component in clinical treatment programs [24,25].

## BEHAVIORAL TREATMENT TECHNIQUES

The specific behavioral strategies found to be most effective in achieving and maintaining lifestyle change include self-monitoring, stimulus control, problem solving, relapse prevention, contingency management, social support, offering choices, and individualizing feedback. Although published reports support the effectiveness of these various behavioral techniques, none stands by itself as a means to promote weight loss and maintenance. Instead, these techniques tend to be used in combination (e.g., in a multicomponent approach as offered through behavioral group therapy meetings). Behavioral weight management treatment strategies focus primarily on maladaptive eating and exercise patterns that lead to positive energy balance and, eventually, weight gain. Environmental antecedents and the consequences of eating behavior are key components of behav-ioral weight programs. Personal and global antecedents are identified, and then participants are instructed in methods to modify these cues for responding. The positive behavioral consequences of specific eating or activity patterns are also explored because they are likely to increase the frequency of these behaviors. Participants are also instructed in the potential negative consequences of their current patterns of behavior in an attempt to decrease the frequency of these behaviors. The following behavioral treatment strategies have been shown to be efficacious in the treatment of overweight and obesity and are designed to increase awareness of eating and activity patterns, to normalize eating patterns, to reduce exposure to cues for maladaptive eating or activity patterns, and to alter the response to problem situations [26–30].

### GOAL SETTING AND ACTION PLANNING

This is often the initial starting point of behavioral programs. Goal setting and action planning involves setting goals for calories, fat, physical activity, and other modifiable behaviors. Because participants are often unrealistic in their weight loss expectations, realistic expectations for short-term and long-term goals are presented to facilitate behavior change.

## SELF-MONITORING

The self-monitoring technique is considered the "cornerstone" of behavioral treatment and involves daily observation and record keeping of eating and exercise behaviors. Monitoring is used to increase awareness of behavior patterns by identifying antecedents or reinforcing consequences that lead to or strengthen faulty eating and activity patterns. Record keeping can also be expanded to include a variety of information about emotions associated with eating, hunger ratings, time of activities, etc.

## STIMULUS CONTROL AND CUE ELIMINATION

Participants are often unaware of how their environment influences their behavior. Stimulus control techniques are used to identify and then modify environmental antecedents that influence eating or activity patterns. The goal is to restrict environmental circumstances that serve as discriminative stimuli for maladaptive eating or sedentary behavior. Techniques typically include instructions such as a specified number of meals and snacks to eat, specified eating times or places, and changing serving and food storage techniques. These procedures are used to decrease the number of conditioned stimuli or situations that may trigger eating behavior.

## MODIFICATION OF EATING AND ACTIVITY PATTERNS

The goal of these modification techniques is to change faulty eating behaviors that may interfere with satiety or lead to excessive calorie intake, as well as those that lead to sedentary behaviors. Typical techniques include slowing pace of eating, reducing portion sizes, measuring food intake, leaving food on plate, improving food choices, and eliminating second servings. In addition, nutrition education on healthy eating is provided. Sedentary behaviors are also targeted, and efforts are made to incorporate increased activity into the daily routine by taking the stairs, parking farther from the building, walking or biking rather than driving.

## CONTINGENCY MANAGEMENT

Positive reinforcement is used to acquire and stabilize new weight management behaviors. Programs focus typically on positive reinforcing consequences for the development or implementation of behavioral changes such as healthier eating or activity patterns rather than weight loss. Punishment or loss of reinforcement, as well as parent-limiting techniques, may also be used to change eating and activity behaviors. Parents are encouraged to eliminate all food rewards and are encouraged to use other methods of motivating or rewarding their children. Monetary incentives have been used in many treatment programs to improve motivation. Behavioral contracting with a therapist or parent may also be used to gain social reinforcements. Behavioral contracting is helpful because it (1) gets the individual involved and invested in treatment, (2) provides a written outline of expected behaviors that reduces forgetfulness and disagreement on goals, and (3) provides an outline of how rewards are obtained based on the fulfillment of a specified goal.

## SOCIAL REINFORCEMENT AND MODELING

Children learn behaviors through observation of others and subsequent reinforcement and punishment of behavior choices, as well as through experiencing the consequences of their own behaviors. In this technique, parents and children are taught to serve as appropriate models for other family/household members and are encouraged to provide positive attention and praise for healthful eating and exercise behaviors.

## RELAPSE PREVENTION AND PROBLEM SOLVING

This technique involves identifying specific problems or potential problems that are interfering with goals. Once problems are identified, possible solutions are brainstormed, pros/cons of the solutions are evaluated, and then a plan is implemented.

## OVERVIEW OF FAMILY-BASED STUDIES

Two recent evidence-based publications have evaluated individual and family-based studies in the treatment of childhood obesity. A position paper by the American Dietetic Association [15] evaluated 40 individual-based and family-based studies. All studies used a combination of diet, exercise/ physical activity, and behavior modification. Findings indicated that the inclusion of the family in counseling sessions improved both short-term and long-term outcomes. In a recent metaanalysis, McLean and colleagues [19] evaluated 16 weight-loss interventions incorporating a family-based component with at least 1-year follow-up data. The authors concluded that (1) few intervention studies with long-term follow-up data exist, (2) there are few studies targeting adolescents, (3) parental involvement is associated with weight loss in children, and (4) a greater range of behavioral techniques improves weight outcomes.

### LITERATURE REVIEW

The primary aim of this chapter is to review randomized controlled trials using individual and group family-based counseling weight management interventions in clinical settings. Forty-nine studies of children and adolescents were identified as containing either a family-based or individual-based behavioral counseling component. Of these 49 studies, 31 were a randomized controlled design that met the following criteria: (1) study duration of greater than 8 weeks, (2) number of participants greater than 30, and (3) use of behavioral counseling techniques (Table 13.1). Two additional randomized controlled trials did not enroll over 30 participants; however, given the robustness of the findings, they were included for discussion (Table 13.1). Of the 33 trials, 30 studies demonstrating significant results included behavioral counseling as a central component [17,18,31–58]. In addition, 16 studies of "other" design or unspecified randomization were also identified (Table 13.2) [59–74].

### FAMILY-BASED COUNSELING INTERVENTIONS

Clinical interventions for the treatment of childhood obesity often use family-based counseling approaches. Research suggests that a family therapy component (minimum of one parent and child) in most obesity treatment programs results in significant reductions in adiposity in children between the ages of 6 and 12 years. Specifically, in 27 of the 30 randomized controlled studies using family-based approaches, children significantly reduced weight status. All of these findings suggest that family involvement is associated with significant weight loss in preadolescent children. Additional studies with children have included one or more components of diet, exercise, and behavior. However, it was unclear from the intervention descriptions in the methods section whether family-based counseling was implemented.

### GROUP TREATMENT

Group treatment with family-based counseling was identified in 27 randomized, controlled trials [16–18,31–37,39–42,44,47–49,51–56] and 10 studies of other design [58,75,76]. All of the treatment interventions addressed the following weight loss strategies: diet and exercise or increased physical activity/reduced sedentary behaviors. For example, Epstein and colleagues examined the effects of mastery criteria and contingent reinforcement for over 2 years in a family-based behavioral weight control program for obese children and their parents [54]. Families were randomly assigned to one of two group conditions. The experimental group was targeted and reinforced for mastery of diet, weight loss, exercise, and parenting skills. The control group was instructed on behavioral techniques and provided noncontingent reinforcement. Both groups received 6 months of family-based behavioral education in a weekly group format, as well as 6 monthly follow-up meetings. Children in the experimental group compared with the control group demonstrated significantly better relative weight change at 6 months and 1 year; however, effects were not maintained at 2 years.

**TABLE 13.1**
**Randomized Controlled Design Family-Based and Individual Intervention Trials**

| Study (Author/Year/Location) | Study Population | Treatment Duration | Study Design and Components | | Outcome Variables and Findings |
|---|---|---|---|---|---|
| Epstein et al., 1981 [16] Location: Pittsburgh, PA | 76 families, with obese children, ages 6–12 years; 55 families at follow-up | 14 sessions over 8 months, 21-month follow-up | D PA B | Three groups Traffic Light Diet, aerobic exercise, and behavior modification for all groups: parent/child target, child target, or nonspecific target (control) | Weight, height, skinfolds, %overweight: no significant difference among groups in decrease of %overweight. |
| Epstein et al., 1990 [17] Location: Pittsburgh, PA | 55 of 76 families with overweight children enrolled initially in the study (72% retention) | Eight weekly sessions, six monthly sessions, 21 months, 5-, and 10-year follow-up | D PA B | Three groups Traffic Light Diet, exercise (aerobic, stretching, spot reducing), and behavioral reinforcements for all groups: child and parent target, child target, or nonspecific target (control) | Weight, height, %overweight: Children in the child and parent group showed significantly greater decreases in %overweight after 5 (−11.2%) and 10 (−7.5%) years than children in the nonspecific control group (+7.9% and +14.3%, respectively). Children in the child-only group showed increases in %overweight after 5 (+2.7%) and 10 (+4.5%) years. |
| Epstein et al., 1994 [18] Location: Pittsburgh, PA | 185 families with overweight children, ages 8–12 years; final sample was 158 (85%) | 8–12 weekly treatment meetings, 6–12 monthly meetings, 10-year follow-up | D PA B | Reports on four randomized studies that included the treatment groups: child only vs. parent–child study; diet only vs. diet plus lifestyle change exercise; lifestyle vs. aerobic and calisthenics; parental weight status; Traffic Light Diet in all studies | Weight, height, BMI, %overweight: Children in parent–child study decreased %overweight by 15.3% and control by 7.6% at 10 years. Child only vs. parent and child were significantly different ($p < 0.025$) at 5 years. %overweight in diet only (−8.4%) vs. diet plus exercise (−10.0%) were both significantly lower at 10 years but not from each other. %overweight decreased significantly at 10 years in lifestyle-exercise (−19.7%) and aerobic (10.9%) but not calisthenics (+12.2%). Change from 5 to 10 years was significantly different as follows: lifestyle ($p < 0.009$) and aerobic ($p < 0.04$) from calisthenics. |

**TABLE 13.1 (continued)**
**Randomized Controlled Design Family-Based and Individual Intervention Trials**

| Study (Author/Year/Location) | Study Population | Treatment Duration | Study Design and Components | | Outcome Variables and Findings |
|---|---|---|---|---|---|
| Golan et al., 1998 [31] Location: Tel Aviv, Israel | 60 overweight children, ages 6–11 years | 12 months, varies among groups | D PA B | Two groups Intervention: parent-only behavioral sessions, 4 weekly, then 4 biweekly, then 6 every 6 weeks; Control: child-only diet and physical activity instruction sessions 8 weekly, then biweekly sessions for 10 months | Weight, height, %overweight: both groups significantly reduced %overweight at 12 months ($p < 0.001$ parent only and $p < 0.01$ child only). Children in the parent-only group had a significantly greater reduction in %overweight at 12 months (14.6%) than children in the child-only group (8.1%; $p < 0.03$). |
| Graves et al., 1988 [32] Location: Memphis, TN | 40 overweight children, ages 6–12 years | 8 weekly sessions with 6-month follow-up | D PA B | Three groups All groups received Traffic Light Diet, physical activity, and problem-solving instruction. Additional treatment based on group assignment: behavioral — 20-minute behavioral therapy during sessions; problem solving — 20-minute problem-solving activity during sessions; instruction only — 15-minutes of exercise during sessions. | Weight, height, %overweight, BMI: Children in problem-solving and behavioral groups decreased weight, %overweight, and BMI ($p < 0.05$) at 8 weeks. Differences were significant among groups: problem solving was greater than behavioral and instruction ($p < 0.05$). Significant differences were maintained at the 3- and 6-month follow-up. Only children in the problem-solving group maintained significant differences in %overweight and BMI at 6 months ($p < 0.05$). |
| DISC Study, 1995 [33] Locations: Baltimore, MD; Chicago, IL; Iowa City, IA; Newark, NJ; New Orleans, LA; Portland, OR | 663 prepubertal overweight children, ages 8–10 years; 623 completed the study | 3 years | D B | Two groups Dietary behavioral intervention: Group and individual sessions, diet- and family-based treatment, personalized counseling based on social learning theory and social action theory Usual care: educational publications provided | BMI, skinfold thickness, waist and hip circumference: no differences between groups in BMI or skinfolds. Intervention group had lower waist–hip ratio at 1 year but no difference at 3 years ($p$ values not specified). The primary aim of the study was to reduce low-density lipoprotein-cholesterol, not adiposity. |

| Reference / Location | Sample | Schedule | Codes | Groups / Intervention | Results |
|---|---|---|---|---|---|
| Epstein et al., 1995 [34] Location: Pittsburgh, PA | Final sample: 113 families with overweight parents, overweight children ages 8–12 years | 8 weekly treatment meetings, monthly meetings for 6–12 months, 5- and 10-year follow-up | D PA B | Three groups Traffic Light Diet, exercise (aerobic, stretching, spot reducing), and behavioral reinforcements for all groups: child and parent target, child target, or nonspecific target (control). | BMI, %overweight: Significant differences in percentage of children vs. adults who had decrease of at least 20%overweight at 6 ($p < 0.001$), 60 ($p < 0.001$), and 120 ($p < 0.001$) months. |
| Epstein et al., 2001 [35] Location: Pittsburgh, PA | 56 of 67 families with overweight children ages 8–12 years (29 boys, 27 girls) | 16 weekly meetings followed by 2 biweekly meetings, 2 monthly meetings, 2-month follow-up | D PA SA B | Two groups Traffic Light Diet and specific behavior change techniques for all participants. Reinforcement provided for either increasing physical activity (control) or increasing activity and decreasing sedentary behavior (combined). | BMI, %overweight: Boys in experimental group had significantly greater %overweight changes than girls ($p < 0.001$ combined group, $p < 0.025$ increase activity group). No sex differences in the control group. |
| Epstein et al., 1986 [36] Location: Pittsburgh, PA | 41 families with overweight children ages 8–12 years; follow-up on 38 families | 8 weekly treatment meetings, 10 monthly meetings, 3-year follow-up. | D PA B | Two groups 1200 kcal diet and lifestyle exercise program point economy to regulate child eating and exercise habits for both parent control and child self-control groups | BMI and %overweight: At 1 year, only children with nonobese parents had %overweight significantly lower than baseline ($p < 0.01$) and had 2.1 times the change in %overweight (16.3%) vs. children with obese parents (7.7%; $p < 0.01$). At 3 years, neither group had %overweight different from baseline. |
| Epstein et al., 1984 [37] Location: Pittsburgh, PA | 53 families with overweight children ages 8–12 years; final sample 47 families at 6 months, 34 families at 1 year | 8 weekly, 3 biweekly, and 4 monthly meetings, 12-month follow-up. | D PA B | Three groups Traffic Light Diet plus lifestyle change exercise; Traffic Light Diet plus point economy system; waiting list control | Weight, height, BMI: Both treatment groups had significantly lower BMI at 6 months than control group ($p < 0.0001$), and they were significantly lower than baseline at 6 months and 1 year. No significant differences were found between treatment groups at 6 months or 1 year. |
| Epstein et al., 1985 [38] Location: Pittsburgh, PA | 35 families with overweight children ages 8–12 years | 8 weekly, 10 monthly sessions, 24-month follow-up | D PA B | Three groups Traffic Light Diet and behavioral change and maintenance techniques for all participants; diet plus programmed aerobic exercise: walk, run, bike, or swim; diet plus lifestyle: lifestyle change exercise program; diet plus calisthenics: six of 12 calisthenics three times per week. | Weight, height, %overweight, BMI: Significant decreases in %overweight were observed at 2, 6, and 12 months in all three groups. No difference in %overweight at 12 months between groups. At 24 months, only the lifestyle group maintained relative weight changes in %overweight. |

**TABLE 13.1 (continued)**
**Randomized Controlled Design Family-Based and Individual Intervention Trials**

| Study (Author/Year/Location) | Study Population | Treatment Duration | Study Design and Components | | Outcome Variables and Findings |
|---|---|---|---|---|---|
| Epstein et al., 1995 [39] Location: Pittsburgh, PA | 61 families with overweight children, ages 8–12 years; complete data for 55 families | Weekly meetings for 4 months, 2 monthly meetings, 1-year follow-up. | Three groups Traffic Light Diet and tailored instruction for behavioral principles for all participants; reinforcement provided for decreasing sedentary activity (sedentary), increasing physical activity (exercise), or increasing physical activity and decreasing sedentary behavior (combined) | D PA SA B | Weight, height, %overweight, percentage body fat, waist–hip ratio: Significant differences between groups in %overweight at 4 months (reducing sedentary < physical activity; $p < 0.05$) and 12 months (reducing sedentary < physical activity and both; $p < 0.05$). |
| Epstein et al., 2000 [40] Location: Pittsburgh, PA | Final sample: 62 parents and 62 overweight children, ages 8–12 years | 16 weekly sessions, 2 monthly sessions, 12- and 24-month follow-up. | Three groups Lifestyle exercise, Traffic Light Diet, behavioral reinforcement for all participants; groups based on problem solving taught to parent and child, problem solving to child only, and no problem solving (control) | D PA B | Weight, height, BMI z-score: No significant differences in BMI z-score between groups at 6 months (all decreased). From baseline to 24 months, both problem-solving to child (.9) and control (1.1) significantly reduced BMI z score > problem-solving parent and child (.5). |
| Israel et al., 1994 [41] Location: Albany, NY | 34 families with overweight children, ages 8–13 years | 8 weekly, 9 biweekly sessions for 26 weeks total treatment, 3-year follow-up | Two groups Both groups followed four-component model of self-regulation standard treatment, with a parental-control focus; enhanced child involvement: child management of weight loss | B | Weight, height, %overweight, triceps skinfolds thickness: All groups significantly decreased %overweight and triceps skinfolds at 26 weeks ($p < 0.01$). %overweight increased above posttreatment levels in all groups at 3-year follow-up. |
| Kirschenbaum et al., 1984 [42] Location: Madison, WI | 40 overweight children, ages 9–13 years; final sample, 23 children | 9 weekly sessions, 3- and 12-month follow-up | Three groups Cognitive behavioral treatment for parent plus child, child only, and waiting list control groups | B | Weight, height, adjusted weight, %overweight: Both parents and children in parent-plus-child group and child-only group significantly reduced weight, %overweight, and weight index compared with the control group ($p < 0.01$) at posttreatment and 3-month follow-up. |

| Study | Subjects | Duration | Design | Outcomes |
|---|---|---|---|---|
| Flodmark et al., 1993 [43] Location: Lund, Switzerland | 94 overweight children, ages 10–11 years | 14–18 month treatment, 1-year follow-up | D PA B | Three groups No intervention (control), conventional treatment (CT), or family therapy; both treatment groups received dietary counseling (1500–1700-kcal diet) and medical checkups, and the family group also received family therapy | Weight, height, BMI, skinfolds: Family group had a significantly lesser increase in BMI than CT group (0.66% vs. 2.31%; $p < 0.042$) and greater decrease in skinfolds (16.8 vs. +6.8%; $p < 0.034$) at the end of treatment. One year following the end of treatment, BMI was significantly less increased ($p < 0.022$) in the family group compared with the control group. BMI did not significantly differ between family and CT or controls and CT at 1-year follow-up. |
| Brownell et al., 1983 [44] Location: Williamsport, PA | 42 obese adolescents, ages 12–16 years | 16 weeks with follow-up session every 2 months for 1 year. | D PA B | Three groups All groups received diet, exercise, behavior modification, and social support instruction; groups were distinguished by session attendance: mother–child together, mother–child separately, or child alone | Weight, %overweight and BMI: %overweight and weight changes were significantly greater in the mother–child separately group compared with other groups at 16 weeks ($p < 0.01$ and $p < 0.04$, respectively) and at 1 year ($p < 0.05$ and $p < 0.01$, respectively). |
| Becque et al., 1988 [45] Location: Ann Arbor, MI | 36 overweight adolescents | 20 weeks | D PA B | Three groups Weekly diet and behavior change sessions for treatment groups: diet, behavior change, and exercise (with exercise sessions three times per week), and diet and behavior only; the control group received no treatment | Weight, percentage fat by hydrostatic weighing: Changes in total number of risk factors, of which percentage fat was included, were significantly greater in the exercise/diet/behavior group ($p < 0.01$). |
| Rocchini et al., 1988 [46] Location: Ann Arbor, MI | 72 obese adolescents, ages 10–17 years; 10 nonobese adolescents ages 10–14 years | 20 weeks | D PA B | Three groups Weekly diet and behavior change sessions for treatment groups: diet, behavior change, and exercise (with exercise sessions three times per week); diet and behavior only; the control group received no treatment | Weight, height, percentage fat by hydrostatic weighing: Compared to overweight control group, both treatment groups reduced body weight and percentage fat significantly ($p < 0.01$). |

**TABLE 13.1 (continued)**
**Randomized Controlled Design Family-Based and Individual Intervention Trials**

| Study (Author/Year/Location) | Study Population | Treatment Duration | | Study Design and Components | Outcome Variables and Findings |
|---|---|---|---|---|---|
| Wadden et al., 1990 [47] Location: Philadelphia, PA | 47 overweight African-American girls, ages 12–16 years; 36 completed, 31 in follow-up | 16 weeks with 6 month follow-up | D PA B | Three groups All received the Weight Reduction and Pride program including 1000–1500 kcal daily, behavioral counseling, increasing physical activity; groups distinguished by session attendance: child alone, mother–child together, and mother–child separately | Weight, height, BMI, body fat by hydrostatic weighing: Weight was significantly reduced in all groups: child alone (1.6 kg), mother–child together (3.7 kg) and mother–child separately (3.1 kg) at 16 weeks. Body fat decreased equally in all subjects (from mean of 37.1 to 35.1 kg; $p < 0.001$). Child alone group increased weight from baseline by 3.0 kg, mother–child together by 1.7 kg, and mother–child separately by 3.5 kg at 6-month follow-up. BMI was not significantly different from baseline in subjects combined. Subjects whose mothers regularly attended treatment sessions lost twice as much weight as those with poor attendance. |
| Coates et al., 1982 [48] Location: Stanford, CA | 31 overweight children, ages 13–17 years | 15 weeks with 9-month follow-up | B | Two groups All subjects attended weekly classes including self-management and weight loss skills; groups distinguished by session attendance: parent or no-parent groups | Weight, height, %overweight: Parent group reduced 5.1% at 15 weeks and 8.2% at 9-month follow-up. No-parent group reduced %overweight by 8.4% at 15 weeks and 9-month follow-up. |
| Mellin et al., 1987 [49] Location: Four sites in northern California | 66 overweight children, ages 12–18 years | 14 weeks, 15-month follow-up | D PA B | Two groups SHAPEDOWN program included 90-minute weekly sessions for 14 weeks including weigh-in, group interaction, and exercise period; control received no intervention | Weight, height, relative weight: SHAPEDOWN group significantly reduced relative weight at 3 months (5.9% at 3 months, $p < 0.001$; –9.9% at 15 months, $p < 0.01$), but not control group (.3% at 3 months; .1% at 15 months). |

| Study / Location | Sample | Duration | Domain | Intervention | Results |
|---|---|---|---|---|---|
| Saelens et al., 2002 [50]<br>Location: Cincinnati, OH | 44 overweight adolescents, ages 12–16 years | 14–16 weeks with 7-month follow-up | D<br>B<br>PA<br>SA | Two groups<br>Behavioral weight control: eight weekly and three biweekly telephone contact sessions 10–20 minutes each, instructed to self-monitor food intake and physical activity; typical care: one physician counseling session | Weight, height, BMI: Typical care group significantly increased mean BMI $z$-scores (1.1) compared with decrease in BMI $z$-score for treatment group (.1) during intervention. |
| Golan and Crow, 2004 [51]<br>Location: Tel Aviv, Israel | 50 of 60 obese children attended; 7-year follow-up | Sessions dependent on group assignment, 7-year follow-up | D<br>PA<br>B | Two groups<br>1500-calorie diet, cognitive restructuring, eating behavior modification, exercise for all participants; parent only: attended four weekly, four biweekly, and six every 6 weeks educational group sessions; child only: attended seven weekly sessions, then biweekly sessions for the remainder of 1 year | Weight, height, %overweight: Weight loss of children in parent-only group significant (13.6%) at 1 year ($p < 0.05$). %overweight reduction in children in parent-only group (15%) at year 2 ($p < 0.01$). %overweight reduction 29% in the parent-only group, and 20.2% in the child-only group at 7 years ($p < 0.05$). |
| Epstein et al., 1987 [52]<br>Location: Pittsburgh, PA | 77 families with obese children ages 6–12 years; 67 at follow-up | 14 sessions over 8 months, 21- and 60-month follow-up. | D<br>PA<br>B | Three groups<br>Traffic Light Diet, aerobic exercise, and behavior modification for all groups: parent/child target, child target, or nonspecific target (control) | %overweight, weight, height: %overweight decrease in children in parent-child group (12.7%), but increased in child-only (4.3%) and control groups (8.2%) at 5-year follow-up. |
| Epstein et al., 1987 [53]<br>Location: Pittsburgh, PA | 77 families with obese children; 49 at follow-up | 14 sessions over 8 months, 5-year follow-up | D<br>PA<br>B | Three groups<br>Traffic Light Diet, Cooper aerobic point system, behavior modification for all groups: parent–child, child alone, or nonspecific target (control); nonparticipating siblings were evaluated at baseline and 5 years | Height, weight, %overweight: Significantly greater %overweight decrease for nonparticipating siblings in parent-child group compared with nonparticipating siblings in child-alone and control groups at 5 years ($p < 0.038$). |

**TABLE 13.1 (continued)**
**Randomized Controlled Design Family-Based and Individual Intervention Trials**

| Study (Author/Year/Location) | Study Population | Treatment Duration | | Study Design and Components | Outcome Variables and Findings |
|---|---|---|---|---|---|
| Epstein et al., 1994 [54] Location: Pittsburgh, PA | 39 families with obese children, ages 8–12 years | 26 weekly and 6 monthly sessions, 2-year follow-up | D PA B | Two groups Traffic Light Diet, lifestyle exercise, and behavioral principles; experimental group: diet, exercise, weight loss, parenting skills; control: behavior change only | Weight, height, %overweight: Experimental group experienced significantly greater decrease in %overweight at 6 months and 1 year ($p < 0.05$). No difference was seen between the groups at 2 years. |
| Israel et al., 1985 [55] Location: Albany, NY | 33 families with overweight children, ages 8–12 years; 20 at follow-up | 9 weekly sessions, 1-year follow-up | D PA B | Three groups Weight-reduction program for weight-reduction-only and parent-training groups; parent-training treatment preceded by parent-only courses; wait list control group | Height, weight, triceps skinfold: At 9 weeks, children in weight-reduction-only group had significantly greater decreases in %overweight compared with parent-training group ($p < 0.025$). Children in parent-trainning group had significantly greater decreases in %overweight when compared with control ($p < 0.01$) at 9 weeks. At 1 year, children in the weight-reduction-only group significantly increased %overweight ($p < 0.001$). |
| Epstein et al., 1985 [56] Location: Pittsburgh, PA | 22 families with overweight girls, ages 8–12 years | 8 weekly intensive and 10 monthly maintenance sessions | D PA B | Two groups Traffic Light Diet, aerobic exercise program, behavioral change techniques; child and parents treated separately in diet only and diet plus 6 weeks of structured exercise conditions | Weight, height, %overweight: Both groups reduced weight and %overweight significantly ($p < 0.01$) at 2 and 6 months. Only diet plus exercise reduced weight significantly ($p < 0.01$) at 12 months; both groups reduced %overweight at 12 months ($p < 0.01$). |
| Ebbeling et al., 2003 [57] Location: Boston, MA | 16 obese adolescents, ages 13–21 years | 6 months (12 sessions), 1-year follow-up | D PA B | Two groups Exercise and behavioral counseling for both groups: reduced glycemic load diet or reduced fat diet | Fat mass by DEXA, BMI: BMI ($p < 0.03$) and fat mass by DEXA ($p < 0.02$) decreased in the low-glycemic load diet group after 12 months, but not in the control, low-fat diet group. |

| Study / Location | Sample | Duration | Type | Groups / Description | Outcomes |
|---|---|---|---|---|---|
| Epstein et al., 2000 [58] Location: Pittsburgh, PA | 90 families with obese children, ages 8–12 | 6 months (16 weekly sessions, 2 biweekly, 2 monthly) | D PA SA B | Four groups Groups varied targeted behaviors (sedentary behaviors vs. physical activity) and treatment dose (low vs. high). All participants given Traffic Light Diet and taught positive reinforcement techniques. | Height, weight, BMI, fat-free body mass, %overweight: significant ($p < 0.001$) decreases in %overweight observed from baseline to 6 months. No significant differences in the rate of change by group were observed for any anthropometric or fitness measure. |
| Obarzanek et al., 2001 [75] Locations: Baltimore, MD; Chicago, IL; Iowa City, IA; Newark, NJ; New Orleans, LA; Portland, OR | 663 prepubertal overweight children, ages 8–10 years; 623 completed treatment, 580 at 7-year follow-up | 3 years with 7-year follow-up | D B | Two groups Dietary behavioral intervention: group and individual sessions, diet- and family-based treatment, personalized counseling based on social learning theory and social action theory; usual care: educational publications provided | BMI was not significantly different between groups; the primary aim of the study was to reduce low-density lipoprotein cholesterol, not adiposity. |
| Epstein et al., 1987 [76] Location: Pittsburgh, PA | 41 obese children, ages 8–12 years; 33 at follow-up | 8 weekly sessions, 10 monthly sessions, 5-year follow-up | D PA B | Two groups 1200-kcal diet for both groups: parent control or child self-control. | %overweight: changes were not significantly different for groups at 6 months or 1, 3, or 5 years. |

*Note:* BMI = body mass index, D = dietary intervention, PA = physical activity intervention, SA = sedentary activity intervention, B = behavioral intervention

**TABLE 13.2**
**Family-Based and Individual Intervention Trials, Non-Randomized Design or Randomization Not Specified**

| Study (Author/Year/Location) | Study Population | Treatment Duration | Study Design and Components | Outcome Variables and Findings |
|---|---|---|---|---|
| Brown et al., 2000 [59] Location: New Orleans, LA | 50 overweight children, ages 7–17 years | Weekly 2-hour sessions for 10 weeks | D PA B — Weight-reduction program including: protein-sparing modified fast diet or balanced hypocaloric diet (based on initial weight status), moderate-intensity progressive exercise, and behavior modification based on social cognitive therapy | Weight, height, %overweight: Both Caucasian and African-American subjects reduced weight and %IBW significantly at 10 weeks ($p < 0.0001$). |
| Chen et al., 1997 [60] Location: Taiwan | 68 obese children, ages 5–18 years; 56 completed 1-year follow-up | Six sessions (three weekly, three biweekly), with a 1-year follow-up | D PA B — Weight-reduction program, focusing on parental/family involvement, that included the five-lamp diet, 25% reduction in energy intake, lifestyle exercise, and behavioral modification | Weight for length index (WLI): Mean WLI declined ($p < 0.0001$); 97% of participants were below baseline WLI at end of treatment, and 80% were below baseline WLI 1 year after treatment. |
| Eliakim et al., 2002 [61] Location: Tel Aviv, Israel | 177 obese children, 6–16 years; 25 obese children matched for age (controls) | 3 or 6 months | D PA SA B — Subjects assigned to a weight-management program including dietary counseling (monthly) and exercise (twice weekly); intervention was tailored to age; 1200–2000-kcal diet, reinforcements to increase physical activity and decrease sedentary behaviors | Weight, height, BMI, BMI percentile: Weight was significantly reduced from 55.8 to 54.9 kg; BMI from 26.1 to 25.4 at 3 months; weight (0.50 kg; $p < 0.05$) and BMI (1.07; $p < 0.01$) reduced significantly greater at 6 months in treatment subjects; control significantly increased body weight at 3 months (54.2–55.8 kg) and at 6 months (+3.23 kg) and BMI at 3 months (25.2–25.6 kg/m$^2$) and (+0.17 kg/m$^2$) at 6 months ($p < 0.005$). |
| Israel, 1984 [62] Location: Albany, NY | 69 children, ages 8–12 and their parents | 9 weekly 90-minute sessions | D PA B — Participants seen in groups of 4–6 families. Parents chose two conditions: engage in concurrent weight loss efforts with their children or serve as only a helper to children's weight loss efforts. Treatment based on CAIR approach (cue control rules, activity, intake, rewards). | Weight, %overweight, triceps skinfold; no significant differences were found for within-treatment effects or follow-up effects. |

| Study / Location | Sample | Duration | | Intervention | Results |
|---|---|---|---|---|---|
| Levine et al., 2001 [63] Location: Pittsburgh, PA | 24 families with obese children, 9–12 years of age; 15 completed treatment | 10–12 sessions, follow-up at 4–13 months (mean 7.8 months) | D PA SA B | Family-based weight-reduction program using the Traffic Light Diet, with reinforcements to increase exercise and decrease sedentary behaviors | Weight, BMI, percentage ideal body weight: Significant amount of weight loss during treatment (2.5 kg, $P =.01$); similar declines in BMI ($P =.003$) and %IBW ($P =.007$). BMI did not change significantly from pretreatment through follow-up ($p = .19$). |
| Nuutinen and Knip, 1992 [64] Location: Finland | 48 obese and 29 nonobese children, ages 6–16 years | 12 months with 5-year follow-up | D PA B | Three groups: Individual counseling, group sessions using behavior counseling, and standard school health setting | Weight, height, relative weight, skinfolds: Groups did not differ significantly in relative weight at 5 years; only 14 children maintained 10% reduction in relative weight at 5 years ($p < 0.001$). |
| Nuutinen & Knip, 1992 [65] Location: Finland | 32 obese children, ages 6–15 | 2 years | D B | Two groups: Groups differed by individual (Group I) or group treatment (Group II) of patients. Group I received dietary counseling with a nutritionist. Group II also received 7 behavioral modification sessions. | Weight, height, relative weight, skinfolds: relative body weight decreased 16.6% in Group I ($p < 0.001$) and 15.8% in Group II ($p < 0.01$). |
| Nuutinen & Knip, 1992 [66] Location: Finland | 48 obese children, ages 6–15 | 2 years | D B | Three groups: Groups differed by individual (Group I) or group treatment (Group II) of patients. Group II treated conventionally in a school healthcare setting. Group I received dietary counseling with a nutritionist. Group II also received 7 behavioral modification sessions. | Weight, height, relative weight, skinfolds: At 1 year, those children who achieved their weight ($p < 0.05$) and less lean body mass ($p < 0.05$). |
| Resnicow et al., 2000 [67] Location: Four inner-city housing projects | 57 overweight African-American girls, ages 11–17 years | 2 years | D PA SA B | Nonrandomized, noncontrolled weight-reduction program involving four 6-month sessions targeting food intake, decreased television viewing, and increased physical activity | BMI, two-site skinfolds, percentage body fat (DEXA): High attenders and low attenders (attended <50% sessions) were compared (due to absence of a control group), and no differences were detected. |

**TABLE 13.2 (continued)**
**Family-Based and Individual Intervention Trials, Non-Randomized Design or Randomization Not Specified**

| Study (Author/Year/Location) | Study Population | Treatment Duration | | Study Design and Components | Outcome Variables and Findings |
|---|---|---|---|---|---|
| Sothern et al., 1999 [68] Location: New Orleans, LA | 73 obese children, ages 7–17 years; 48 completed entire program | Phases vary by treatment, 1-year follow-up | D PA B | Three groups: phase I (30 weeks) for severely obese, phase II (20 weeks) for moderately obese, phase III (10 weeks) for mildly obese, phase IV "maintenance" phase; protein-sparing modified fast diet, behavior modification, and progressive exercise program used | Weight, %IBW, BMI, relative fat (%), and fat-free mass (using skinfolds): Body weight, %IBW, BMI, and percentage fat decreased significantly in all three groups by 10 weeks compared with baseline ($p < 0.001$). Percentage fat, BMI, and %IBW remained decreased at 52-week follow-up ($p < 0.001$). |
| Sothern et al., 2000 [69] Location: New Orleans, LA | 50 overweight children, ages 7–17 years, 29 girls, 21 boys | Weekly 2-hour sessions for 10 weeks | D PA B | Treatment included protein-sparing modified fast diet, home-based exercise program, and behavior modification based on social cognitive therapy (Committed to Kids and Trim Kids approach). | Weight, height, BMI, %IBW, percentage fat by skinfolds: Both males and females reduced weight (females $p < 0.05$, males $p < 0.0004$), %IBM ($p < 0.0001$ for both), and BMI (females $p < 0.01$, males $p < 0.0001$) significantly from baseline to 10 weeks. |
| Sothern et al., 2000 [70] Location: New Orleans, LA | 67 overweight children, ages 7–17 years; 32 completed 1 year | 10 weekly 2-hour sessions, 1-year follow-up | D PA B | Multidisciplinary weight-management program of aerobic exercise alone or aerobic exercise plus resistance training, with protein-sparing modified fast diet and behavior modification | Weight, height, %IBW, BMI, percentage fat by skinfolds (resistance training only): BMI and %IBW decreased significantly at 10 weeks and 1 year in both groups ($p < 0.0001$); weight was significantly lower at 10 weeks in both groups but only in resistance training group at 1 year ($p < 0.001$); in resistance training subjects, percentage body fat decreased significantly at 10 weeks and at 1 year ($p < 0.0001$). |

| Reference/Location | Subjects | Schedule | Intervention | Components | Outcome measures/results |
|---|---|---|---|---|---|
| Sothern et al., 2000 [71] Location: New Orleans, LA | 56 overweight children, ages 7–17 years; 52 completed intervention, 35 completed 1 year | Weekly 2-hour sessions for 12 months | Very low calorie diet, home-based exercise program (tailored to severity of obesity), and family behavior modification based on social cognitive therapy (Committed to Kids and Trim Kids approach) | D, PA, B | Weight, height, %IBW, percentage fat by skinfolds: Weight (9.4 kg), %IBW (25.6%), and percentage fat (7.3%) reduced significantly at 10 weeks compared with baseline ($p < 0.0001$); weight (6 kg), %IBW (20.2%), BMI (3.9), and percentage fat (9.1%) reduced significantly at 1 year compared with baseline ($p < 0.0001$). |
| Sothern et al., 2002 [72] Location: New Orleans, LA | 93 adolescents ages 13.1–17.7 years; 56 completed study | Weekly 2-hour sessions for 12 months | Protein-modified fast diet or hypocaloric diet (based on initial weight status), moderate-intensity progressive exercise, and behavior modification for all participants | D, PA, B | Weight, height, %overweight, BMI: Subjects reduced BMI from 32.3 to 29.3 and percentage IBW from 177% to 156% at 10 weeks. BMI was further reduced to 28.2 and %IBW to 141.9% at 1 year ($p < 0.001$). |
| Spieth et al., 2000 [73] Location: Boston, MA | 107 obese children | 4 months | Comprehensive medical evaluation, dietary and lifestyle counseling (increase activity, decrease sedentary behavior), and low–glycemic index (LGI) diet or reduced-fat (RF) diet based on food guide pyramid; problem-focused behavior therapy, if needed | D, PA, SA, B | Weight, height, BMI: BMI was reduced significantly by 1.53 in the LGI diet group compared with 0.06 in the RF group ($p < 0.001$); weight changes were similar, 2.03 kg in LGI vs. +1.31 kg in RF ($p < 0.01$). |
| Suskind, 1993 [74] Location: New Orleans, LA | 50 obese children, ages 7–17 | 1 year (10-week cohorts) | Participants stratified by obesity: severely obese, moderately obese, mildly obese. All received dietary and behavior modification intervention | D, PA, B | Height, weight, %overweight, BMI: An average weight loss of 9 kg was observed in 40 subjects who completed the program and weight maintenance observed at 26 weeks. |

*Note:* D = dietary intervention, PA = physical activity intervention, SA = sedentary activity intervention, B = behavioral intervention; %IBW = .

Of the 49 studies reviewed for this chapter, two controlled studies and four of other design used group treatment approaches without a family-based counseling component (e.g., parental involvement) [45,46,64–67]. The two randomized controlled studies demonstrated that adolescents receiving diet and exercise interventions significantly decrease body weight or percentage fat compared with an obese control group. In one of the studies of other design, Nuutinen and Knip demonstrated significant reductions in body weight among children ages 6 to 16 years with weight maintenance effects at 5 years posttreatment [64].

## WEIGHT MAINTENANCE

The effects of maintaining weight loss after the end of intensive treatment are promising. McLean et al. identified eight randomized clinical trials of children and adolescents with 1-year follow-up data that included a family involvement component [19]. Studies in children under the age of 13 years have consistently illustrated significant reductions in weight status over 6-month to 2-year time periods when parents were included in behavioral counseling. Several randomized controlled family-based trials and one controlled, clinical observation [16–18,34,51–53,64,77] have demonstrated maintenance of reductions in adiposity over 5 to 10 years. Specifically, in a study of long-term maintenance effects, Epstein and colleagues have followed the effects of an intensive weight loss program over a 10-year period [17]. This randomized controlled design examined the effects of a family-based behavioral treatment program on weight and growth across a 10-year period in obese 6 to 12 year olds. Children and their parents were randomized to one of three experimental groups. Each was provided similar diet, exercise, and behavior management skills training. However, the groups differed in reinforcement for weight loss and behavior change. Specifically, the child-and-parent condition reinforced both the parent's and child's weight loss and behavior change. The child-only condition reinforced only the child's weight loss and behavior change. The non-specific control group reinforced families for attendance. Children in the child-and-parent condition demonstrated significantly greater decreases in percent overweight after 5 and 10 years compared with children in the nonspecific control group (e.g., 11.2% and 7.5% at 5 and 10 years, respectively, compared with +7.9% and +14.3%). The child-only group showed increases in percentage overweight after 5 and 10 years (+2.7% and +4.5%); however weight changes were not statistically different from the other two groups. Notably, at 10 years, there were no differences in height between groups.

In another study, children had significantly lower percentage of overweight and triceps skinfolds at 6 months. However, at 3-year follow-up, weight reductions were not maintained [41]. Interestingly, a 3-year study focusing on improvement in lipid profiles, with weight loss as a secondary outcome measure, showed no significant changes in adiposity at 7-year follow-up [33,75].

## ADOLESCENTS

Few studies focused solely on adolescents have been conducted. There are two randomized controlled trials that evaluated family-based therapy in adolescents 12 years of age and older [44,47]. Brownell and colleagues reported that weight loss was significantly greater in older youth (i.e., 12 to 16 years) who participated in counseling separate from parents than in those treated together with parents or treated alone [44]. Specifically, this study was a 16-month controlled trial that examined weight and blood pressure changes among three methods that involved mothers in the treatment. The treatments were (1) Mother–Child Separately, in which the adolescents and their mothers attended separate groups; (2) Mother–Child Together, in which the children and mothers were in the same group; and (3) Child Alone, in which the children met in groups alone and without any mother involvement. Techniques included in the program were nutritional education, exercise, social support, and behavior modification. The Mother–Child Separately group lost more weight during treatment than the other two groups, and differences between the groups increased at 1-year follow-up. Brownell and colleagues suggested that with adolescents, a program of behavior modification and parent involvement could lead to significant weight losses. However, the nature of parent involvement may be a critical component.

Wadden and colleagues investigated the efficacy of a behavioral weight control program in overweight African-American female adolescents [47]. All adolescents participated in the same 16-week program; however, they differed with regard to level of parent participation (e.g., child-alone, mother-and-child treated together, and mother and child treated separately). Adolescents in all three conditions lost weight. However, there were no statistical differences among conditions. Interestingly, results revealed that the greater the number of sessions attended by mothers, the greater their daughters' weight loss.

Coates and others evaluated the effect of a group multidisciplinary weight loss program for adolescents aged 13 to 17 years [48]. Teenagers were assigned to either a parent or a no-parent participation group. All of the classes incorporated weight loss training and self-management skills. In the parent participation group, parents learned skills for assisting their children in losing weight. The parent participation group showed the greater decreases in percentage above ideal weight, suggesting that parent participation enhanced the weight loss of adolescents at 15 weeks. However, at 9-month follow-up, weight loss was similar between the groups, with no significant differences.

## COMPONENT ANALYSIS OF BEHAVIORAL TECHNIQUES

Most weight loss studies in the clinical environment have not evaluated the independent impact that a particular behavioral technique may have on adiposity reduction. Only two studies have systematically assessed the separate influence that a specified behavioral technique (e.g., problem-solving) had on weight loss compared with other techniques. The independent contribution of problem solving–skills training among 6- to 12-year-old children enrolled in a multi-disciplinary weight management intervention (e.g., "the Traffic Light Diet," self-monitoring, stimulus control, cognitive restructuring, diet and exercise information, family support, peer relations, games and stories, and maintenance strategies) was examined [32]. The inclusion of problem-solving techniques to the intervention significantly improved weight loss and maintenance of weight loss at 3 and 6 months follow-up. Interestingly, Epstein and colleagues found no significant differences between groups when problem solving was added to their behavioral interventions after 6 months. However, in the problem solving plus parent-and-child intervention, BMI was significantly lower than the child-only problem solving and no problem solving groups at 24-month follow-up.

## SUMMARY

All of these family-based counseling studies consistently demonstrated reductions in weight post-treatment and at follow-up. Evidence is limited in older children; however, family-based counseling may result in significant adiposity reductions.

## PARENT TRAINING OR MODELING INTERVENTIONS

Parent training or modeling is often an integral part of a family-based counseling clinical intervention. Thirty randomized clinical trials and 12 studies of other design were identified that included parental involvement, training, or modeling in the counseling interventions. Nineteen studies of randomized design examined child-only versus parent-only interventions, or child-only versus parent and child combined counseling. The results of the studies are fairly consistent. Parent-only or parent-plus-child interventions are typically superior to child-only interventions on weight reductions in children. However, there are three exceptions. Specifically, Kirschenbaum and colleagues found nonsignificant differences at 9 weeks and at 3- and 12-month follow-up among 9- to 13-year-old children participating in parent-plus-child versus child-only group interventions [42]. In another study of 12- to 16-year-old African-American adolescents, Wadden and colleagues found no significant differences when adolescents participated in counseling alone, with their mothers, or when the mothers and adolescents were seen separately [47]. Epstein and colleagues found no difference in weight loss at 1 year among 6- to 12-year-old children who participated in a child self-control condition versus those who participated in a parent self-control condition [36]. Interestingly, only those children with overweight parents reduced weight status significantly.

## WEIGHT MAINTENANCE

Epstein and colleagues have published a series of findings demonstrating the importance of parent training or modeling in child weight management. In a long-term study by Epstein and others, weight maintenance was superior among children whose parents participated in the intervention program versus those children treated alone [17]. In another study, weight loss of children compared with that of their parents after 6 months and at 10 years was evaluated [34]. Results were limited by the absence of control groups; however, children maintained the original weight reductions, whereas parents did not. Interestingly, Eliakim et al. examined the influence that parental overweight had in the maintenance of weight loss in a sample of overweight children between the ages of 6 and 16 years [61]. Children with normal-weight parents maintained their original weight loss better than those with either one or two overweight parents. This finding demonstrates the importance of parental contribution in the ability of overweight children to maintain initial weight loss.

## PARENTS AS THE FOCUS OF TREATMENT

Parents as a focus of treatment have been noted in a few studies. Several studies by Epstein and colleagues [16,52–54,76] targeted both the parent and the child for weight loss. Typically, both the parent and the child contracted for weight loss and had contingencies placed on them for successful weight loss. In a study by Golan and colleagues, enhanced weight loss occurred when the parents, as opposed to the overweight children, were targeted with nutritional education and counseling [31]. However, generalizations from this study should be made with caution because there was a high drop-out rate in the control groups. Interestingly, 7-year follow-up data revealed that mean reductions in percentage overweight were significantly greater in the parent condition compared with the child-only condition [51]. Additionally, parental overweight [61] and parental attempts at concurrent weight loss [62] have been found to significantly influence weight-loss maintenance efforts in children.

## SUMMARY

In summary, all 42 intervention studies that incorporated parental involvement, training, or modeling showed positive changes in child weight status. Three studies in younger children and one in adolescents demonstrated no difference in weight reduction between child-only versus child-plus-parent interventions. Family-based counseling that incorporates parent training or modeling as part of a clinical intervention program results in significant weight reductions in preadolescent children. Therefore, sufficient evidence exists to recommend parent training and modeling techniques as part of weight-management programs for children. Parent training or modeling for adolescent-based interventions has shown inconsistent and inconclusive results. Thus, whether parent training or modeling in overweight adolescents should be recommended needs further investigation.

# INDIVIDUAL TREATMENT APPROACHES

There is a dearth of data available on individual treatment for obesity in children and adolescents in a nongroup format. Saelens and colleagues evaluated the efficacy of a 4-month-long behavioral weight control intervention in a primary care setting with extended follow-up through telephone and mail contact [50]. Specifically, overweight adolescents were randomly assigned to either a multiple-component behavioral weight control intervention (e.g., physical activity education and nutritional education) or a single session of physician weight counseling (usual care). Notably, participant satisfaction and behavioral skills use were also measured. Adolescents receiving the multiple-component intervention demonstrated a better change in BMI than did adolescents receiving usual care. Adolescents in the treatment condition demonstrated higher use of behavioral skills, and higher behavioral skills use was related to better weight outcome. The results revealed that a physician-based, individual counseling program that included physical activity education and nutritional education was superior to a usual care approach in overweight teenagers. Furthermore, this study suggests that innovative delivery approaches (e.g., telephone contacts and mailed materials) may improve weight management skills in an adolescent overweight population.

In another randomized study of adolescents, Ebbeling and colleagues [57] evaluated the effects of a reduced–glycemic load diet compared with an energy-restricted, reduced-fat diet. The study yielded significant reductions in fat mass and BMI for both diet conditions. However, the glycemic load diet condition resulted in significantly lower decreases in fat mass and BMI compared with the reduced fat diet at 12-month follow-up.

## SUMMARY

Overall, family-based behavioral counseling is shown to be an effective method for changing eating and activity patterns in overweight children in clinical settings. Diet, exercise/ physical activity, and behavioral counseling are common components of efficacious studies of family-based weight loss interventions in children younger than 13 years of age. These studies demonstrate that the inclusion of the family in counseling sessions (e.g., targeting the parent) improves both short-term and long-term weight outcomes. Parental education is strongly recommended, particularly if the parents are obese. Weight losses appear to be similar regardless of which dietary counseling approach is implemented. The health benefits of family-based weight management programs in a clinical environment are well established in 9- to 12-year-old overweight children. Specifically, benefits in lipid profiles and body composition have been documented in these children 10 years posttreatment. Therefore, there is sufficient evidence to support recommending family-based counseling in children under 12 years of age.

The majority of studies in children over the age of 12 years indicate that group behavioral approaches focused on nutritional and physical activity education are most effective. However, family-based interventions and long-term studies in adolescents are lacking and have shown inconsistent results. There is mixed evidence to support recommending family-based, group behavioral counseling in children over the age of 12 years. Specifically, it is unclear whether parents and adolescents should be provided behavioral counseling alone or together. Therefore, there is a need for individualized, age-appropriate, overweight treatment programs for adolescents.

## ACKNOWLEDGMENT

The authors would like to thank Brooke L. Barbera for her hard work and attention to detail in preparation of this chapter.

## REFERENCES

1. Falkner B, Michel S. Obesity and other risk factors in children. *Ethn Dis.* 1999;9(2):284–289.
2. Hill J, Throwbridge F. The causes and health consequences of obesity in children and adolescents. *Pediatrics.* 1998;101(3):497–575.
3. Rippe JM, Hess S. The role of physical activity in the prevention and management of obesity. *J Amer Diet Assoc.* 1998;98(10 Suppl 2):S31–S38.

4. Zannolli R, Rebeggiani A, Chiarelli F, Morgese G. Hyperinsulinism as a marker in obese children. *Amer J Dis Children*. 1993;147(8):837–841.

5. Witchel SF, Smith R, Tomboc M, Aston CE. Candidate gene analysis in premature pubarche and adolescent hyperandrogenism. *Fertil Steril*. 2001;75(4):724–730.

6. Bideci A, Cinaz P, Hasanoglu A, Elbeg S. Serum levels of insulin-like growth factor-I and insulin-like growth factor binding protein-3 in obese children. *J Pediatr Endocrinol Metabol*. 1997;10(3):295–299.

7. Must A. Morbidity and mortality associated with elevated body weight in children and adolescents. *Amer J Clin Nutr*. 1996;63(3 Suppl):445S–447S.

8. Tershakovec AM, Weller SC, Gallagher PR. Obesity, school performance and behaviour of black, urban elementary school children. *Intl J Obes Rel Metabol Disord*. 1994;18(5):323–327.

9. Latner JD, Stunkard AJ. Getting worse: the stigmatization of obese children. *Obes Res*. 2003;11(3):452–456.

10. Strauss RS, Pollack HA. Social marginalization of overweight children. *Arch Pediatr Adolesc Med*. 2003;157(8):746–752.

11. Bouchard C. Obesity in adulthood — the importance of childhood and parental obesity. *New Engl J Med*. 1997;337(13):926–927.

12. Whitaker RC, Wright JA, Pepe MS, Seidel KD, Dietz WH. Predicting obesity in young adulthood from childhood and parental obesity. *New Engl J Med*. 1997;337(13):869–873.

13. Simic B. Childhood obesity is a risk factor in adulthood. In: Collip PJ, Ed. *Childhood Obesity*. 2nd ed. Littleton, MA: PSG Publishing; 1980.

14. Dietz W. Childhood Obesity. In: Cheung L, Richmand J, Eds. *Child Health Nutrition and Physical Activity*. Champaign, IL: Human Kinetics; 1995.

15. Crawford P, Sothern M, Riche L, Hoest, D. Evidence-based analysis of childhood overweight prevention and treatment programs: a position paper for the American Dietetic Association. *J Amer Diet Assoc*. In press.

16. Epstein LH, Wing RR, Koeske R, Andrasik F, Ossip DJ. Child and parent weight loss in family-based behavior modification programs. *J Consult Clin Psychol*. 1981;49(5):674–685.

17. Epstein LH, Valoski A, Wing RR, McCurley J. Ten-year follow-up of behavioral, family-based treatment for obese children. *JAMA*. 1990;264(19):2519–2523.

18. Epstein LH, Valoski A, Wing RR, McCurley J. Ten-year outcomes of behavioral family-based treatment for childhood obesity. *Health Psychol*. 1994;13(5):373–383.

19. McLean N, Griffin S, Toney K, Hardeman W. Family involvement in weight control, weight maintenance and weight-loss interventions: a systematic review of randomised trials. *Intl J Obes*. 2003;27:987–1005.

20. St Jeor ST, Perumean-Chaney S, Sigman-Grant M, Williams C, Foreyt JP. Family-based interventions for the treatment of childhood obesity. *J Amer Diet Assoc*. 2002;102(5):639–644.

21. Nutzinger DO, Cayiroglu S, Sachs G, Zapotoczky HG. Emotional problems during weight reduction: advantages of a combined behavior therapy and antidepressive drug therapy for obesity. *J Behav Therap Exper Psychiatr*. 1985;16(3):217–221.

22. Brownell KD, Kramer FM. Behavioral management of obesity. *Med Clin N Amer*. 1989;73:185–201.

23. Foreyt JP, Goodrick GK. Impact of behavior therapy on weight loss. *Amer J Health Promotion*. 1994;8(6):466–468.

24. Epstein LH, Wing RR, Steranchak L, Dickson B, Michelson J. Comparison of family-based behavior modification and nutrition education for childhood obesity. *J Pediatr Psychol*. 1980;5(1):25–36.

25. Johnson WG, Hinkle LK, Carr RE, Anderson DA, Lemmon CR, Engler LB, Bergeron KC. Dietary and exercise interventions for juvenile obesity: long-term effect of behavioral and public health models. *Obes Res*. 1997;5(3):257–261.

26. Wadden TA, Sarwer DB, Berkowitz RI. Behavioural treatment of the overweight patient. Bailliere's best practice and research. *Clin Endocrinol Metabol*. 1999;13(1):93–107.

27. Poston WSC, Hyder ML, O'Byrne KK, Foreyt JP. Where do diets, exercise, and behavior modification fit in the treatment of obesity? *Endocrine*. 2000;13(2):187–192.

28. Foreyt JP, Poston WSC. The role of the behavioral counselor in obesity treatment. *J Amer Diet Assoc*. 1998;10(Suppl 2):S27–S30.

29. Foreyt JP, Poston WSC. What is the role of cognitive-behavior therapy in patient management? *Obes Res*. 1998;6(Suppl 1):18S–22S.

30. Foster GD, Wadden TA, Vogt RA, Brewer G. What is a reasonable weight loss? Patients' expectations and evaluations of obesity treatment outcomes. *J Consult Clinl Psychol.* 1997;65:79–85.

31. Golan M, Weizman A, Apter A, Fainaru M. Parents as the exclusive agents of change in the treatment of childhood obesity. *Amer J Clin Nutr.* 1998;67:1130–1135.

32. Graves T, Meyers AW, Clark L. An evaluation of parental problem-solving training in the behavioral treatment of childhood obesity. *J Consult Clin Psychol.* 1988;56(2):246–250.

33. The Writing Group for the Dietary Intervention Study in Children (DISC) Collaborative Research Group. Efficacy and safety of lowering dietary intake of fat and cholesterol in children with elevated low-density lipoprotein cholesterol. *JAMA.* 1995;273(18):1429–1435.

34. Epstein LH, Valoski AM, Kalarchian MA, McCurley J. Do children lose and maintain weight easier than adults: a comparison of child and parent weight changes from six months to ten years. *Obes Res.* 1995;3(5):411–417.

35. Epstein LH, Paluch RA, Raynor HA. Sex differences in obese children and siblings in family-based obesity treatment. *Obes Res.* 2001;9(12):746–753.

36. Epstein LH, Wing RR, Koeske R, Valoski A. Effect of parent weight on weight loss in obese children. *J Consult Clin Psychol.* 1986;54:400–401.

37. Epstein LH, Wing RR, Koeske R, Valoski A. Effects of diet plus exercise on weight change in parents and children. *J Consult Clin Psychol.* 1984;52(3):429–437.

38. Epstein L, Wing R, Koeske R, Valoski A. A comparison of lifestyle exercise, aerobic exercise, and calisthenics on weight loss in obese children. *Behav Ther.* 1985;16:345–356.

39. Epstein LH, Valoski AM, Vara LS, McCurley J, Wisniewski L, Kalarchian MA et al. Effects of decreasing sedentary behavior and increasing activity on weight change in obese children. *Health Psychol.* 1995;14(2):109–115.

40. Epstein LH, Paluch RA, Gordy CC, Saelens BE, Ernst MM. Problem solving in the treatment of childhood obesity. *J Consult Clin Psychol.* 2000;68(4):717–721.

41. Israel AC, Guile CA, Baker JE, Silverman WK. An evaluation of enhanced self-regulation training in the treatment of childhood obesity. *J Pediatr Psychol.* 1994;19(6):737–749.

42. Kirschenbaum DS, Harris ES, Tomarken AJ. Effects of parental involvement in behavioral weight loss therapy for preadolescents. *Behav Ther.* 1984;15:485–500.

43. Flodmark C-E, Ohlsson T, Ryden O, Sveger T. Prevention of progression to severe obesity in a group of obese schoolchildren treated with family therapy. *Pediatrics.* 1993;91(5):880–885.

44. Brownell KD, Kelman JH, Stunkard AJ. Treatment of obese children with and without their mothers: changes in weight and blood pressure. *Pediatrics.* 1983;71:515–523.

45. Becque MD, Katch VL, Rocchini AP, Marks CR, Moorehead C. Coronary risk incidence of obese adolescents: reduction by exercise plus diet intervention. *Pediatrics.* 1988;81(5):605–612.

46. Rocchini AP, Katch V, Anderson J, Hinderliter J, Becque D, Martin M, Marks C. Blood pressure in obese adolescents: effect of weight loss. *Pediatrics.* 1988;82(1):16–23.

47. Wadden TA, Stunkard AJ, Rich L, Rubin CJ, Sweidel G, McKinney S. Obesity in black adolescent girls: a controlled clinical trial of treatment by diet, behavior modification, and parental support. *Pediatrics.* 1990;85(3):345–352.

48. Coates TJ, Kilien JD, Slinkard L. Parent participation in a treatment program for overweight adolescents. *Intl J Eating Disord.* 1982;1(3):37–49.

49. Mellin LM, Slinkard LA, Irwin CE, Jr. Adolescent obesity intervention: validation of the SHAPEDOWN program. *J Amer Diet Assoc.* 1987;87(3):333–338.

50. Saelens BE, Sallis JF, Wilfley DE, Patrick K, Cella JA, Buchta R. Behavioral weight control for overweight adolescents initiated in primary care. *Obes Res.* 2002;10(1):22–32.

51. Golan M, Crow S. Targeting parents exclusively in the treatment of childhood obesity: long-term results. *Obes Res.* 2004;12(2):357–361.

52. Epstein LH, Wing RR, Koeske R, Valoski A. Long-term effects of family-based treatment of childhood obesity. *J Consult Clin Psychol.* 1987;55(1):91–95.

53. Epstein LH, Nudelman S, Wing RR. Long-term effects of family-based treatment for obesity on nontreated family members. *Behav Ther.* 1987;18(2):147–152.

54. Epstein LH, McKenzie SJ, Valoski A, Klein KR, Wing RR. Effects of mastery criteria and contingent reinforcement for family-based child weight control. *Addictive Behav.* 1994;19(2):135–145.

55. Israel AC, Stolmaker L, Andrian CA. The effects of training parents in general child management skills on a behavioral weight loss program for children. *Behav Ther.* 1985;16(2):169–180.

56. Epstein LH, Wing RR, Penner BC, Kress MJ. Effect of diet and controlled exercise on weight loss in obese children. *J Pediatr.* 1985;107(3):358–361.

57. Ebbeling CB, Leidig MM, Sinclair KB, Hangen JP, Ludwig DS. A reduced-glycemic load diet in the treatment of adolescent obesity. *Arch Pediatr Adol Med.* 2003;157(8):773–779.

58. Epstein LH, Paluch RA, Gordy CC, Dorn J. Decreasing sedentary behaviors in treating pediatric obesity. *Archiv Pediatr Adolesc Med.* 2000;154(3):220–226.

59. Brown R, Sothern M, Suskind R, Udall J, Blecker U. Racial differences in the lipid profiles of obese children and adolescents before and after significant weight loss. *Clin Pediatr* (Phila). 2000;39(7):427–431.

60. Chen W, Chen SC, Hsu HS, Lee C. Counseling clinic for pediatric weight reduction: program formulation and follow-up. *J Formosan Med Assoc.* 1997;96(1):59–62.

61. Eliakim A, Kaven G, Berger I, Friedland O, Wolach B, Nemet D. The effect of a combined intervention on body mass index and fitness in obese children and adolescents — a clinical experience. *Eur J Pediatr.* 2002;161(8):449–455.

62. Israel AC, Stolmaker L, Sharp JP, Silverman WK, Simon LG. An evaluation of two methods of parental involvement in treating obese children. *Behav Therap.* 1984;15:266–272.

63. Levine MD, Ringham RM, Kalarchian MA, Wisniewski L, Marcus MD. Is family-based behavioral weight control appropriate for severe pediatric obesity? *Intl J Eating Disord.* 2001;30:318–328.

64. Nuutinen O, Knip M. Long-term weight control in obese children: persistence of treatment outcome and metabolic changes. *Intl J Obes.* 1992;16:279–287.

65. Nuutinen O, Knip M. Weight loss, body composition and risk factors for cardiovascular disease in obese children: long-term effects of two treatment strategies. *J Amer Coll Nutr.* 1992;11(6):707–714.

66. Nuutinen O, Knip M. Predictors of weight reduction in obese children. *Europ J Clin Nutr.* 1992;46(11):785–794.

67. Resnicow K, Yaroch AL, Davis A Wang DT, Carter S, Slaughtr L, et al. GO GIRLS! Results from a nutrition and physical activity program for low-income, overweight African American adolescent females. *Health Educ Behav.* 2000;27(5):616–631.

68. Sothern MS, Hunter S, Suskind RM, Brown R, Udall JN, Blecker U. Motivating the obese child to move: the role of structured exercise in pediatric weight management. *South Med J.* 1999;92(6):577–584.

69. Sothern MS, Despinasse B, Brown R, Suskind RM, Udall JN Jr., Blecker U. Lipid profiles of obese children and adolescents before and after significant weight loss: differences according to sex. *South Med J.* 2000;93(3):278–282.

70. Sothern MS, Loftin JM, Udall JN, Suskind RM, Ewing TL, Tang SC, Blecker. Safety, feasibility, and efficacy of a resistance training program in preadolescent obese children. *Amer J Med Sci.* 2000;319(6):370–375.

71. Sothern, Udall JN, Jr., Suskind RM, Vargas A, Blecker U. Weight loss and growth velocity in obese children after very low calorie diet, exercise, and behavior modification. *Acta Paediatr.* 2000;89(9):1036–1043.

72. Sothern M, Schumacher H, von Almen K, Carlisle K, Udall J. Committed to kids: an integrated, four-level team approach to weight management in adolescents. *J Amer Diet Assoc.* 2002;102(3):S81–S85.

73. Spieth LE, Harnish JD, Lenders CM, Raezer LB, Pereira MA, Hangen SJ, Ludwig DS. A low-glycemic index diet in the treatment of pediatric obesity. *Arch Pediatr Adolesc Med.* 2000;154(9):947–951.

74. Suskind RM, Sothern MS, Farris RP et al. Recent advances in the treatment of childhood obesity. *Ann NY Acad Sci.* 1993;699:181–199.

75. Obarzanek E, Kimm SYS, Barton BA et al. Long-term safety and efficacy of a cholesterol-lowering diet in children with elevated low-density lipoprotein cholesterol: seven-year results of the dietary intervention study (DISC). *Pediatrics.* 2001;107(2):256–264.

76. Epstein LH, Wing RR, Valoski A, Gooding W. Long-term effects of parent weight on child weight loss. *Behav Ther.* 1987;18:219–226.

77. Epstein L. Methodological issues and ten-year outcomes for obese children. *Ann NY Acad Sci.* 1993;699:237–249.

# Section 7

## Exercise and Physical Activity

# 14 Increasing Physical Activity in Overweight Youth in Clinical Settings

*Melinda S. Sothern, Connie VanVrancken-Tompkins, Courtney Brooks, and Camille Thélin*

## CONTENTS

## INTRODUCTION

Unfortunately, today's American youth exhibit unhealthy lifestyle attitudes and practices toward physical activity [1–3]. Children of all ages are heavier and less active and are thus less physically fit [4–6]. Overweight children are caught in a vicious cycle because excess fat will, in turn, reduce activity because of joint discomfort and distressed breathing [7–9]. Once activity is reduced, body fat will continue to increase, creating even more aversion to exercise.

Educational studies indicate that physical fitness improves students' self image and promotes a positive school environment. Students who are physically fit are shown to be absent less often and illustrate higher academic achievement than nonfit students [10]. Children's feelings of self-worth or self-esteem begin developing in the early elementary years [11]. Some types of exercise training may improve self-esteem in prepubescent youth [12]. Furthermore, regular physical training may promote the attainment of self-esteem during the elementary years, which may transfer to improved self-worth in the later, more difficult, pubertal and postpubertal years. Exercise programs must be goal-oriented with easily attainable outcomes to ensure individual student success. Exercise techniques must be appropriate to the physical development level of the student.

Because children today are becoming more overweight and less active, it is important to establish baseline information regarding the child's performance before providing recommendations to increase physical activity or incorporate a structured exercise routine. This is particularly important for overweight children. Childhood is a critical time in which children's physical activity behaviors are formed and in which they develop healthy attitudes toward physical activity. Physicians and health care professionals should be actively involved in promoting physical activity to their patients [13]. There are several ways physicians and health care professionals can help their patients adopt a healthier and more physically active lifestyle. It is important that physicians and health care professionals take the time to assist their patients in developing physical activity programs, particularly for their overweight or obese patients [14].

## DETERMINANTS OF PHYSICAL ACTIVITY

Many factors are described as determinants of increased physical activity and adherence to exercise programs. Research conducted over the last decade has produced a vast amount of information concerning known determinants to physical activity adherence [15]. For example, biomedical status has been identified as a personal attribute that affects physical activity adherence. Conditions such as obesity promote resistance to the adoption of regular physical activity. However, research indicates that biomedical status, as a single factor, is not a powerful predictor of human behavior [15].

Environmental factors such as a perceived lack of time have been proposed as primary deterrents to physical activity. Although individuals report a lack of available time for physical activity, other complex issues affect this perception. Poor behavioral skills, that is, limit setting and time management, may contribute more to the lack of opportunity for physical activity, or the individual may lack adequate motivation to be physically active. Lack of time then becomes a perceived determinant as opposed to an environmental one. These fluctuations in context disable the prescription of appropriate physical activity interventions [15–17]. It may be important to observe these physical activity determinants with respect to specific races, genders, ages, and health status or fitness levels, and the different environments and orders in which these occur and interact.

Dishman suggests that past physical activity history may be a more reliable predictor of exercise adherence than the individual's intention to exercise [15]. Measuring self variables, such as perceived competence, self-efficacy, and self-esteem, may describe the psychological benefits associated with physical activity [16]; however, these variables do not predict behavior unless incentives are present or past history is considered [15].

Stucky-Ropp and DiLorenzo [18] explored factors among fifth and sixth graders that influenced their level of physical activity. Child enjoyment of physical activity was the most prominent predictor of exercise behavior. It was found, for both boys and girls, that the mothers' perception of barriers to exercise and their report of family social support were important predictors as well. On the contrary, only boys reported that the perception of modeling and support of exercise behavior from friends and family was important. In addition, only girls were highly influenced by the number of exercise-related pieces of equipment at home and parental modeling of exercise. The authors concluded that children are influenced by important socialized family variables. Furthermore, families serve as important learning environments for enhancing health-related behavior, including physical activity, in children. Perhaps targeting families rather than individuals may provide more of a beneficial effect. This has certainly been shown to be effective in multidisciplinary weight management [19–22]

Duncan et al. observed similar findings of social support for youth ages 10 to 14 years [23]. A positive correlation was observed with physical activity and youth who received parent, sibling, and friend support. In particular, youth who perceived a greater level of support from friends had higher levels of physical activity. Another positive correlation was observed between parents, siblings, and friends watching a game and the youth's level of physical activity [23].

Taylor et al. examined the relationship between specific components of physical activity during childhood and adolescence and exercise habits in adulthood [24]. An interesting finding was the inverse relationship between adult physical activity and those who were forced to exercise as preteens and during teen years. Also, there was an inverse correlation between adult physical activity and those who were encouraged to exercise during preteen years. These results indicate that being forced and encouraged during childhood may facilitate negative attitudes toward physical activity that may extend into adulthood [24].

Recent research, primarily within sport psychology studies, indicates that the concept described as "flow state" may give insight into factors which enhance the exercise experience [25]. A flow state is achieved during activities that totally absorb the individual. Qualitative descriptions by athletes of this condition indicate that achieving a flow state is an extremely enlightening and positive experience [25]. For the average individual engaged in exercise, achieving a flow state of some magnitude may enhance future exercise adherence. How achieving this state affects formerly sedentary individuals is another question worthy of investigation.

Young children are easily distracted and are incapable of focused activity for long periods of time. This contributes to the sporadic nature of their physical activity. Adults can engage in long-duration exercise easily because of their enhanced ability to concentrate. In addition, it may be possible for adults to achieve the semi-trance flow state, which allows them to participate without much mental effort. Although most individuals engage in activity because they enjoy the effort, children need activity to be fun for them to continue. Adults are more able to engage in challenging activities that may be slightly painful to reach performance or aesthetic goals. Young children, in contrast, are not concerned with appearance and are not overly concerned with winning or competition [26–28].

The idea of learned helplessness has been indicated as a probable reason for lack of motivation to participate in healthy behaviors [29]. Learned helplessness is a maladaptive habit of withdrawing from definable, manageable adversities through succumbing to everyday problems [30]. A learned helplessness response is shown by cognitive, motivational, and emotional deficits that follow exposure to uncontrollable events [31]. Learned helpless children justify the causes of bad events in their lives as stable in time, global in effect, and internal to themselves. Such children develop a cluster of helplessness deficiencies. These deficiencies include passivity/nonassertiveness, cognitive flaws/inability to recognize existing opportunities to control outcomes (e.g., unaware or unable to see alternatives), sadness, lowered self-esteem, lowered competitiveness/achievement oriented behaviors, and lack of initiative and persistence [32]. This conclusion is derived from studies reporting that deprived subjects display a sense of personal inadequacy, negative self-image, self-blame, pessimism, low achievement motivation [33], and the expectation of future incompetence compared with nondeprived counterparts.

Both children and adults avoid situations that they believe exceed their capabilities and make them feel helpless. They will, however, undertake and perform with self-confidence behaviors they believe they can do, and they will derive benefit. Given appropriate skills and incentives, personal efficacy beliefs are some major determinants of children's choice of behaviors. Personal efficacy beliefs can help determine how much effort children will expend, and how long they will sustain effort in dealing with uncomfortable or new situations [34]

## MOTIVATIONAL THEORIES AND MODELS

Modern strategies for chronic disease prevention and treatment include a variety of social learning theories and health promotion models. Many of these theories and models are based on the results of behavioral research. Because diseases related to poor lifestyle choices can be altered by changes in individual behavior patterns, the physician or health care professional should possess a thorough knowledge of these behavioral theories and models [35].

## THE THEORY OF PLANNED BEHAVIOR

The Theory of Planned Behavior attempts to clarify many of the issues that surround negative behavior patterns [36,37]. Because previous research in human behavior patterns failed to provide good predictors for behavior change, this theory was developed to account for many of the variables associated with alterations in behavior. These variables include individual attitude and disposition and specific personality traits [36]. The Theory of Planned Behavior, using central concepts from the behavioral sciences, provides a framework that allows the understanding and prediction of individual behavior patterns in specific situations and across a wide variety of personality types. This framework moderates the relationship of intention to behavior from perceived behavioral control. For instance, if perceived behavioral control is high, then the intention will convert to behavior. In contrast, if the perceived behavioral control is low, then it is not likely that the intention will convert to behavior [38].

Mummery et al. examined the Theory of Planned Behavior in predicted physical activity in a nationwide sample of Canadian school youth in grades 3, 5, 8, and 11 [39]. Measures included physical activity intention, attitude, subjective norm, and perceived behavioral control. Results of these specific measures explained 47% of the variability in predicting physical activity intention. In particular, perceived behavioral control made the largest contribution to predicting physical activity intention. Conversely, Trost et al. [40] observed that similar components of the Planned Behavior Theory could not account for a substantial portion of the variance in intentions or moderate-to-vigorous physical activity in sixth-grade youths. Further research is needed to determine the role of the Theory of Planned Behavior within the context of diet, physical activity, and obesity in children [38].

## THE HEALTH BELIEF MODEL

The Health Belief Model is based on the premise that people will perceive the severity and susceptibility of an issue/disease and be motivated to change (also called "readiness to act"). The Health Belief Model has been criticized because it was developed originally with a concern for public health issues. This model has not been received well in the pediatric community because children and adolescents typically perceive themselves as immortal. It is suggested that other outcomes other than disease prevention may motivate individuals to adopt an active lifestyle [38].

## SOCIAL COGNITIVE THEORY

Bandura suggests that before people alter their current lifestyle to that of a healthy one, they must have a knowledge of health risks associated with their present condition [41]. Because people self-evaluate their behavior, they abstain from behaviors that breed self-dissatisfaction. A challenge facing physicians and health care professionals is helping people believe they can, in fact, adapt a healthier lifestyle and help strengthen their belief in themselves that they do have the power and ability to make these changes.

According to Social Cognitive Theory, children are motivated to behave a certain way if they believe that the targeted behavior will benefit them and if they believe that they can do the intended behavior. Self-efficacy beliefs influence goals and shape the outcomes that individuals expect will be produced by their efforts. A person with high self-efficacy usually expects to see favorable results, whereas people with low self-efficacy tend to expect poor outcomes. Those people with low self-efficacy tend to give up easily, whereas those with high self-efficacy tend to overcome difficulties that they may encounter. Chronic disease treatment intervention programs for youth may be enhanced through the application of the training concepts of social cognitive theory.

Although individuals may know the health risks associated with negative behaviors, it is self-efficacy that governs whether they will translate that knowledge into a more healthful behavior. For instance, those with low self-efficacy, although aware of the health risks, still will take no action, whereas those with high levels of self-efficacy will combine their beliefs with positive outcome expectations. Stated simply, individuals with high levels of self-efficacy believe that the benefits of adapting a healthy lifestyle will outweigh the disadvantages of the lifestyle change. Sonstroem suggests that no matter what model is used to analyze physical activity behaviors, it is vital that it is used repeatedly over time and as a complete and whole intervention [16]. In Chapter 5, Schwimmer provides a detailed summary of other related motivational theories and models.

## MOTIVATIONAL TECHNIQUES TO INCREASE PHYSICAL ACTIVITY

### INITIAL EVALUATION

Before prescribing any type of physical activity program, physicians and health care professionals should evaluate their patient's level of self-efficacy. Those patients with a high level of self-efficacy need minimal guidance and can succeed in changing their behavior in most situations; however, those with little to no self-efficacy beliefs need a great deal of personal guidance and structure. Positive reinforcement and progressive successes will build belief in the patients' abilities and help with any difficulties or setbacks they may encounter.

Because physical activity without caloric restriction may yield only small reductions in weight, particularly in obese patients, physicians and health care professionals should encourage their patients to adjust their dietary habits as well. The physician and health care professional should make aware the benefits of slow, modest weight loss including significant reductions in cardiovascular morbidity and mortality, decrease of fat, increase of muscle mass, and an enhanced sense of psychological well-being [14]. To provide safe exercise guidelines, the American College of Sports Medicine recommends an evaluation of coexisting cardiovascular risk factors or musculoskeletal conditions for patients; however, most overweight or obese patients can begin an exercise program with a gradual increase in physical activity [42,43]

In addition to evaluating a patient's level of self-efficacy, the individual's readiness to begin a physical activity program should be assessed [44]. The physician or health care professional should consider whether the patient has come to them seeking help and whether they recognize the need for weight loss. The patient's motivation and stress levels should be assessed and discussed, along with the subject's relationship with food, as this may warrant other forms of counseling as well. Both the physician or health care professional and the patient should play an active role in developing a physical activity program with activities that the patient feels that he or she can perform successfully. In addition, the physician or health care professional and patient should develop achievable goals together [45].

To achieve greater physical activity compliance, the physician or health care professional should take the time to understand and discuss any social or physical barriers the patient might encounter that would be associated with being physically active. These barriers can include an overweight or obese parent, feeling uncomfortable exercising in public, or thinking that certain exercises have to be painful or extremely vigorous to be beneficial [46]. In promoting physical activity with their patients, physicians or health care professionals should help establish realistic expectations and correct overly pessimistic or optimistic attitudes. Both long- and short-term goals should be established, as well as routine times and places for physical activity. The physician or health care professional should relay the benefits of social support and prepare patients for situations that may present challenges to exercising (i.e., holidays). The patient should develop some sort of contract with the health professional and practice self-reinforcement with rewards [47]. In addition to a physical activity program, daily lifestyle activities should be emphasized as a way to increase overall physical activity levels and energy expenditure [47,48].

Research indicates that children have an intrinsic natural need to be physically active. Young animals, including humans, are inherently active [26]. Therefore, children will be active if given encouragement and opportunity. Childhood activity is often intermittent and sporadic in behavior

[49]. Thus, children will not likely do prolonged exercise without rest periods. Physical activity patterns vary with children of different developmental and ability levels. Young children may not be attracted to high-intensity sports performance activities; older children may be [27]. The amount of total daily activity (volume) is a good indicator of childhood activity. If given the opportunity, young children will perform relatively large volumes of intermittent physical activity [26,49].

## Music as a Motivational Tool

Priest et al. investigated the presence of music as a motivational tool for exercise [50]. It was found that motivational qualities of music are heightened when the music is delivered at a higher volume and that females reported that music was of higher importance than did males. In addition, the participants reported that the music facilitated their performance on cardiovascular equipment more so than on any other equipment. The researchers also found an effect of music compared with age. Whereas older adults (36 to 45 years) preferred noncurrent music, the youngest age group (16 to 26) preferred current music and dance music [50].

## Team (Group) versus Individual Physical Activity

Researchers suggest that a task-orientation approach to physical activity and sport will promote higher levels of moral reasoning in children [51]. With this approach, outcome goals such as winning or scoring are replaced with individual self-referenced criteria and mastery of specific skills. Individual goal setting in sport and exercise has been shown to be a reliable motivational technique and may improve exercise and sport performance [51,52]. The use of cooperative team concepts such as buddy systems can enhance the safety and effectiveness of exercise programs. Teacher and health care professionals should focus the student's attention toward achieving personal goals as opposed to team competitive goals.

## Individualizing Physical Activity Programs

King and colleagues suggest that exercise-promoting interventions be specifically tailored to the individual needs of each participant, especially as these needs relate to age, race, and gender [53]. For example, overweight children are physiologically and emotionally different from children of normal weight [29]. Therefore, successful intervention may depend on the use of specialized exercise programs designed to meet the overweight child's specific needs [54]. If the student is cognitively ready to receive the information and physiologically capable of performing the physical task, then the instructor should experience success in motivating the obese child to participate in the physical activity, encouraging the child to maintain increased physical activity patterns, and promoting the student's acquisition of educational concepts that support the physical activity [55].

In the last few years, researchers have unanimously adopted the multidisciplinary intervention model as a viable treatment for childhood obesity. The term *multidisciplinary* may be defined as that which includes more than two interactions from individuals, and treatment or interventions from different areas of study, expertise, or disciplines. The term is used loosely in medical research, referring to any treatment intervention in which professionals from different medical fields collaborate [56,57]. This model allows for the blending of behavioral techniques that promote increased self-efficacy recommendations individualized to the participant.

## Application of Social Cognition Theory to Promote Physical Activity in Multidisciplinary Settings

Social cognition theory [34] provides training ideas that influence motivation to adopt any behavior (e.g., diet modification and physical activity) based on individual self-efficacy beliefs. Self-efficacy beliefs are learned from four separate sources: knowledge transfer, emotional or physiological responses when associated with behavioral performance, clear success or failure events or mastery experiences, and vicarious experiences through observational learning or through modeling and imitation [29]. Social cognitive theory recognizes a shared blend of these self-efficacy beliefs, which are interacting determinants of each other. An example of the use of these four separate sources of self efficacy is found in an intervention by Sothern and colleagues [55,58–60] as follows.

## Increasing Daily Energy Expenditures: The Moderate Intensity Progressive Exercise Program Step

The initial class sets the stage for subsequent lessons in increasing daily energy expenditures. The Moderate Intensity Progressive Exercise Program (MPEP) step (Appendices A3.1, A3.3) is a fitness-/behavior-modeling tool that provides immediate motivational instruction during the very first class. Students are instructed to stand erect, hold their shoulders back, and walk briskly around the room. Using Bandura's concepts described earlier, this session provides an example of his theory that may be applied to the exercise setting.

### Mastery Experience and Role Modeling

The participant becomes energized and feels taller, slimmer, and more in control through the action of lifting the chin, pulling the shoulders back, keeping the tummy tight, and taking quick, long steps. Additional motivation is derived from the fact that more calories will be burned, weight will be lost even before the diet is begun, and the participants will feel and look fitter, taller, and healthier.

### Knowledge Transfer

Information on the value of increasing daily activity patterns is transferred through the illustration of the term *work*: work = force × distance; force = weight moved (simplified); distance = area covered in one step. When more space is covered in a step, more work is performed in the same amount of time, and thus more calories are burned. Sitting in a chair burns approximately 35–50 calories per hour, standing burns approximately 60–65 calories per hour, and just walking casually burns 150 to 300 calories per hour. For verbal cues please refer to Appendix A1.

### Physiologic Feedback

Participants are instructed to observe their muscles as they contract, relax, and stretch. The patients are told that diets will quickly take off weight; however, unless the amount of activity each day is increased, the weight will be back in a very short time. Any time an individual moves a body part, one or more muscles contract or become shorter. The human body needs energy or "calories" to make the muscles do this. The body gets these calories either from the food that is eaten or from the stored fat in the body. The metabolic systems of the body and cardiopulmonary, aerobic exercise are listed in Table 14.1 and detailed in Chapter 20 and Appendices A3.1 and A3.3.

## Muscular Strength & Endurance: The MPEP Pump! (Chapter 20; Appendices A3.1, A3.3)

Another objective within the MPEP program is the improvement of body movement awareness. The objective is based on the assumption that if an individual becomes competent at knowing which part of the body is responsible for a particular movement, he or she will then be able to identify safe and effective exercise. A balanced, symmetrical physique will promote long-term health in several ways. Injury will be deterred by the prevention of weak areas in the muscles. Balanced training will improve posture, resulting in a taller appearance. Through an improved perception of body size, the individual will experience increased self-esteem. He or she will be able to discriminate between movement that will enhance fitness and appearance, and that which may injure. This body

**TABLE 14.1**

**Illustrations of the Six Basic Areas of the Exercise Component and Examples in Each of the Four Concepts**

| Physical Activity Lessons | Mastery | Knowledge | Role Models | Physiological Feedback |
|---|---|---|---|---|
| The MPEP step: increasing daily energy | Participant becomes energized, feels taller and thinner | Movement burns calories; definition of work | Individuals who walk briskly | Body parts moving as muscles contract. Brisk pace is energizing |
| Body locomotion: The engines of the body; metabolic systems: aerobic and anaerobic | The concept of the body as an engine is easily understood | Anaerobic and aerobic metabolism | Olympic power lifters; marathon runners, track and field stars, basketball stars | Rate of perceived exertion: student can identify vigorous or mild activity |
| Cardiorespiratory endurance: aerobic exercise | Low-impact aerobics are easy to perform | Many activities are aerobic; how to take a heart rate | Sport celebrities, mother and father, teacher | Students feel different muscles working, feel the heart rate pulse |
| The MPEP pump: muscular strength and endurance | Student's muscles control movement; strength exercises are easy to execute | Trained muscles are stronger and burn calories. | Television and movie celebrities; the muscles of the body; negative: fat tissue model. | Feeling muscles shorten to move limb; visualizing muscles as tight, strong |
| Stretch and flex: muscular flexibility | Posture is enhanced — feeling of well-being | Balanced posture and body symmetry. | Negative: poor posture, lordosis, kyphosis | Observe personal body imbalance |
| Body composition | Students will feel successful after losing fat weight | Healthy ranges of fat in the body | Athletes and people who exercise frequently | Clothes feel loose; muscles feel tight |

movement awareness will contribute to a feeling of control over the student's near environment, enabling him or her to know precisely which muscles are responsible for certain movements. With this knowledge comes the power to gain self-control, self-discipline, and a healthy mind and body.

Young children should be provided opportunities to safely climb, run, and jump to encourage the development of muscular strength and endurance [60]. The health benefits of strength training in children include the following: improved strength, increased power, improved muscular endurance, increased bone density and tendon–bone interface strength, improved motor performance, enhanced self-satisfaction, increased self-esteem, and positive body image. The prepubescent child in particular is at an increased risk of injury as a result of a reduction in joint flexibility caused by rapid growth in the long bones. The results of strength training provide additional resistance to sports injury in the prepubescent child and reduce the incidence of overuse injury.

Moderate aerobic exercise combined with high-repetition resistance training and behavioral modification is most efficacious for reducing body composition variables in overweight children. A metaanalysis examined 30 childhood obesity treatment studies that included an exercise intervention. Significant decreases in body composition were associated with programs that combined low-intensity aerobic with high-repetition strength training [60,61].

Muscular strength and endurance are discussed as the instructor passes around plastic models of lean tissue and fat tissue for the students to observe and feel. The function of the muscle as a shortening unit to lift and lower body parts is illustrated (Chapter 20, Appendix A3.3).

## Mastery

Mastery is achieved immediately as students realize the muscular control they possess, naturally, to move the individual body parts. Likewise, there is instantaneous physiological feedback as the students "feel" the muscles shorten and lengthen. The strength circuit exercises are easy to execute when performed with the recommended amount of weight or resistance. Students are amazed at how easily they can achieve the prescribed number of repetitions with the hand and leg weights.

## Knowledge Transfer and Physiological Feedback

Knowledge of how the muscles function is transferred through the class discussion. The importance of practice or repeating the movement to "teach the muscles" to become stronger, more dense, and tighter achieves both knowledge transfer and physiological feedback.

## Role Modeling

The plastic fat and lean tissue models serve as desired and undesired outcomes. Positive role models such as television and movie celebrities are used to motivate the students. The muscles themselves become role models, taking on an animated character of their own through the verbal cues described above. The remaining topics, muscular flexibility and body fat composition, are summarized in Table 14.1 and detailed in Chapter 20 and Appendices A3.1, A3.3.

The lessons described above are examples from a specialized program called MPEP by Sothern et al. [55,58–60] that consists of a system of knowledge that organizes the educational content according to social cognitive theory [62]. It is designed to ensure that the recommended physical activities may be successfully performed by individuals with various overweight conditions. In addition, the educational content is organized in a developmentally appropriate manner that is easily comprehended by students of all ages. Therefore, the program is designed to better serve the emotional and cognitive, as well as physiologic, needs of obese individuals. By providing activities that illicit initial success, it is proposed that the program will improve mastery concepts, thereby increasing self-efficacy beliefs. Because knowledge of the positive outcome of the desired behavior change is central to the application of social learning theories ("learning" is even in the title), the specialized program is also designed according to established curriculum design principles, follows behavioral learning and cognitive/developmental theories, and is based on well-accepted instructional methodologies. The specialized exercise curriculum design provides content knowledge in health and fitness through participation in physical activities and instructional sessions. By using a specialized exercise curriculum design, the concepts of social cognitive theory are implemented.

When designing exercise programs for obese children, the instructor should consider activities that are easily mastered. Such activities will ensure that students experience initial success when participating in physical activity if adherence to the program is desired [55,59]. Competitive programs with nonobese counterparts may not be appropriate because of the limited physiologic capacity of the obese child and the additional risk of injury resulting from excess weight on the premature musculoskeletal system [63–65]. The Moderate Intensity Progressive Exercise Program by Sothern et al. [55,58–60] provides guidelines for duration, frequency, and intensity of exercise for at risk for overweight, overweight, and severely overweight children (Figure 14.1, Figure 14.2, Figure 14.3). These guidelines are conservative and progressive, increasing gradually over time. This is to ensure safety and to promote the attainment of mastery in the overweight students.

The MPEP program is specific to the different levels of overweight (i.e., initially the severely overweight students have shorter beginning durations and frequencies than do the overweight or at risk for overweight students) (Figure 14.1, Figure 14.2). In addition, because excess fat weight places an increased burden on an individual's cardiorespiratory and musculoskeletal systems, the recommended exercise activities for the moderate and severely obese children are arm specific and less weight bearing. Students are allowed to choose the type of aerobic activity from an extensive list provided by the instructor. The guidelines are discussed in greater detail in Chapter 20.

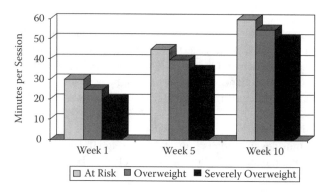

**FIGURE 14.1** Moderate intensity progressive exercise, prescribed duration of exercise.

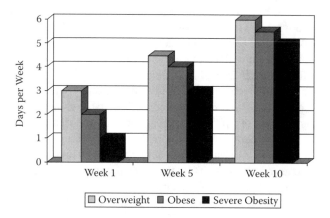

**FIGURE 14.2** Moderate intensity progressive exercise, prescribed frequency of exercise.

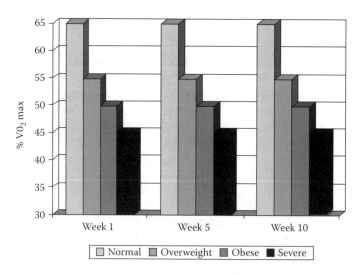

**FIGURE 14.3** Moderate intensity progressive exercise, prescribed intensity of exercise.

A recent study examined changes in self-reported physical activity versus prescribed MPEP physical activity guidelines in children with increasing levels of BMI [66] (Figure 14.4, Figure 14.5, Figure 14.6, Figure 14.7). Eighteen overweight children were enrolled in the Louisiana State University Health Sciences Center pediatric weight management program. Measures of weight and

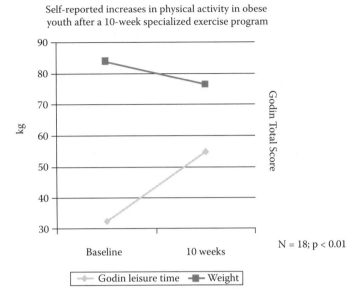

FIGURE 14.4 Reduction in body weight and increase in physical activity.

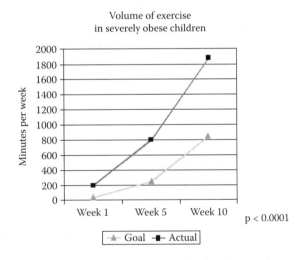

FIGURE 14.5 Self-reported (actual) vs. prescribed (goal) exercise in severely overweight (≥ 99th %BMI) youth.

height were obtained at both baseline and 10 weeks. The program, based on social cognitive theory [62], included the MPEP program and a low-calorie diet, supplemented with extra fluid, minerals, and vitamins. Subjects were given a Godin Leisure-Time Exercise Questionnaire [67]. After completion, each was scored accordingly: total number of 15-minute intervals of strenuous, moderate, and mild exercise completed for each week. The subjects met weekly to evaluate progress and also completed exercise report cards, listing individual daily activity volume (frequency × duration). From baseline to 10 weeks, weight and BMI significantly decreased (Figure 14.4). In addition, there was a significant increase in the Godin coded scores and self-reported exercise volume from baseline to 10 weeks (Figure 14.4). More important, when the prescribed volume of exercise was compared with that self-reported by the overweight children, significant differences were observed in at-risk, overweight, and especially severely overweight youth (Figure 14.5, Figure 14.6, Figure 14.7).

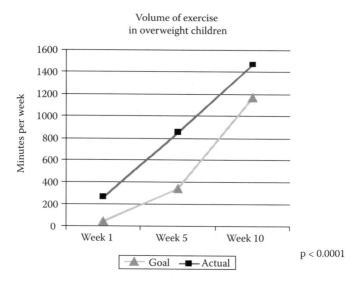

**FIGURE 14.6** Self-reported (actual) vs. prescribed (goal) exercise in overweight (≥ 95% BMI) youth,

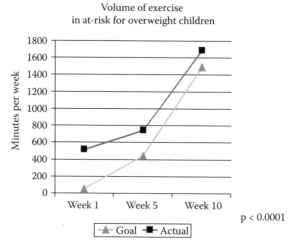

**FIGURE 14.7** Self-reported (actual) vs. prescribed (goal) exercise in at-risk for overweight (≤ 85% BMI) youth.

Children consistently self-reported a significantly greater volume of exercise than what was prescribed. These results reinforce the concept that exercise programs for overweight youth should first seek to increase mastery concepts by establishing clear, attainable goals that gradually increase in volume over time. In these physically inactive youth, an incremental approach with increases of approximately 10% per week is recommended [68]. Progressing too quickly is counter-productive and leads to injury.

## SUMMARY

Changing health habits requires both motivation and self-regulatory skills. Individuals must learn to monitor their health behavior and use proximal goals to motivate themselves. Realistic, attainable goals are desired, and therefore, information concerning the initial health, abilities, fitness levels, and interests of the patients are essential. Social support from family and peers will help sustain

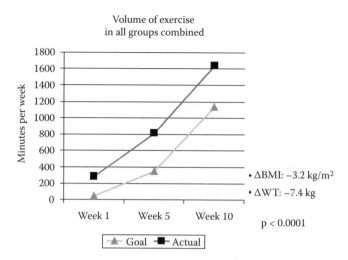

**FIGURE 14.8** Self-reported (actual) vs. prescribed (goal) exercise in overweight youth.

their efforts as long as it provides the type of support that enhances their self-efficacy. The health care professional must provide ongoing supervision and guidance. Individuals with increasing levels of overweight conditions will respond differently to exercise of differing modalities and intensities. In specialized populations such as these, clinicians and educators are at a great disadvantage when attempting to prescribe appropriate activities and deliver educational interventions. By implementing specialized programs that address these issues, successful prevention and treatment of pediatric obesity may be possible. Clinical treatment intervention programs designed to promote behavior change should contain activities structured to the specific physical, emotional, and cognitive needs of the participants. Physical activities for overweight individuals should be appropriate to their specific physiologic needs. Educational activities should be based on well-established curriculum design principles to ensure successful motivation and a positive learning environment.

## REFERENCES

1. Baranowski, T., C. Bouchard, O. Bar-Or et al. Assessment, prevalence, and cardiovascular benefits of physical activity and fitness in youth. *Med Sci Sports Exerc.* 24:S237–S247, 1992.
2. Strong, W. B. Physical activity and children. *Circulation.* 81:1697–1701, 1990.
3. Armstrong, N., J. Balding, P. Gentle, and B. Kirby. Estimation of coronary risk factors in British schoolchildren: a preliminary report. *Br J Sports Med.* 24:61–66, 1990.
4. Centers for Disease Control and Prevention. Update: prevalence of overweight among children, adolescents, and adults — United States, 1988-1994. *Morb Mortal Wkly Rep.* 46:198–202, 1997.
5. Sallis, J. F. Epidemiology of physical activity and fitness in children and adolescents. *Crit Rev Food Sci Nutr.* 33:403–408, 1993.
6. Sallis, J. F., B. G. Simons-Morton, E. J. Stone et al. Determinants of physical activity and interventions in youth. *Med Sci Sports Exerc.* 24:S248–S257, 1992.
7. McGoey, B. V., M. Deitel, R. J. Saplys, and M. E. Kliman. Effect of weight loss on musculoskeletal pain in the morbidly obese. *J Bone Joint Surg Br.* 72:322–323, 1990.
8. Taylor, W. and T. Baranowski. Physical activity, cardiovascular fitness, and adiposity in children. *Res Q Exerc Sport.* 62:157–163, 1991.
9. Lusky, A., V. Barell, F. Lubin, G. Kaplan, V. Layani, Z. Shohat, B. Lev, and M. Wiener. Relationship between morbidity and extreme values of body mass index in adolescents. *Intl J Epidemiol.* 25:829–834, 1996.
10. Hennessy, B. Administrative exercises to shape up a school fitness program. *Thrust.* 18:8–11, 1988.
11. O'Brien, S. J. How can I help my preadolescent? *Childhood Educ.* 66:35–36, 1989.

12. Metcalf, J. A. and S. O. Roberts. Strength training and the immature athlete: an overview. *Pediatr Nurs.* 19:325–332, 1993.

13. McWhorter, J. W., H. W. Wallmann, and P. T. Alpert. The obese child: motivation as a tool for exercise. *J Pediatr Health Care.* 17:11–17, 2003.

14. McInnis, K. J., B. A. Franklin, and J. M. Rippe. Counseling for physical activity in overweight and obese patients. *Am Fam Physician.* 67:1249–1256, 2003.

15. Dishman, R. K. The measurement conundrum in exercise adherence research. *Med Sci Sports Exerc.* 26:1382–1390, 1994.

16. Sonstroem, R. J. Physical self-concept: assessment and external validity. *Exerc Sport Sci Rev.* 26:133–164, 1998.

17. Chalip, L., Csikszentmihalyi, M., Kleiber, D., Larson, R. Variations of experience in formal and informal sport. *Res Q Exerc Sport.* 35:109–116, 1984.

18. Stucky-Ropp, R. C. and T. M. DiLorenzo. Determinants of exercise in children. *Prev Med.* 22:880–889, 1993.

19. Epstein, L. H., K. R. Klein, and L. Wisniewski. Child and parent factors that influence psychological problems in obese children. *Intl J Eat Disord.* 15:151–158, 1994.

20. Epstein, L. H., A. Valoski, R. Koeske, and R. R. Wing. Family-based behavioral weight control in obese young children. *J Am Diet Assoc.* 86:481–484, 1986.

21. Epstein, L. H., A. Valoski, R. R. Wing, and J. McCurley. Ten-year follow-up of behavioral, family-based treatment for obese children. *JAMA.* 264:2519–2523, 1990.

22. Epstein, L. H., R. R. Wing, R. Koeske, and A. Valoski. Effect of parent weight on weight loss in obese children. *J Consult Clin Psychol.* 54:400–401, 1986.

23. Duncan, S. C., T. E. Duncan, and L. A. Strycker. Sources and types of social support in youth physical activity. *Health Psychol.* 24:3–10, 2005.

24. Taylor, W. C., S. N. Blair, S. S. Cummings, C. C. Wun, and R. M. Malina. Childhood and adolescent physical activity patterns and adult physical activity. *Med Sci Sports Exerc.* 31:118–123, 1999.

25. Jackson, S. A. Athletes in flow: a qualitative investigation of flow states in elite figure skaters. *J Appl Sport Psychol.* 4:161–180, 1992.

26. French, S. A., C. L. Perry, G. R. Leon, and J. A. Fulkerson. Food preferences, eating patterns, and physical activity among adolescents: correlates of eating disorders symptoms. *J Adolesc Health.* 15:286–294, 1994.

27. Borra, S. T., N. E. Schwartz, C. G. Spain, and M. M. Natchipolsky. Food, physical activity, and fun: inspiring America's kids to more healthful lifestyles. *J Am Diet Assoc.* 95:816–823, 1995.

28. Moore, L. L., U. S. Nguyen, K. J. Rothman, L. A. Cupples, and R. C. Ellison. Preschool physical activity level and change in body fatness in young children. The Framingham Children's Study. *Am J Epidemiol.* 142:982–988, 1995.

29. Hunter, S., Johnson, C.C., Little-Christian, S. et al. Heart Smart: a multifactorial approach to cardio-vascular risk reduction for grade school students. *Am J Health Promot.* 4:352–360, 1990.

30. Braden, C. J. Learned self-help response to chronic illness experience: a test of three alternative learning theories. *Sch Inq Nurs Pract.* 4:23–41; discussion 43–25, 1990.

31. Garber, J. and S. D. Hollon. Universal versus personal helplessness in depression: belief in uncontrollability or incompetence? *J Abnorm Psychol.* 89:56–66, 1980.

32. Nolen-Hoeksema, S., J. S. Girgus, and M. E. Seligman. Learned helplessness in children: a longitudinal study of depression, achievement, and explanatory style. *J Pers Soc Psychol.* 51:435–442, 1986.

33. Fincham, F. D., A. Hokoda, and R. Sanders, Jr. Learned helplessness, test anxiety, and academic achievement: a longitudinal analysis. *Child Dev.* 60:138–145, 1989.

34. Bandura, A. *Social Foundations on Thought and Action: A Social Cognition Theory.* Englewood Cliffs, NJ: Prentice-Hall, Inc., 1986.

35. Blair, J. E. Social learning theory: strategies for health promotion. *J Amer Assoc Occup Hlth Nurses.* 41:245–249, 1993.

36. Ajzen, I. The theory of planned behavior. *Organiz Behav Hum Decision Processes.* 50:179–211, 1991.

37. Crawley, F. E., Koballa, R.R. Attitude research in science education: contemporary models and methods. *Sci Educ.* 78:35–55, 1994.

38. Baranowski, T., K. W. Cullen, T. Nicklas, D. Thompson, and J. Baranowski. Are current health behavioral change models helpful in guiding prevention of weight gain efforts? *Obes Res.* 11 Suppl:23S–43S, 2003.

39. Mummery, W. K., J. C. Spence, and J. C. Hudec. Understanding physical activity intention in Canadian school children and youth: an application of the theory of planned behavior. *Res Q Exerc Sport.* 71:116–124, 2000.

40. Trost, S. G., R. Saunders, and D. S. Ward. Determinants of physical activity in middle school children. *Am J Health Behav.* 26:95–102, 2002.

41. Bandura, A. Health promotion by social cognitive means. *Health Educ Behav.* 31:143–164, 2004.

42. Pollock, M. G. Gaesser, J. Butcher, J. Despres, R. Dishman, B. Franklin et al. American College of Sports Medicine Position Stand. The recommended quantity and quality of exercise for developing and maintaining cardiorespiratory and muscular fitness, and flexibility in healthy adults. *Med Sci Sports Exerc.* 30:975–991, 1998.

43. American College of Sports Medicine. *ACSM's Guidelines for Testing and Prescription*, 6th ed. Baltimore, MD: Lippincott, Williams & Wilkins, 2000.

44. Barriers to guideline adherence. Based on a presentation by Michael Cabana, MD. *Am J Manag Care.* 4:S741–S744; discussion S745–S748, 1998.

45. Kushner, R. F. and R. L. Weinsier. Evaluation of the obese patient. Practical considerations. *Med Clin North Am.* 84:387–399, 2000.

46. Albright, C. L., S. Cohen, L. Gibbons, S. Miller, B. Marcus, J. Sallis, K. Imai, J. Jernick, and D. G. Simons-Morton. Incorporating physical activity advice into primary care: physician-delivered advice within the activity counseling trial. *Am J Prev Med.* 18:225–234, 2000.

47. Gordon, P. M., G. W. Heath, A. Holmes, and D. Christy. The quantity and quality of physical activity among those trying to lose weight. *Am J Prev Med.* 18:83–86, 2000.

48. Jakicic, J. M., R. R. Wing, B. A. Butler, and R. J. Robertson. Prescribing exercise in multiple short bouts versus one continuous bout: effects on adherence, cardiorespiratory fitness, and weight loss in overweight women. *Int J Obes Relat Metabol Disord.* 19:893–901, 1995.

49. Bailey, R. C., J. Olson, S. L. Pepper, J. Porszasz, T. J. Barstow, and D. M. Cooper. The level and tempo of children's physical activities: an observational study. *Med Sci Sports Exerc.* 27:1033–1041, 1995.

50. Priest, D. L., C. I. Karageorghis, and N. C. Sharp. The characteristics and effects of motivational music in exercise settings: the possible influence of gender, age, frequency of attendance, and time of attendance. *J Sports Med Phys Fitness.* 44:77–86, 2004.

51. Kylo, B. and D. Landers. Goal setting in sport and exercise: a research synthesis to resolve the controversy. *J Sport Exercise Psychol.* 17:117–137, 1995.

52. Lerner, B. and E. Locke. The effects of goal setting, self-efficacy, competition, and personal traits on the performance of an endurance task. *J Sport Exercise Psychol.* 17:138–152, 1995.

53. King, A. C., C. B. Taylor, W. L. Haskell, and R. F. DeBusk. Influence of regular aerobic exercise on psychological health: a randomized, controlled trial of healthy middle-aged adults. *Health Psychol.* 8:305–324, 1989.

54. Neiman, D. *Fitness and Sports Medicine: An Introduction.* Palo Alto, CA: Bull Publishing Co., 1990

55. Sothern, M. S., S. Hunter, R. M. Suskind, R. Brown, J. N. Udall Jr., and U. Blecker. Motivating the obese child to move: the role of structured exercise in pediatric weight management. *South Med J.* 92:577–584, 1999.

56. Figueroa-Colon, R., T. K. von Almen, F. A. Franklin, C. Schuftan, and R. M. Suskind. Comparison of two hypocaloric diets in obese children. *Am J Dis Child.* 147:160–166, 1993.

57. Tuiten, A., A. Jansen, and H. P. Koppeschaar. Anorexia, bulimia, and exercise-induced amenorrhea: multidisciplinary approach. *Curr Ther Endocrinol Metabol.* 5:12–15, 1994.

58. Sothern, M. S., H. Schumacher, T. K. von Almen, L. K. Carlisle, and J. N. Udall. Committed to kids: an integrated, 4-level team approach to weight management in adolescents. *J Am Diet Assoc.* 102:S81–S85, 2002.

59. Sothern, M. S. Exercise as a modality in the treatment of childhood obesity. *Pediatr Clin North Am.* 48:995–1015, 2001.

60. Sothern, M., T. K. von Almen, and H. Schumach. *Trim-Kids: The Proven Plan That Has Helped Thousands of Children Achieve a Healthier Weight.* New York: Harper Collins, 2001.

61. LeMura, L. M. and M. T. Maziekas. Factors that alter body fat, body mass, and fat-free mass in pediatric obesity. *Med Sci Sports Exerc.* 34:487–496, 2002.

62. Bandura, A., D. Cioffi, C. B. Taylor, and M. E. Brouillard. Perceived self-efficacy in coping with cognitive stressors and opioid activation. *J Pers Soc Psychol.* 55:479–488, 1988.

63. Van Itallie, T. Health implications of overweight and obesity in the United States. *Ann Intern Med.* 103:983–988, 1992.

64. Felson, D. T., Y. Zhang, J. M. Anthony, A. Naimark, and J. J. Anderson. Weight loss reduces the risk for symptomatic knee osteoarthritis in women. The Framingham Study. *Ann Intern Med.* 116:535–539, 1992.

65. Davis, M. A., W. H. Ettinger, and J. M. Neuhaus. Obesity and osteoarthritis of the knee: evidence from the National Health and Nutrition Examination Survey (NHANES I). *Semin Arthritis Rheum.* 20:34–41, 1990.

66. Reed, J., C. Van Vrancken, M. Loftin, C. Singley, J. Udall and M. Sothern. Self reported increases in physical activity in obese youth after a 10-week specialized moderate intensity exercise program. *Obes Res.* 9(3), 159S, 2001.

67. Godin, G. and R. J. Shephard. Gender differences in perceived physical self-efficacy among older individuals. *Percept Mot Skills.* 60:599–602, 1985.

68. Strong, W., R. Malina, C. Blimkie, S. Daniels et al. Evidence-based physical activity for school-aged youth. *J Pediatr.* 146:732–737, 2005.

# 15 Exercise and Physical Activity: Exercise Training Programs and Metabolic Health

*Scott Owens*

## CONTENTS

## INTRODUCTION

Pediatric obesity is often associated with a poor metabolic profile. Data from the third National Health and Nutrition Examination Survey indicate that although the prevalence of metabolic syndrome in 12 to 19 year olds of normal body weight (body mass index [BMI] < 85th percentile) was relatively low (<1%), nearly 30% of overweight adolescents (BMI ≥ 95th percentile) met criteria for metabolic syndrome [1]. Accordingly, health care professionals involved in pediatric obesity management are interested in monitoring not only changes in the obesity status of their clients but also to changes in their patients' metabolic status as well. Interventions that positively affect the metabolic profile of obese youths are therefore of considerable interest.

This chapter examines the effects of exercise interventions on metabolic health in pediatric obesity. A brief discussion of the components of metabolic health usually targeted in exercise programs is presented first. Next, the effects of exercise on the individual components of metabolic health are presented. That discussion is followed by summary observations regarding the components of successful exercise interventions relative to mode, intensity, duration, frequency of exercise, and length of intervention.

## COMPONENTS OF METABOLIC HEALTH IN THE PEDIATRIC OBESITY/EXERCISE LITERATURE

Research on the effects of exercise on metabolic health in pediatric obesity has tended to focus on components of the metabolic syndrome as described in adults — that is, dyslipidemia, hyperglycemia, hypertension, and abdominal obesity. Although a uniform definition of the metabolic syndrome has yet to be established for the pediatric population [2], recent reviews on the topic have recommended measurements in youths that mirror those used with adults and include triglycerides and high-density lipoprotein-cholesterol (HDL-C) to characterize dyslipidemia, fasting glucose (or a glucose tolerance test) to characterize hyperglycemia, resting systolic and diastolic blood pressure to characterize hypertension, and waist circumference to characterize abdominal obesity [1,2]. This chapter focuses primarily on these components of metabolic health, with the effects of exercise on fasting insulin (a risk factor for the development of type II diabetes) and on visceral adipose tissue (a more precise measure of abdominal obesity risk) also being presented.

## EFFECTS OF EXERCISE ON COMPONENTS OF METABOLIC HEALTH

There have been relatively few training studies reporting on the effects of exercise on the metabolic health of obese youths. Table 15.1 summarizes the studies most pertinent to this discussion. These studies involved obese children or adolescents; included an exercise intervention lasting at least 6 weeks; provided details relative to exercise mode, frequency, intensity, and duration; and reported on changes in at least one of the components of the metabolic syndrome, as described above. Only five of the studies examined the effects of exercise alone on components of metabolic health [3–7]. More frequently, the interventions included some combination of exercise, caloric restriction, and behavior modification. These multicomponent interventions, although considered the preferred approach to pediatric obesity management [8,9], tended to make more difficult the task of determining the effects of exercise per se on changes in metabolic parameters. Nevertheless, examination of the available data supports the notion that exercise interventions can have beneficial effects on the metabolic health of obese children and adolescents.

### EXERCISE AND DYSLIPIDEMIA

#### Exercise and Triglycerides

Reduced triglycerides in obese youths following exercise training have been reported by several research groups. In studies conducted at the Medical College of Georgia, subjects attending after-school exercise programs for either 4 months (7- to 11-year-old boys and girls) or 8 months (13- to 16-year-old boys and girls) had significantly lower fasting triglyceride concentrations following training, as compared with nonexercising control group subjects [10,11]. In both studies, the supervised exercise programs were offered 5 days per week at the Medical College's indoor gym and included free transportation to the facility for the subjects. The exercise program for the obese (mean percentage body fat = 44.3 ± 9.4 via dual-energy x-ray absorptiometry [DEXA]) 7- to 11-year-old boys and girls consisted of 40 minutes of aerobic activities (20 minutes on exercise machines such as treadmills, cycle ergometers, and rowers and 20 minutes of continuous-movement games) [10]. The 73 subjects who completed the 4-month program (out of the original 79) averaged 4 days of attendance per week and exercised at an average heart rate of 157 beats per minute (subjects wore heart rate monitors each day). Estimated energy expenditure per exercise session was 233 kcal. No dietary intervention was involved. Fasting triglyceride concentrations were 21%

**TABLE 15.1**
**Studies Examining Exercise and Metabolic Health in Pediatric Obesity**

| Study | Ex Only | Ex + Diet | Ex + Diet + Beh | Diet Only | Con | Mean Age | Obesity Status | Mode | Int | Dur Min | Freq d/wk | Length Wks | TG | HDL | Glu | SBP | DBP | WC |
|---|---|---|---|---|---|---|---|---|---|---|---|---|---|---|---|---|---|---|
| Becque et al. [19] | — | — | 11 M/F | 11 M/F | 14 M/F | 13 | 40% BF | Various aerobic | 60–80% max HR | 50 | 3 | 20 | NS | +22% | — | → | → | — |
| Ferguson et al. [10] | 40 M/F | — | — | — | 39[a] M/F | 9 | 44% BF | Various aerobic | 157 bpm | 40 | 5 | 16 | 21% | NS | NS | — | — | — |
| Gutin et al. [3] | 13 F | — | — | — | 12 F[b] | 9 | 43% BF | Various aerobic | 163 bpm | 30 | 5 | 10 | NS | NS | NS | — | — | — |
| Kahle et al. [4] | 7 M | — | — | — | — | 13 | 39% BF | Various aerobic | 60–70% max HR | 45 | 3 | 15 | NS | NS | 15% | → | NS | — |
| Kang et al. [11] | 41[c] M/F | — | — | — | 18[d] M/F | 15 | 44% BF | Various aerobic | 138 bpm[e] 154 bpm[f] | 43[g] 29[h] | 5 | 32 | | NS | NS | NS | ↓[i] | VAT[j] |
| Owens et al. [5] | 27 M/F | — | — | — | 32 M/F | 9 | 44% BF | Various aerobic | 157 bpm | 40 | 5 | 16 | — | — | — | — | — | VAT[k] |
| Rocchini et al. [21] | — | — | 25 M/F | 26 M/F | 22 M/F | 13 | 44% BF | Various aerobic | 70–85% max HR | 40 | 3 | 20 | — | — | — | ↓[l] | ↓[m] | — |
| Sasaki et al. [6] | 41 M/F | — | — | — | 48[n] M/F | 11 | >20% excess weight | Running | 70% VO$_2$ max | 20 | 7 | 104 | ↓[o] | +16%[p] +19%[q] | | — | — | — |
| Sothern et al. [13] | — | — | 50 M/F | — | — | 12 | 183% IBW | Aerobic + strength | 45–55% VO$_2$ max | — | — | 10 | 32% | NS | | — | — | — |
| Treuth et al. [7] | 12 F | — | — | 11 F | — | 9 | 39% BF | Circuit strength training | 12–15 Reps | 20 | 3 | 20 | NS | NS | | — | — | NS |
| Wabitsch et al. [20] | — | 116 F | — | — | — | 15 | 31.3 BMI | Various aerobic | — | 60–120 | 7 | 6 | 8% | NS | | → | → | 8.1 cm |
| Woo et al. [15] | — | 41 M/F | — | 41 M/F | — | 10 | 38% BF | Aerobic + strength | 60–70% max HR | 40 | 3 | 6 | NS | NS | | — | — | — |

## TABLE 15.2 (continued)
## Studies Examining Exercise and Metabolic Health in Pediatric Obesity

[a] Nonexercise group during months 1–4, exercise group during months 5–8.

[b] Received lifestyle education program.

[c] Number of subjects assigned to either the moderate- or high-intensity exercise group and provided with postintervention data. Subjects also received lifestyle education.

[d] Number of subjects assigned to the lifestyle education group and who were provided postintervention data.

[e] Moderate-intensity exercise group.

[f] High-intensity exercise group.

[g] Moderate-intensity exercise group.

[h] High-intensity exercise group.

[i] High-intensity exercise group significantly lower than lifestyle-only group.

[j] Visceral adipose tissue significantly lower in the exercise groups compared with the lifestyle-only group.

[k] Significantly lower increase in VAT; the exercise group compared with the nonexercise group.

[l] Significantly lower in the exercise group than in diet or control group.

[m] Significantly lower in the exercise group than in the control group.

[n] Nonobese controls.

[o] Significant decrease in girls only.

[p] In boys.

[q] In girls.

*Note:* Ex = Exercise; Beh = Behavioral; Con = Control group; Int = Intensity of exercise; Dur = Duration of exercise; Freq = Frequency of exercise sessions; TG = Triglycerides; HDL = High-density lipoprotein cholesterol; Glu = Glucose; SBP = Systolic blood pressure; DBP = Diastolic blood pressure; WC = Waist circumference; M = Male; F = Female; BF = Body fat; HR = Heart Rate; Reps = repetitions; NS = not statistically significant; ↓ = significant decrease; bpm = Beats per minute; VAT = Visceral adipose tissue; IBW = Ideal body weight; BMI = Body mass index; dash (—) = variable not reported.

lower following 4 months of exercise training as compared with after 4 months of nontraining. Significant reductions in percentage body fat also occurred following training.

In the obese (mean percentage body fat = 44.5 ± 12.8 via DEXA) 13- to 16-year-old boys and girls, the after-school exercise program lasted 8 months [11]. The 80 adolescents were randomly assigned to one of three groups: moderate-intensity exercise plus lifestyle education, high-intensity exercise plus lifestyle education, or lifestyle education only. The exercise program again consisted of a combination of aerobic exercise on machines and continuous-movement activities. Across the 8 months, attendance at the exercise sessions averaged 2 to 3 days per week in the two exercise groups. The moderate-intensity exercise group averaged 43 minutes of exercise per session at an average heart rate of 138 beats per minute. The high-intensity group exercised for an average of 29 minutes per session at 154 beats per minute. The estimated exercise energy expenditures for the two groups were similar, averaging 250 kcal/session for the moderate-intensity group and 236 kcal/session for the high-intensity group. Pre- to posttraining change scores indicated a significant reduction in triglyceride concentrations in the high-intensity exercise group (0.22 ± 0.08 mmol·L$^{-1}$) as compared with the lifestyle education-only group (0.13 ± 0.08 mmol·L$^{-1}$). Triglycerides also declined in the moderate-intensity exercise group (0.04 ± 0.08 mmol·L$^{-1}$), but the comparison with the lifestyle-only group was not statistically significant. The changes in percentage body fat among the three groups were not significantly different.

The authors also conducted an analysis in which the high- and moderate-intensity exercise groups were combined into a single exercise group and then compared with the nonexercise lifestyle group [11]. This analysis indicated a significant interaction between the baseline triglyceride value and group assignment, indicating that exercise was especially effective in reducing triglyceride values in subjects with high baseline values. This finding is encouraging because obese children and adolescents tend to display elevated triglyceride values [12]. The analysis also indicates the exercise group reduced percentage body fat to a significantly greater extent than the nonexercise lifestyle group (3.57 ± 0.80 vs. 0.19 ± 0.62) [11].

In another exercise-only intervention, Japanese researchers reported that a 2-year program of in-school aerobic exercise significantly reduced triglyceride levels in obese (>120% of ideal body weight) 11- to 13-year-old girls, but not in obese boys [6]. The exercise program consisted primarily of running for 20 minutes at 70% of VO$_2$ max four mornings and three afternoons per week for 2 years. Compliance with the exercise program was nearly 100%. Triglyceride levels declined 27% in girls and 13% in boys, but only the difference in girls was statistically significant. The reason for the gender difference in triglyceride response was unclear. Significant decreases in body fat were observed in both sexes.

Researchers at the Louisiana State University School of Medicine and the Children's Hospital of New Orleans reported significant reductions in triglycerides in a group of 50 obese (BMI = 35.4 ± 6.98) boys and girls (mean age = 12.3 ± 2.7 years) following 10 weeks of diet and exercise intervention [13]. The diet involved a protein-sparing modified fast supplying approximately 800 kcal per day. A home-based exercise program was used (including an instructional video) that was individualized according to the degree of obesity. The program included moderate intensity (45 to 55% VO$_2$ max) aerobic activities as well as strength and flexibility exercises [14]. The duration and frequency of exercise were gradually increased through the 10 weeks of the program. In addition, subjects engaged in supervised exercise classes of 30 to 40 minutes during weekly group meetings. After 10 weeks of intervention, BMI declined an average of 12.7% from 35.4 ± 7.0 to 30.9 ± 6.5, and triglyceride values declined 32% from 96.3 mg·dL$^{-1}$ to 65.7 mg·dL$^{-1}$. Although the individual contributions of the diet and exercise components of the intervention were not parceled out, the authors have suggested that the reduced triglycerides were probably a result of the combined effects of diet and exercise [14].

Not all exercise interventions have been associated with significant reductions in triglyceride levels. Kahle et al. reported that a 15-week school-based exercise program that included participation in various aerobic activities 3 days per week, 45 minutes per session, at 60 to 70% of maximum heart rate, failed to result in a significant change in triglyceride values in a group of seven obese (mean percentage body fat = 38.8 ± 5.5 via hydrostatic weighing) boys 11 to 14 years of age [4]. Woo et al. examined changes in triglycerides in 82 obese (mean percentage body fat = 37.6 ± 3.7 via DEXA) boys and girls 10 years of age who were randomly assigned to interventions that involved either diet alone (900 to 1200 kcal per day) or diet plus exercise [15]. The exercise program consisted of 30 minutes of resistance and 10 minutes of aerobic exercises 2 days per week in a hospital setting. No significant changes in triglyceride concentrations were observed in either group after 6 weeks of training.

Despite the negative findings in some studies, the majority of the pediatric obesity studies have reported favorable changes in triglycerides following interventions involving exercise (Table 15.1).

## Exercise and HDL Cholesterol

Although increased HDL-C following exercise training has been observed in several obese adult populations [16–18], reports involving obese youths have been somewhat inconsistent. In a University of Michigan study, changes in HDL-C were examined in 36 obese (mean percentage body fat = 40.3 via hydrostatic weighing) adolescents following a 20-week intervention that involved random assignment to one of three groups: diet plus behavior change, diet plus behavior change plus exercise, or control [19]. The exercise component consisted of three 40-minute aerobic activity sessions (walking, jogging, swimming, dance, soccer, and continuous-play activities) per week with heart rates maintained between 60% and 80% of age-predicted maximum. Increases in HDL-C following the intervention were significantly greater in the group engaged in aerobic training (+23%) as compared with either the diet plus behavior change group (+11%) or the control group (+8%). The observation that the greater increase in HDL-C for the exercise group occurred despite a somewhat greater reduction in percentage body fat in the diet plus behavior change group (44.0 to 40.5% vs. 38.3 to 35.3%) prompted the authors to suggest that an exercise training effect, independent of change in body fat, was primarily responsible for the improvement in HDL-C.

In the study of obese Japanese children mentioned above [6], 2 years of daily 20-minute jogging without dietary intervention was associated with significant increases in HDL-C in boys (62.6 to 69.2 mg·dL$^{-1}$) and in girls (57.5 to 65.3 mg·dL$^{-1}$). Kahle et al. reported that HDL-C increased from 0.89 ± 0.12 to 1.04 ± 0.29 mmol·L$^{-1}$ following 15 weeks of aerobic training in seven obese boys, although the increase was not statistically significant [4]. The Medical College of Georgia studies with obese children and adolescents have failed to observe significant increases in HDL-C following exercise training programs [3,10,11], although in their study of 13- to 16-year-old boys and girls, a significant improvement in the total cholesterol/HDL-C ratio was observed in the subjects engaged in 8 months of after-school exercise as compared with nonexercising controls [11]. The Louisiana State University group also found only nonsignificant increases in HDL-C (41.3 to 42.0 mg·dL$^{-1}$) following 10 weeks of exercise and dietary intervention in 50 obese boys and girls [13]. Likewise, a 6-week program of dietary intervention (~1000 kcal/day) and 1 to 2 hours of daily controlled exercise (swimming, jogging, ball games) resulted in a less than 2% increase in HDL-C in a group of 116 obese (>120% ideal body weight) adolescent girls [20]. The 6-week exercise intervention by Woo et al. also failed to produce changes in HDL-C [15].

Thus, it appears the HDL-C responses to exercise programs in pediatric obesity are less predictable than those in obese adults. The short duration of some of the pediatric studies (6 to 10 weeks) may partially explain the negative findings. Whether future research with obese children and adolescents will be able to identify the optimal exercise dose for positively influencing this particular risk factor remains to be seen.

## Exercise and Hyperglycemia/Hyperinsulinemia

### Exercise and Glucose

Only a few studies have reported on the effects of exercise training on fasting glucose concentrations in pediatric obesity, with mixed results. In their 15-week aerobic training study, Kahle et al. reported that fasting serum glucose decreased from $5.24 \pm 0.25$ to $4.45 \pm 0.44$ mmol·L$^{-1}$ in obese 11- to 14-year-old boys [4]. Woo et al. reported that glucose decreased significantly in obese children after 6 weeks of diet plus exercise training, whereas decreases in glucose were not statistically significant in the diet-only group [15].

Others have failed to observe decreases in fasting glucose. Treuth et al. examined the effects of a 5-month resistance training program on fasting glucose in 11 obese (mean percentage body fat = $38.9 \pm 6.6$ via DEXA) 7- to 10-year-old girls [7]. The resistance training program took place at an elementary school and consisted of 20-minute sessions, three times per week, for 5 months, with subjects completing six upper-body exercises and one lower-body exercise using a circuit training approach. Fasting glucose values were similar before and after training ($5.0 \pm 0.03$ vs. $4.8 \pm 0.18$ pmol·L$^{-1}$). Likewise, the Medical College of Georgia group failed to observe significant changes in fasting glucose concentrations after 4 months of after school exercise in obese 7- to 11-year-old subjects or following 8 months of after-school exercise in subjects aged 13 to 16 years [10,11].

### Exercise and Insulin

The picture appears somewhat different relative to insulin. Although 5 months of resistance training failed to alter fasting insulin levels significantly in 7- to 10-year-old obese girls [7], the Georgia group found that 4 months of after-school aerobic exercise reduced fasting insulin significantly (~15%) in obese 7- to 11-year-old boys and girls [10]. In another exercise-only study, Kahle et al. reported that after 15 weeks of aerobic exercise, peak insulin response and total insulin area following a test meal were significantly lower than before training and were independent of changes in body weight or body fat [4]. Also, 6 weeks of dietary intervention (~1000 kcal/day) and 1 to 2 hours of daily swimming, jogging, and ball games resulted in a 21% decrease in fasting insulin levels in a group of 116 obese adolescent girls [20]. Thus, some experimental data support the efficacy of exercise for reducing fasting insulin levels in obese youths. Additional research on this component of metabolic health is clearly needed.

### EXERCISE AND HYPERTENSION

There are several reports of significantly reduced resting blood pressure following exercise programs in obese youths. Rocchini et al. randomly assigned 72 obese (mean percentage body fat = $44 \pm 7$ via hydrostatic weighing) adolescents to one of three treatment groups: diet plus behavior change, diet plus behavior change plus exercise, and no intervention control [21]. The diet was designed to produce a weight loss of approximately 1 to 2 lb per week. The exercise program included 40 minutes of aerobic activities (walking, jogging, swimming, dancing, and other recreational activities) at 70 to 75% of maximum heart rate 3 days per week for 20 weeks. After 20 weeks, both intervention groups experienced significantly greater decreases in resting systolic and diastolic blood pressure as compared with the control group. Because both intervention groups also lost significant amounts of body weight, the authors performed a secondary analysis in which change in body weight was included as a covariate. This analysis revealed that the group that combined caloric restriction and exercise experienced the greatest decrease in resting systolic blood pressure.

The study by Wabitsch et al. that included a 6-week program of dietary intervention (~1000 kcal/day) and 1 to 2 hours of daily controlled exercise (swimming, jogging, ball games) resulted in significant declines in systolic ($125 \pm 11$ mm Hg to $116 \pm 10$ mm Hg) and diastolic ($65 \pm 9$ mm Hg to $60 \pm$ mm Hg) blood pressure in a group of 116 obese (>120% ideal body weight) adolescent girls [20]. The Medical College of Georgia group reported that obese 13- to 16-year-old subjects who engaged in 8 months of lifestyle education and after-school exercise experienced a significantly greater reduction in resting diastolic blood pressure than the group that participated in lifestyle education only [11]. Changes in resting systolic blood pressure were also greater in the exercise group as compared with the lifestyle-only group ($6 \pm 3$ mm Hg vs. $+ 2 \pm 3$ mm Hg), but the differences did not achieve statistical significance. Kahle et al. observed a significant reduction in systolic, but not diastolic, blood pressure following 15 weeks of aerobic training in obese 11- to 14-year-old boys [4].

## EXERCISE AND ABDOMINAL OBESITY

### Exercise and Waist Circumference

Data are limited on the effects of exercise on waist circumference in pediatric obesity. Wabitsch et al. observed a mean reduction of 8.1 cm in waist circumference in a group of 116 obese adolescent girls following 6 weeks of dietary intervention (~1000 kcal/day) and 1 to 2 hours of daily controlled aerobic exercise [20].

### Exercise and Visceral Adipose Tissue

Two research groups have reported on the favorable effects of exercise, without dietary intervention, on visceral adipose tissue in obese youths. The Medical College of Georgia group observed an attenuation in the rate at which visceral adipose tissue accumulated in 7- to 11-year-old subjects who participated in 4 months of after-school exercise, as compared with the nonexercising control subjects. That is, the accumulation of visceral adipose tissue was significantly less after 4 months in the exercise group as compared with the nonexercise group (1.3 cm$^3$ vs. 20.9 cm$^3$) [5]. In their study of obese adolescents, the Georgia group reported that those who attended after-school exercise classes at least 2 days per week for 8 months showed a significantly greater reduction in visceral adipose tissue than did those attending lifestyle-education-only classes (42.0 ± 9.3 cm$^3$ vs. 11.0 ± 10.0 cm$^3$) [22].

Treuth et al. reported that a resistance training program (20-minute sessions, three times per week for 5 months) attenuated the expected increase in visceral adipose tissue in 11 obese 7- to 10-year-old girls [7]. The authors noted that although the exercise did not reduce visceral adipose tissue, prevention of an increase can be considered a favorable outcome because an increase in this adipose tissue depot is of primary health importance as a result of its association with cardiovascular risk in children.

## SUMMARY OF COMPONENTS OF SUCCESSFUL EXERCISE PROGRAMS

### MODE OF EXERCISE

A variety of modes of aerobic exercise have been employed to improve the metabolic health of obese children and adolescents, including walking, jogging, swimming, rope skipping, aerobic dance, and various continuous-movement games [4,5,11,13,19]. Stationary exercise machines such as treadmills, cycle ergometers, and rowers have been employed successfully with children as young as 7 years of age, although it appears that also including play-oriented aerobic activities with younger age groups is advisable [23]. Providing a choice of aerobic activities appears to relate to the "likeability" young people have for various modes of exercise [24].

The data also indicate that successful alteration of metabolic health components through exercise is not limited to aerobic type activities. Sothern et al. [13] and Woo et al. [15] employed strength training as part of their exercise programs, and Treuth et al. reported that resistance training three times per week for 5 months appeared to attenuate the expected increase in visceral fat in 7- to 10-year-old girls [7].

### INTENSITY OF EXERCISE

Exercise intensities for the aerobic component of successful interventions have tended to fall within the "moderate to vigorous" category; that is, 60 to 80% of maximum age-related heart rate [4,10,15,19,21]. This intensity is in keeping with the recent Scientific Statement of the American Heart Association's Committee on Atherosclerosis, Hypertension, and Obesity in the Young that recommended at least 30 minutes of moderate to vigorous physical activity on most, and preferably all, days of the week [25].

The effect of exercise intensity on metabolic health outcomes was directly tested by the research group at the Medical College of Georgia. After 8 months of after-school exercise in 13- to 16-year-old obese subjects randomly assigned to either the moderate-intensity exercise group (average heart rate of 138 beats per minute, 69% of age-predicted maximum) or the high-intensity exercise group (154 beats per min, 77% of age-predicted maximum), the researchers found little evidence that high-intensity training was more effective than moderate-intensity training in enhancing the metabolic health of obese adolescents [11].

## DURATION OF EXERCISE

Durations of individual training sessions in successful exercise interventions have varied widely, ranging from as little as 20 minutes per session [6] to as long as 2 hours [20]. Most of the studies, however, reported durations falling within the 30- to 50-minute range [4,5,13,19,21,22], which would meet the American Heart Association's recommendation that obese youths engage in at least 30 minutes of moderate to vigorous physical activity daily [25].

## FREQUENCY OF EXERCISE

Two successful interventions included exercise 7 days per week [6,20], although one of these studies occurred in association with a 6-week weight-loss camp [20]. After-school exercise programs were offered 5 days per week in the Medical College of Georgia studies, with attendance averaging 4 days per week across 4 months in the 7- to 11-year-old children and 2 to 3 days per week over 8 months in the 13- to 16-year-old subjects [5,22]. Greater exercise frequency was associated with less increase in body mass in the 7- to 11-year-old children [26], whereas in the 13- to 16-year-old subjects, the combination of increased attendance, exercise heart rate, and energy expenditure was associated with greater reductions in percentage body fat [22]. Exercise frequencies of 3 days per week were associated with improved metabolic profiles in several studies [4,7,19,21].

## LENGTH OF EXERCISE TRAINING PROGRAM

It is not clear from the limited number of studies in this area whether there exists a minimum length of exercise training for improving metabolic health in pediatric obesity. As discussed here, improvements in the metabolic health of obese youths were reported for training studies as short as 6 weeks [20] and as long as 2 years [6]. Practical considerations associated with clinical obesity management in terms of staffing, availability of exercise space and equipment, and the nature of parental involvement will likely play a major role in determining the length of a structured exercise component of an obesity management program.

## REFERENCES

1. Cook S, Weitzman M, Auinger P, Nguyen M, Dietz WH. Prevalence of a metabolic syndrome phenotype in adolescents: findings from the third National Health and Nutrition Examination Survey, 1988-1994. *Arch Pediatr Adolesc Med.* 2003;157:821–827.
2. Cruz ML, Goran MI. The metabolic syndrome in children and adolescents. *Curr Diab Rep.* 2004;4:53–62.
3. Gutin B, Cucuzzo N, Islam S, Smith C, Stachura ME. Physical training, lifestyle education, and coronary risk factors in obese girls. *Med Sci Sports Exer.* 1996;28:19–23.
4. Kahle EB, Zipf WB, Lamb DR, Horswill CA, Ward KM. Association between mild, routine exercise and improved insulin dynamics and glucose control in obese adolescents. *Inter J Sports Med.* 1996;17:1–6.
5. Owens S, Gutin B, Allison J, Riggs S, Ferguson M, Litaker M, Thompson W. Effect of physical training on total and visceral fat in obese children. *Med Sci Sports Exer.* 1999;31:143–148.

6.  Sasaki J, Shindo M, Tanaka H, Ando M, Arakawa K. A long-term aerobic exercise program decreases the obesity index and increases the high density lipoprotein cholesterol concentration in obese children. *Inter J Obesity.* 1987;11:339–345.

7.  Treuth MS, Hunter GR, Figueroa-Colon R, Goran MI. Effects of strength training on intra-abdominal adipose tissue in obese prepubertal girls. *Med Sci Sports Exer.* 1998;30:1738–1743.

8.  Epstein LH, Myers MD, Raynor HA, Saelens BE. Treatment of pediatric obesity. *Pediatrics.* 1998;101:554–570.

9.  Suskind R, Blecker U, Udall J, Jr., Von Almen T, Schumacher H, Carlisle L, Sothern M. Recent advances in the treatment of childhood obesity. *Pediatr Diab.* 2000;1:23–33.

10. Ferguson MA, Gutin B, Le NA, Karp W, Litaker M, Humphries M et al. Effects of exercise training and its cessation on components of the insulin resistance syndrome in obese children. *Inter J Obes Rel Metab Disor.* 1999;22:889–895.

11. Kang HS, Gutin B, Barbeau P, Owens S, Lemmon CR, Allison J, Litaker MS, Le NA. Physical training improves insulin resistance syndrome markers in obese adolescents. *Med Sci Sports Exer.* 2002;34:1920–1927.

12. Smoak CG, Burke GL, Webber LS, Harsha DW, Srinivasan SR, Berenson GS. Relation of obesity to clustering of cardiovascular disease risk factors in children and young adults. The Bogalusa Heart Study. *Am J Epidemiol.* 1987;125:364–372.

13. Sothern MS, Despinasse B, Brown R, Suskind RM, Udall JN, Jr., Blecker U. Lipid profiles of obese children and adolescents before and after significant weight loss: differences according to sex. *South Med J.* 2000;93:278–282.

14. Suskind RM, Sothern MS, Farris RP, von Almen TK, Schumacher H, Carlisle L et al. Recent advances in the treatment of childhood obesity. *Ann NY Acad Sci.* 1993;699:181–199.

15. Woo KS, Chook P, Yu CW, Sung RY, Qiao M, Leung SS et al. Effects of diet and exercise on obesity-related vascular dysfunction in children. *Circulation.* 2004;109:1981–1986.

16. Williams PT, Stefanick ML, Vranizan KM, Wood PD. The effects of weight loss by exercise or by dieting on plasma high-density lipoprotein (HDL) levels in men with low, intermediate, and normal-to-high HDL at baseline. *Metabolism.* 1994;43:917–924.

17. Thompson PD, Yurgalevitch SM, Flynn MM, Zmuda JM, Spannaus-Martin D, Saritelli A et al. Effect of prolonged exercise training without weight loss on high-density lipoprotein metabolism in overweight men. *Metabolism.* 1997;46:217–223.

18. Nicklas BJ, Katzel LI, Busby-Whitehead J, Goldberg AP. Increases in high-density lipoprotein cholesterol with endurance exercise training are blunted in obese compared with lean men. *Metabolism.* 1997;46:556–561.

19. Becque MD, Katch VL, Rocchini AP, Marks CR, Moorehead C. Coronary risk incidence of obese adolescents: reduction by exercise plus diet intervention. *Pediatrics.* 1988;81:605–612.

20. Wabitsch M, Hauner H, Heinze E, Muche R, Bockmann A, Parthon W et al. Body-fat distribution and changes in the atherogenic risk-factor profile in obese adolescent girls during weight reduction. *Amer J Clin Nutr.* 1994;60:54–60.

21. Rocchini AP, Katch V, Anderson J, Hinderliter J, Becque D, Martin M, Marks C. Blood pressure in obese adolescents: effect of weight loss. *Pediatrics.* 1988;82:16–23.

22. Gutin B, Barbeau P, Owens S, Lemmon CR, Bauman M, Allison J et al. Effects of exercise intensity on cardiovascular fitness, total body composition, and visceral adiposity of obese adolescents. *Amer J Clin Nutr.* 2002;75:818–826.

23. Gutin B, Riggs S, Ferguson M, Owens S. Description and process evaluation of a physical training program for obese children. *Res Q Exer Sport.* 1999;70:65–69.

24. Epstein LH, Valoski AM, Vara LS, McCurley J, Wisniewski L, Kalarchian MA et al. Effects of decreasing sedentary behavior and increasing activity on weight change in obese children. *Health Psychol.* 1995;14:109–115.

25. Williams CL, Hayman LL, Daniels SR, Robinson TN, Steinberger J, Paridon S, Bazzarre T. Cardiovascular health in childhood: A statement for health professionals from the Committee on Atherosclerosis, Hypertension, and Obesity in the Young (AHOY) of the Council on Cardiovascular Disease in the Young, American Heart Association. *Circulation.* 2002;106:143–160.

26. Barbeau P, Gutin B, Litaker M, Owens S, Riggs S, Okuyama T. Correlates of individual differences in body-composition changes resulting from physical training in obese children. *Amer J Clin Nutr.* 1999;69:705–711.

# Section 8

## Internet-Based Approaches

# 16 Internet-Based Treatment for Pediatric Obesity

*Donald A. Williamson, Heather Walden, Emily York-Crowe, and Tiffany M. Stewart*

## CONTENTS

## BACKGROUND

Advances in technology and the emphatic increase in the use of the Internet for shopping, making reservations, education, therapy, and live communication has radically changed modern communication. The use of Internet applications and electronic forms of communication continues to increase. Of all users, children and teenagers appear to use the Internet more than any other age group. About 90% of children between the ages of 5 and 17 years (47 million individuals) now use computers, and about 59% (31 million individuals) use the Internet [1].

Clinic-based treatments for weight loss can involve high costs and time commitments (e.g., travel to appointments, missed appointments because of illness, and missed school or work), which often result in poor adherence or increased attrition rates. Recent research has investigated the use of alternative means of delivering weight-loss interventions (e.g., interventions delivered via mail, telephone, or television) to remove some of these obstacles; however, few studies have tested using computers for the delivery of weight-loss or obesity treatment. There has also been little research investigating the efficacy of Internet-based treatment for weight loss. The capabilities of an Internet approach far exceed those of previous alternative methods, in which high-speed interaction and dissemination of large amounts of information is not possible. In addition, this method substantially increases accessibility to treatment for individuals who may not have the time or means to participate in clinic-based programs. Such a program used alone, or in addition to a clinic-based program with fewer face-to-face contact hours, can remove some of the obstacles related to standard behavioral programs and can improve compliance. This chapter reviews the results of studies that have tested the efficacy of Internet-based weight-loss programs and describes in detail one recent study that tested this approach for pediatric obesity.

## USING THE INTERNET FOR WEIGHT MANAGEMENT

Six papers, including two related to pediatric obesity, have reported the use of the Internet for the purpose of delivering a weight-management program. Four of the six studies focused exclusively on adults. The samples for all four adult studies were predominantly white, and all participants had Internet access at home or work before beginning the study. The research designs of two of the studies compared the efficacy of interactive Internet-based interventions with health education Web sites [2,3]. Both studies found a 2.5-kg difference between the two treatments at the end of 6 to 12 months. A third study tested the efficacy of an Internet-based intervention as a weight-maintenance strategy for adults who had lost weight using a face-to-face behavioral counseling approach [4]. The study reported negative results in that the Internet-based intervention did not yield good weight maintenance in comparison with face-to-face contact. A recent study reported no differences in weight-maintenance results between face-to-face contact and Internet support [5]. Thus, mixed evidence has been found for the efficacy of using the Internet as a means for yielding long-term weight maintenance.

A fifth study, reported by Baronowski et al., tested the efficacy of an 8-week Internet-based intervention for overweight 8-year-old African-American girls [6]. The study did not yield significant weight changes in comparison with a control group. The sixth study, the Health Information Program for Teens (HIPTeens) project, is the only study that has reported the use of an Internet-based approach for weight loss in children or adolescents. The parents of these children were also overweight and were also targets of the Internet-based treatment. This study yielded body fat loss for the adolescent girls and greater weight loss for their parents, providing further support for Internet-based interventions for weight loss. The next section describes this Internet-based intervention and the preliminary results of the study that have been reported by White et al. [7].

## HIPTEENS

### PROGRAM DESCRIPTION

The HIPTeens project was designed to evaluate the efficacy of an Internet-based intervention for weight loss in overweight African-American girls in a randomized clinical trial. The intervention tested in the study was planned as a secondary prevention study for overweight African-American girls. The study enrolled 57 African-American adolescent girls (ages 11 to 15 years) who were overweight (body mass index [BMI] > 85th percentile for girls) and had at least one biological parent who was obese (BMI > 30). The participants were randomly assigned to an interactive, behavioral, Internet-based program or to a passive (noninteractive) Internet-based health education program, which served as the control condition. Parents of the girls were also participants in the study. All but one of the parents was the mother. Participants in both treatment groups met in face-to-face therapy sessions on four occasions over the first 12 weeks. In this project, two Web sites were developed: an interactive, behavioral, Internet-based program, and an Internet-based health education program. Data collection for HIPTeens has now spanned two consecutive years, and findings from the full 2-year period are currently being analyzed. To control for potential biases related to owning a computer and having access to the Internet, each family enrolled in the study was required to purchase a new computer at a greatly reduced cost and was provided free Internet access as long as they were active participants in the study. Individuals who were still unable to afford the computer at the reduced cost were eligible for an additional monetary scholarship toward the computer.

**TABLE 16.1**
**Description of the HIPTeens Web Site**

Components

Online treatment sessions on health/nutrition, each including a quiz to assess comprehension
Links to educational, health-related Web sites
Interactive graph to track weight loss
Interactive graph to track physical activity
Behavioral contracts
Interactive food monitoring worksheets with instant feedback on food choices
Healthy menu ideas, including recipes
Ability to e-mail case manager from site
Treatment strategies emphasizing problem-solving, goal setting, and behavioral contracting
Components promoting low-fat, low-calorie diet high in fruits and vegetables
Structured programs to increase physical activity

## DESCRIPTION OF INTERNET COMPONENT

The HIPTeens program is an Internet-based intervention that was designed to promote weight loss and long-term weight maintenance in overweight students (BMI > 85th percentile). An Internet/e-mail account was established for each participant after enrollment in the study. Participants recorded food intake, nutrient goals, physical activity, and behavioral goals on electronic forms that were then sent by e-mail to the research team. Parents and children were able to participate in the interactive program from home or from other places with Internet access. Each student was assigned an Internet counselor who provided support and instruction for health-related behavior change. The primary form of participant–counselor contact was e-mail messaging. The Web site included the following components: 52 lessons about healthy nutrition and exercise, problem-solving, eating patterns, and so on; links to other health Web sites related to nutrition, physical fitness, and health; automated interactive components (e.g., a self-monitoring program that provides immediate feedback about the quality of food choices made by the participant, based on the caloric and fat content of the food and number of servings within each Food Guide Pyramid category that is represented by each food); interactive components that allow the participant to graph body weight and minutes of physical activity over time by entering these values into the computer program; recipes for low-calorie/low-fat meals; school menus for each day of the next week, with instructions on healthy foods that should be selected; and a calendar that describes upcoming local recreational events for children and adolescents during the next month that promote healthy eating and activity behavior. The basic components for the Internet-based behavioral intervention and the alternative health education intervention are outlined in Table 16.1.

## MEASUREMENT OF PARTICIPATION IN THE INTERNET-BASED INTERVENTIONS

The computer server automatically tracked use of the Web sites (by adolescents and parents). For both interventions, overall participation was measured by the number of "hits" per person to the Web site during the 6-month intervention. A "hit" was recorded each time the participant clicked (refreshed) to another page of the Web site. For the behavioral intervention, using the specific components of the program was also tracked. These components included completion of quizzes at the end of each weekly chapter, percentage of correct answers for each quiz, number of e-mails to Internet counselors, submission of body weight data to the weight graph component, and submission of number of minutes of physical activity to the physical activity graph component.

### Non-Internet Aspects of the Study

## Computer Training and Counseling Sessions

During the first 12 weeks of the program, the adolescent participant and her overweight/obese parent (in both treatment conditions) were scheduled to attend four face-to-face counseling sessions, at weeks 1, 3, 6, and 12. Participants in both treatment arms were reinforced (with small gifts) for attendance at face-to-face therapy sessions. At this time, participants and parents in both groups received additional training and help with problem solving, related to use of their computers and their access and using the Web site appropriate for treatment assignment (e.g., control or experimental). Participants in the behavioral treatment group also learned how to complete and submit monitoring records, quizzes, and graphs that were administered over the Internet. For the behavioral group, these four sessions focused on introduction to food monitoring and goal setting for nutrient intake, introduction to monitoring of physical activity and goal setting to yield a minimum of 150 minutes of physical activity per week by week 20, introduction to behavioral contracting with a goal of modeling appropriate strategies for behavioral contracting, and review of progress and problem solving to address poor adherence. Each of these sessions was coordinated with a module on the Web site that corresponded to the same goals. Participants in the control group received nutrition education from a registered dietitian but were not prescribed behavioral tasks to yield weight loss.

## Measurement of Body Weight at Home

At the first face-to-face session, families in both treatment arms received an electronic scale that could be used to measure the body weight of the adolescent and participating parent every week. Participants were instructed to weigh at the same time of day (on awakening in the morning), with the same clothing, and after voiding to minimize extraneous influences on the measurement of total body weight. The participants in both treatment groups were prompted (via e-mail) to weigh at least once every 2 weeks and to send a record, via e-mail, of their body weight to the research team. Although the participants in both groups were able to plot their weight information on an individualized weight graph that provided visual feedback about the pattern of weight loss over time; only the behavioral group was provided with a similar graph to record minutes of physical activity.

### Initial Findings from the First 6 Months

The initial results of the HIPTeens project are summarized in Figure 16.1. These data depict change scores from baseline. An intent-to-treat statistical methodology was used to test the hypothesis that the interactive behavioral program would yield greater fat/weight loss in comparison with the control arm for both adolescents and parents. During the first 6 months, seven participants dropped out of treatment (five behavioral and two control), and the baseline values for body weight (kg), body mass index (BMI–parents; BMI percentile–adolescents), and percentage body fat as measured by dual x-ray absorptiometry were carried forward to the 6-month period (i.e., no fat/weight changes were recorded). Over the course of the first 6 months of treatment, adolescents and parents in the behavioral treatment lost greater body fat/weight relative to the control condition. As can be seen in the graphs for BMI percentile and body weight, adolescents in the control group tended to gain weight, and these changes were greater than those for adolescents in the behavioral group. The BMI percentile of adolescents in the control condition also increased relative to baseline, whereas the BMI percentile of adolescents in the experimental condition decreased. Parents in both groups tended to lose weight, but this weight loss was statistically significant only for parents in the behavioral group. In summary, the hypothesis that the behavioral group would be more effective for fat/weight loss was supported by these preliminary findings.

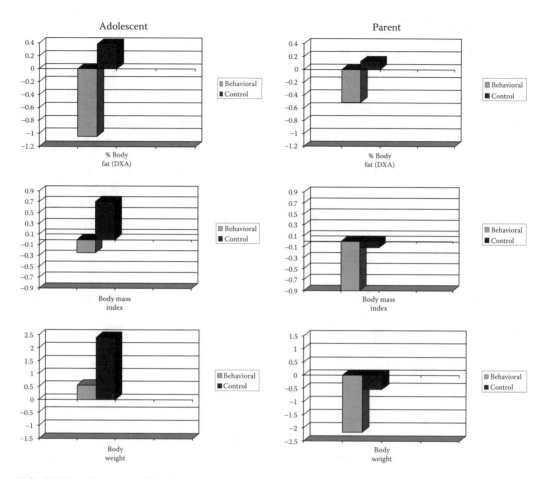

**FIGURE 16.1** Summary of the initial results of the HIPTeens study.

Using the Internet-based behavioral intervention was associated with decreased adiposity of the adolescents in the behavioral treatment group. Furthermore, parental use of the Web site and adolescent use of the Web site were positively correlated. In addition, a supportive family environment was positively correlated with both weight and fat loss in adolescents. For parents, reduction in dietary fat in the behavioral treatment group mediated weight loss. In general, the preliminary findings of this study indicated that adolescent weight loss was associated with a supportive family environment and with a parent who actively used the Internet-based weight management program.

Consumer satisfaction with the HIPTeens program was high. Preliminary consumer satisfaction ratings at the end of 2 years indicated that 95% of the participants in both treatment arms reported that they enjoyed being in the HIPTeens program. Also, 100% of the participants in the behavioral arm and 96% of those in the health education arm had recommended the program to others.

In summary, the HIP-Teens Internet-based behavioral intervention yielded positive initial results in terms of weight and fat loss. These results are comparable with findings from previous studies using minimal contact behavioral interventions in a primary care setting [8]. However, when comparing results of this study with results of more intensive, clinic-based weight-loss studies, the clinic-based approach appears to be more effective [9]. Additional studies are needed to investigate the applicability of this type of weight-loss approach for populations other than overweight adolescent African-American girls and their parents.

## SUMMARY AND CONCLUSIONS

### PROS AND CONS FOR USING THE INTERNET

At present, the study of Internet-based interventions for weight loss or prevention of weight gain in pediatric obesity is limited to two investigations. Thus, this area of research is still in its infancy. There are numerous advantages of the Internet approach over a more traditional clinic-based approach, including the capability for rapid dissemination of health information, tracking of program use, live chats, and e-mail contacts with dieticians and therapists, as well as electronic recording and submission of participant's weight, physical activity, and dietary data to clinic staff. In addition, this approach allows the researcher and clinician to reach a larger population because of the reduction in travel time and clinic visits, and the increased flexibility of program utilization. The reductions in travel time and clinic visits potentially serve to increase the cost-effectiveness of this approach. Finally, results from existing research indicate that participants appreciate and respond to this type of approach.

Although an Internet-based approach for weight loss offers some unique opportunities and benefits, there are also some costs associated with having fewer face-to-face contact hours. For the Internet-based program, participants may need a high level of motivation and commitment, as there is less opportunity for motivational enhancement than in traditional face-to-face sessions. Furthermore, as there are fewer in-person contact hours with a therapist, it may be more difficult to establish rapport, and the participant may therefore feel less accountable for behavioral change.

### FEASIBILITY OF INTERNET-BASED INTERVENTIONS

Research to date investigating the efficacy of Internet-based approaches has yielded mixed results. Recent data from the HIPTeens project indicate that this approach can be efficacious, albeit less so than a more intensive, clinic-based program. Therefore, this type of approach may be more effective for people who need to lose smaller amounts of weight, rather than larger amounts, and may be most useful as a strategy for the prevention of weight gain in children, adolescents, and adults. Several important factors should be considered before proceeding with Internet-based weight-loss or weight-gain-prevention programs, including problems with and barriers to Internet access, computer and Internet literacy, and level of motivation of the intended population. To increase the likelihood of commitment and adherence by the children, it is essential that parents or other caregivers also become involved. Despite the greater accessibility of weight-loss interventions associated with an Internet-based approach, if the participant is inexperienced with this technology or is limited in motivation and support, such an approach may not be successful without additional training and motivational enhancement before program implementation.

Another vital component of success for using the Internet for the delivery of weight-loss treatment is use by the participant. The participant must log onto the Web site for the intervention to be delivered and to increase the likelihood that the intervention will be effective. The HIPTeens program included a few face-to-face sessions but relied heavily on the individual to access the Web site from home. Incentives are sometimes necessary to motivate participants to use the Internet program, as well as perform certain behaviors that are in line with treatment goals. For this reason, participants in the HIPTeens program were awarded gift certificates for completion of clinic visits and questionnaires. Although these incentives were generally handed out in session or mailed to the participant, Internet technology allows for the delivery of on-line gift certificates via e-mail, which can be used to enhance program adherence and motivation. The overall effectiveness of on-line incentives to improve Web site utilization in an environmental approach to weight management is currently being investigated by our research team. Thus far, we have found that although it is possible to reinforce Web site utilization with on-line incentives, participants do not always redeem the gift certificates. The reasons for not redeeming certificates have included, but are not limited to, participants not wanting to use their credit cards on-line to order merchandise (to subsidize the amount of the gift certificate), and participants not wanting to go through the "trouble" of redeeming the gift certificates (going through the steps of redeeming the gift certificates online). Several participants also reported that although instructions were clearly presented and simple to follow, they did not fully understand how to redeem the gift certificate and, as a result, did not follow through. However, through online surveys, we are able to identify such problems and are able to aid participants in overcoming simple obstacles to redeeming their certificates; we can also assist them if they desire to redeem certificates they have earned in the past.

## FUTURE DIRECTIONS

To maximize the effectiveness of any intervention, it is ideal to include any physical and social environments that may influence the behavior of the individual (e.g., parents, teachers, school, home environment). Our ideas for future research include investigating the efficacy of an Internet-based approach for weight management and health promotion delivered in a classroom setting. This type of program could be developed and implemented in a school setting by creating a program that uses the Internet for presentation and education about weight loss or weight gain prevention behaviors, developing a classroom curriculum-based program to accompany the Internet program, training teachers to present this information to the children, and allowing the children to log on to the Internet to use the program at school and at home. We hope that this approach might empower children to become "agents" of behavioral change, resulting in a carryover of the newly learned behaviors from the school environment to the home environment. In summary, we suspect that the use of Internet-based interventions may be only part of the solution for pediatric obesity and that more broad-based environmental programs may be required to curtail the current rates of obesity. Nevertheless, there appears to be a place for Internet-based approaches, and these approaches may be quite useful for widespread dissemination of health information and for Internet counseling for children and adolescents who need to lose weight but find attending clinics unfeasible or impractical because of time or travel constraints.

## REFERENCES

1.  U.S. Department of Education, National Center for Education Statistics. Computer and Internet Use by Children and Adolescents in 2001, NCES 2004-014. Washington, DC, 2003. Available at http://nces.ed.gov/pubsearch/pubsinfo.asp?pubid=2004014.
2.  Tate, DF, Wing, RR, & Winett, RA. Using Internet technology to deliver a behavioral weight loss program. *JAMA*. 2001;285:1172–1177.
3.  Tate, DF, Jackvony, EH, & Wing, RR. Effects of Internet behavioral counseling on weight loss in adults at risk for type 2 diabetes: a randomized trial. *JAMA*. 2003; 289:1833–1836.
4.  Harvey-Berino, J, Pintauro, S, Buzzell, P, DiGiulio, M, Casey Gold, B, Moldovan, C, & Ramirez, E. Does using the Internet facilitate the maintenance of weight loss? *Int J Obes Metabol Dis*. 2002;26:1254–1260.
5.  Harvey-Berino J, Pintauro S, Buzzell P, & Gold EC. Effect of Internet support on the long-term maintenance of weight loss. *Obes Res*. 2004;12:320–329.
6.  Baronowski, T, Baronowski, JC, Cullen, KW, Thompson, DI, Nicklas, T, Zakeri, IE, & Rochon, J. The Fun, Food, and Fitness Project (FFFP): The Baylor GEMS pilot study. *Ethnicity Dis*. 2003;13:S30–S39.
7.  White, MA, Davis Martin, P, Newton, RL, Walden, HM, York-Crowe, EE, Gordon, ST et al. Mediators of weight loss in a family-based intervention presented over the Internet. *Obes Res*. 2004;12:1–10.
8.  Saelens BE, Sallis JF, Wilfley DE, Patrick K, Cella JA, Buchta R. Behavioral weight control for overweight adolescents initiated in primary care. *Obes Res*. 2002;10:22–32.
9.  Berkowitz RI, Wadden TA, Tershakovec AM, Cronquist JL. Behavior therapy and sibutramine for the treatment of adolescent obesity: a randomized controlled trial. *JAMA*. 2003;289:1805–1812.

# Section 9

## Pharmacology

# 17 Pharmacologic Treatment of Adolescent Obesity

*Canice E. Crerand, Thomas A. Wadden, and Robert I. Berkowitz*

## CONTENTS

## INTRODUCTION

The prevalence of obesity in children and adolescents is increasing at an alarming rate. According to the most recent data, 16% of American children ages 6 to 19 years are overweight (defined as body mass index [BMI] ≥ 95th percentile), and 31% are considered to be at risk for overweight (defined as BMI ≥ 85th percentile) [1]. Equally alarming, the incidence of weight-related comorbidities, such as type 2 diabetes, has also increased in youth [2,3]. Investigators fear that the progression of such diseases may be hastened by their early age of onset [4]. Furthermore, up to 80% of obese adolescents will become obese adults [5,6], thus placing them at risk for developing obesity-related comorbidities, including cardiovascular disease, hyperlipidemia, cancer, sleep disorders, and gallbladder disease [7,8]. In addition to its adverse effects on physical health, obesity in youth frequently has a negative psychosocial effect. One study reported that women who had been obese as adolescents were poorer, less educated, and less likely to be married than were women who had been normal weight as teenagers [9]. Quality of life in obese teens and children has been found to be comparable to that of children with cancer [10].

These disturbing statistics leave little doubt that effective treatments for adolescent obesity are now needed more than ever. Even with the best behavioral treatments, however, only about half of children maintain their weight losses long-term [11,12]. These findings have led to continuing interest in pharmacologic treatment of adolescent obesity.

As with the management of adult obesity, pharmacotherapy for the treatment of adolescent obesity has had a checkered history. Many agents, although initially promising, were later found to do more harm than good. For example, amphetamines were once considered to be effective treatments for obesity. However, concerns about abuse and tolerance arose, and the American Academy of Pediatrics issued a statement discouraging the use of such medications in children and adolescents [13]. In 1997, fenfluramine, which had shown promise in treating adult and adolescent obesity, was removed from the market because of its association with valvular heart disease [14,15]. More recently, a randomized, placebo controlled trial of ephedrine combined with caffeine appeared to improve weight loss in obese adolescents [16]. However, ephedrine was removed from the market in 2004 because of concerns about dangerous short- and long-term cardiovascular effects [17,18].

Thus, the use of pharmacotherapy in adolescents remains controversial, principally because of concerns about side effects and the unknown long-term effect of pharmacological agents on growth, metabolism, and development. Nonetheless, pharmacotherapy still holds promise as an adjunctive treatment for adolescent obesity. This chapter reviews the literature on the pharmacological treatment of adolescent obesity, offers suggestions for clinical practice, and concludes with priorities for future research.

## PHARMACOLOGICAL AGENTS FOR THE TREATMENT OF OBESITY

At present, two medications, orlistat and sibutramine, have been approved by the Food and Drug Administration (FDA) for the induction of weight loss in adults. Orlistat (Xenical®) is a gastric and pancreatic lipase inhibitor that causes weight loss by blocking the absorption of dietary fat, which is excreted in stool [19–21]. Orlistat is not centrally absorbed, and side effects are primarily gastrointestinal in nature. They include production of oily, fatty stools; increased flatulence; and fecal leakage. Sibutramine (Meridia®) is a combined norepinephrine-serotonin reuptake inhibitor that is associated with increased satiation and a resulting reduction in food intake [22–24]. Side effects include constipation, headache, and dry mouth. Of greater concern are increases in blood pressure and pulse rate.

Randomized, controlled trials of these medications in adults have demonstrated weight losses of 7 to 10% when combined with an energy-deficit diet [19,20,22,25]. However, sibutramine is only indicated for use in individuals ages 16 years and older. In December 2003, the FDA approved the use of orlistat in children between the ages of 12 and 16 years, thus making it the only FDA-approved medication for use in adolescents. To date, few studies have investigated the use of these medications in treating adolescent and childhood obesity.

Other agents of interest for the treatment of adolescent obesity include metformin (Glucophage®), a medication that inhibits hepatic glucose production, and recombinant leptin replacement therapy, a treatment for congenital leptin deficiency. Metformin is currently indicated for the treatment of type 2 diabetes in adults and children ages 10 years and older [26]. In addition to regulating glucose levels, metformin appears to induce weight loss (typically about 2 kg), even in nondiabetic adults [27,28]. Side effects of metformin include nausea, flatulence, bloating, diarrhea, vitamin B12 deficiencies, and in rare cases, lactic acidosis. Few studies to date have investigated the efficacy of metformin for the treatment of adolescent obesity.

Congenital leptin deficiency has been identified as the cause of severe, early onset obesity in a handful of children [29]. Recombinant leptin therapy has been found to result in substantial weight loss among children with this disorder [30,31]. However, recombinant leptin therapy for obese children and adolescents who do not suffer from congenital leptin deficiencies has yet to be investigated. Studies of adults have shown modest weight losses of 4 to 8% of initial weight [32].

## USE OF ORLISTAT WITH ADOLESCENTS AND CHILDREN

### SAFETY AND EFFICACY TRIALS

The largest study of orlistat with obese adolescents was conducted by the makers of orlistat, Roche Pharmaceuticals [33]. This 1-year, randomized, placebo-controlled, double-blind study evaluated the safety and efficacy of the medication in 539 obese adolescents. Following a 2-week placebo run-in phase, participants were randomly assigned to receive either orlistat (120 mg, TID) or placebo. All participants were instructed to consume a reduced-calorie diet that provided no more than 30% of calories from fat. They received nutritional and behavioral counseling throughout the study and were instructed to take a daily multivitamin.

Adolescents treated with orlistat plus diet had a significantly reduced BMI compared with patients who received placebo plus diet. According to Roche, 27% of participants who received orlistat achieved a 5% or greater reduction in BMI, compared with 16% of subjects on placebo; 13% of those treated with orlistat and 4.5% of the placebo group attained a 10% or greater reduction in baseline BMI [33,34]. Gastrointestinal events (e.g., fatty/oily stool, oily spotting, and oily evacuation) were the most commonly reported adverse events, with 50% of the orlistat group and 8% of the placebo group reporting symptoms [33]. No deaths occurred during the course of this study. The results of this trial led the FDA to approve orlistat for use in persons 12 to 16 years of age.

## OPEN-LABEL TRIALS

An open-label study of obese adolescents provides further evidence of the safety and tolerability of orlistat. McDuffie and colleagues evaluated the medication in 20 obese adolescents (10 males, 10 females) who had at least one obesity-related comorbid condition, such as hyperinsulinemia, hyperlipidemia, hypertension, type 2 diabetes, or impaired glucose tolerance [35]. Participants had a mean age of 14.6 ± 2.0 years (range of 12 to 17.9 years) and BMI of 44.1 ± 12.6 kg/m$^2$. Orlistat treatment was provided for 12 weeks as an adjunct to a behavioral weight loss program. Adolescents and their parents received nutritional counseling and were instructed to adhere to a 500-calorie-deficit diet that provided no more than 30% of calories from fat. Participants were instructed to take orlistat (120 mg) three times per day with meals. They were also instructed to take a daily multivitamin.

Eighty-five percent of participants completed the 3-month study. Participants lost 4.4 ± 4.6 kg, equal to 3.8 ± 4.1% of initial weight. Improvements were noted in low-density lipoprotein and total cholesterol levels, fasting glucose and insulin levels, and insulin sensitivity. Participants reported taking 80% of prescribed doses of orlistat, and only one participant withdrew because of side effects. Nearly all participants reported at least two side effects, and more than 50% of the sample reported increased defecation, soft stools, fatty or oily stools, oily spotting on clothing, and increased flatus [35].

McDuffie et al. recently published a 6-month follow-up of this sample [36]. After completing the first 3 months of behavior modification and orlistat, participants continued the medication and returned for assessments at three monthly follow-up visits. Fifteen of the 20 participants completed 6 months of treatment. At this time, participants had lost 3.5 ± 6.0% of initial body weight. Similar to the 3-month outcome data, improvements in total and low-density lipoprotein cholesterol were noted, as well as improvements in fasting glucose and insulin levels and insulin sensitivity.

At 6 months, an 81% medication adherence rate was reported. According to pill counts, participants took an average of 75% of possible doses. Participants attributed nonadherence to skipping meals, eating fat-free meals, snacking instead of eating a full meal, and concerns about taking the medication at school. Two participants discontinued orlistat on their own before the completion of the study.

Caucasian adolescents lost significantly more weight than African-American participants (7.3 vs. 0.8 kg, respectively, after 6 months of orlistat). The authors noted that this finding could be, in part, a result of known differences in resting energy expenditure in African Americans and Caucasians. Further studies are needed to confirm the smaller losses in African Americans. The authors also noted that more gastrointestinal side effects were reported in these younger participants compared with the number typically reported by adults [35]. The authors speculated that this finding may reflect greater difficulty in adolescents in adhering to a low-fat diet. Participants in this sample reported skipping doses when consuming high-fat meals to prevent unwanted side effects.

Additional randomized, placebo-controlled trials of orlistat with larger samples of adolescents are needed to determine whether the medication is more effective than a comprehensive behavioral program used alone. Studies of longer duration also are needed to further assess the long-term safety, tolerability, and efficacy of orlistat in adolescents.

## ORLISTAT AND VITAMIN AND MINERAL ABSORPTION

An industry-sponsored trial investigated the effect of orlistat on mineral balance over 3 weeks of treatment in 27 obese adolescents [37]. This double-blind, randomized, placebo-controlled study found that orlistat inhibited dietary fat by 27%. This inhibition of fat absorption, however, did not significantly affect mineral balance (e.g., calcium, phosphorus, magnesium, zinc, and copper) compared with placebo. These findings support the safety of orlistat's use with adolescents, although longer-term studies are needed.

Another study examined the effects of orlistat on fat-soluble vitamins (e.g., vitamins A, D, E, and K) over a 3- to 6-month period in a sample of 17 obese adolescents [38]. Acute absorption of vitamin A was not altered by orlistat treatment; however, absorption of vitamin E decreased significantly over the course of the study. Serum levels of vitamins A and E remained similar from baseline to the end of treatment, and serum levels of vitamin K decreased by the end of treatment, although not significantly. Finally, serum vitamin D levels decreased from baseline following 1 month of treatment. However, this finding may be in part a result of the consistently lower levels of vitamin D among African-American participants. Three African-American participants required vitamin D supplementation after 1 month, in addition to taking a multivitamin. Results indicate that vitamin D concentrations should be monitored, particularly among African-American adolescents [38].

## ORLISTAT'S USE IN CHILDREN

One study to date has examined orlistat's tolerance, safety, and psychosocial effects in a sample of 11 healthy, obese, prepubertal children [39]. In this open-label, 12-week clinical trial, the median age of participants was 10.7 years (range, 8.3 to 12.3 years). Children were treated with a standard dose of 120 mg orlistat, taken three times daily. Parents or guardians were provided with information regarding dietary sources of fat and recommendations for their child's fat intake while taking orlistat. No other dietary or behavioral intervention was provided.

At the end of the 12 weeks, the median weight loss was 4.0 kg (range, 12.7 to +2.5 kg). Over 98% of the capsules were taken (as measured by self-report and pill counts). Children reported increased control over their eating and greater avoidance of high-fat foods, as measured by the Children's Eating Attitudes Test. All children reportedly experienced loose stools. Four children reported frequent diarrhea or increased flatulence. However, no participants discontinued treatment because of side effects. Levels of vitamin A decreased significantly with orlistat, although they were still in the normal reference interval.

This study's findings appear to be positive. However, they must be viewed in light of several limitations, principally the small sample size, open-label design, and short duration. Randomized, placebo-controlled trials of orlistat are needed in obese children before the medication can be recommended for use in this population.

## USE OF SIBUTRAMINE WITH ADOLESCENTS

Experimental studies indicate that sibutramine may be of potential benefit in the treatment of obese adolescents. At present, however, the medication is not approved for persons younger than 16 years of age.

## Safety and Efficacy Trials

Berkowitz and colleagues conducted the first randomized, double-blind, placebo-controlled study of sibutramine in a sample of 82 adolescents ages 13 to 17 years with a BMI range of 32 to 44 kg/m$^2$ [40]. Exclusion criteria for this trial included the presence of cardiovascular disease, types 1 or 2 diabetes, major psychiatric disorders, or pregnancy; cigarette smoking; use of medications not recommended with sibutramine; and use of medications known to induce weight gain (e.g., oral steroids). For the first 6 months of the study, participants were assigned to a sibutramine plus behavior or a placebo plus behavior therapy. Those randomly assigned to sibutramine received a 5 mg/day dose, which was gradually increased to 15 mg/day by week 7. Adolescents treated with sibutramine plus behavior therapy lost an average of 7.8 ± 6.3 kg (i.e., 8.5 ± 6.8% reduction in BMI) whereas those assigned to placebo lost a significantly smaller 3.2 ± 6.1 kg (i.e., 4.0 ± 5.4% reduction in BMI). Sibutramine-treated participants also reported significantly greater reductions in hunger, as measured by the Eating Inventory, than adolescents assigned to placebo. Nineteen of the 43 participants treated with sibutramine initially experienced significant increases in blood pressure and pulse rate, which led to dose reductions. The medication was discontinued in five participants who experienced significant, sustained increases in blood pressure.

During months 7 to 12, all participants received sibutramine in an open-label fashion. Adolescents who were initially assigned to placebo lost an additional 1.3 kg, whereas those assigned to sibutramine maintained their weight loss through month 12. From baseline to month 12, participants originally assigned to sibutramine lost 7.0 ± 9.3 kg (i.e., 8.6 ± 9.9% of initial BMI), compared with 4.5 ± 8.8 kg (i.e., 6.4% ± 8.3% of initial BMI) for those initially assigned to the placebo and later converted to sibutramine.

Godoy-Matos and colleagues also conducted a randomized, placebo-controlled trial of sibutramine with adolescents [41]. This study included 60 Brazilian youth who were 14 to 17 years of age, were free of weight-related comorbidities, and had a BMI range of 30 to 45 kg/m$^2$. Participants were initially prescribed placebo and an energy-deficit diet for a 1-month run-in period. They received dietary counseling and instructions to increase their physical activity to a minimum of 30 minutes per day. Participants were then randomly assigned to either placebo or sibutramine (10 mg/day) for the next 6 months. No additional behavioral counseling was provided. At 6 months, adolescents assigned to sibutramine had lost 10.3 ± 6.6 kg, compared with 2.4 ± 2.5 kg in the placebo group. Aside from constipation, no serious adverse events were reported, including any events related to increased blood pressure or pulse rate. No participants discontinued the trial because of cardiovascular changes.

Weight loss reported in this study was greater than that obtained by Berkowitz et al. [40], although sibutramine was administered in a lower dose and without behavioral treatment. The authors suggested that their finding of greater weight loss might be a result of cultural and ethnic differences in the food environment in Brazil compared with that found in the United States. Differences in cardiovascular side effects in the two studies may have been caused by the lower dose of sibutramine used in the Brazilian investigation.

A multisite, randomized, placebo-controlled trial designed to further investigate the safety and efficacy of sibutramine in 498 obese adolescents is currently underway [42]. Safety and efficacy findings appear to be similar to those reported by Berkowitz et al. [40], with statistically significant improvements in BMI in the sibutramine-treated participants.

Data indicate that obese adolescents' response to sibutramine is similar to that of adults, including side effects of increased blood pressure and pulse rate. Further study is needed of the optimal dose of sibutramine (with adolescents) to induce weight loss but minimize these cardiovascular side effects. Similarly, further investigation is needed of the amount of behavioral counseling required with sibutramine, given the disparate protocols used by Berkowitz et al. and Goydos-Matos et al. Studies of the long-term (>1 year) risks and benefits with adolescents also are needed.

## METFORMIN

An early study investigated metformin with nine nondiabetic obese children (ages 8 to 14 years) [43]. In this open-label trial, participants received metformin (500 mg, TID) and dietary counseling. After 3 months, they lost 10.9 ± 4.1 kg. These promising results, however, should be viewed in light of methodological limitations that include a small sample size and an open-label design.

More recently, Freemark and Bursey conducted a 6-month, randomized, placebo-controlled study of the effects of metformin (500 mg, BID) on BMI [44]. Participants were 29 obese adolescents, ages 12 to 19 years, who had a BMI greater than 30 kg/m², hyperinsulinemia, and a family history of type 2 diabetes. Participants were not instructed to make any dietary modifications. At 6 months, BMI fell 1.3% in metformin-treated participants, compared with an increase of 2.3% in the placebo group. Metformin-treated participants experienced significant reductions in fasting glucose and insulin levels compared with those treated with placebo. Seven metformin-treated participants reported abdominal discomfort and diarrhea. However, these side effects were mild and resolved over time. Persistent nausea led to a dose reduction in one participant, but no adolescents discontinued treatment because of side effects.

Kay and colleagues conducted an 8-week, randomized, placebo-controlled trial of metformin (850 mg, BID) in 24 adolescents (ages 14 to 16 years, mean BMI of 41 kg/m²) [45]. All participants were instructed to consume a 1500 to 1800 kcal/day diet. Those treated with metformin and diet lost 6.5 ± 0.8% of initial weight, compared with 3.8 ± 0.4% in the placebo group. Significantly greater decreases in fasting insulin, plasma leptin, cholesterol, triglycerides, and free fatty acids also were found in metformin-treated adolescents. Minimal side effects (e.g., mild nausea) were reported in five participants, but no adolescents discontinued participation because of these complaints.

Results of these trials indicate that metformin, in combination with a low-calorie diet, may provide modest weight losses and reductions in fasting glucose and insulin levels for adolescents with obesity and risk factors for type 2 diabetes. Metformin appears to be well tolerated in this age group. However, larger studies of longer duration are needed.

## CLINICAL IMPLICATIONS AND CONCLUSIONS

Pharmacotherapy appears to be a promising tool to aid in the treatment of adolescent obesity. Orlistat is currently the only antiobesity agent with an indication for use in adolescents (12 to 16 years of age). Sibutramine also appears to be beneficial with adolescents, but its use must be considered experimental, at this time, in persons below the age of 16 years. Studies of metformin demonstrate modest weight reductions in samples of adolescents with insulin resistance. However, metformin is not currently indicated for weight reduction in this population.

Studies indicate that these medications are fairly well tolerated in adolescents. However, sibutramine has not been studied in adolescents with obesity-related comorbidities, and it may be inappropriate for adolescents with hypertension or other complications. Because orlistat does not have systemic side effects, it may be considered to be a "safer" medication compared with sibutramine and metformin. However, orlistat's gastrointestinal side effects may be intolerable and potentially embarrassing for teenagers.

At present, no long-term data (i.e., beyond 1 year) exist regarding the safety, efficacy, and tolerability of weight-loss medications in adolescents. In addition, there have been no head-to-head comparisons of the medications. Thus, although sibutramine appears to induce greater weight losses in adolescents compared with orlistat or metformin, additional studies are needed to confirm these observations. Additional investigations are needed to assess the risk–benefit profile of different doses of these medications, such that weight loss is maximized without causing undue risk of side effects. Data regarding the potential additive benefit of combining pharmacotherapy with behavioral treatments are especially needed. Long-term medication adherence and the role of pharmacotherapy in promoting weight maintenance also require further empirical attention.

Investigators have suggested that intensive treatments, such as pharmacotherapy, may be appropriate for seriously obese adolescents with comorbidities [46,47], particularly as these individuals are likely to become obese adults. However, with the exception of orlistat, antiobesity agents should be viewed as experimental until safety and effectiveness are further established [48]. In light of the history of pharmacological agents in the treatment of obesity, it is likely best to proceed with caution in using these agents in young persons, and as Dietz [49] suggests, to use them only as "adjuncts to behavior modification, family therapy, and increased activity" (p. 55).

## REFERENCES

1. Hedley AA, Ogden CL, Johnson CL, Carroll MD, Curtin LR, Flegal, KM. Prevalence of overweight and obesity among US children, adolescents, and adults, 1999-2002. *JAMA* 2004; 291:2847–2950.
2. Rosenbloom AL, Joe JR, Young RS, Winter WE. Emerging epidemic of type 2 diabetes in youth. *Diabetes Care* 1999; 22:345–354.
3. Pinhas-Hamiel O, Dolan LM, Daniels SR, Standiford D, Khoury PR, Zeitler P. Increased incidence of non-insulin-dependent diabetes mellitus among adolescents. *J Pediatr* 1996; 128:608–615.
4. Styne DM. Childhood and adolescent obesity. *Pediatr Clin North Am* 2001; 48:823–847.
5. Casey VA, Dwyer JT, Coleman KA, Valadian I. Body mass index from childhood to middle age: a 50-year follow-up. *Am J Clin Nutr* 1992; 56:14–18.
6. Garn SM, Sullivan TV, Hawthorne VM. Fatness and obesity of the parents of obese individuals. *Am J Clin Nutr* 1989; 50:1308–1313.
7. Pi-Sunyer F. Medical hazards of obesity. *Ann Intern Med* 1993; 119:655–660.
8. National Research Council Committee on Diet and Health. *Diet and Health: Implications for Reducing Chronic Disease Risk*. Washington, DC: National Academy Press, 1989.
9. Gortmaker SL, Must A, Perrin JM, Sobol AM, Dietz WH. Social and economic consequences of overweight in adolescence and young adulthood. *New Engl J Med* 1993; 329:1008–1012.
10. Schwimmer JB, Burwinkle TM, Varni JW. Health-related quality of life in severely obese children and adolescents. *JAMA* 2003; 289:1812–1819.
11. Epstein LH, Valoski A, Wing RR, McCurley J. Ten-year follow-up of behavioral, family-based treatment for obese children. *JAMA* 1990; 264:2519–2523.
12. Epstein LH, Valoski A, Wing RR, McCurley J. Ten-year outcomes of behavioral, family-based treatment for childhood obesity. *Health Psychol* 1994; 13:373–383.
13. American Academy of Pediatrics, Committee on Nutrition. Factors affecting food intake. *Pediatrics* 1964; 33:135–143.
14. Connolly HM, Crary JL, McGoon MD, Hensrud DD, Edwards BS, Edwards WD, Schaff HV. Valvular heart disease associated with fenfluramine-phentermine. *N Engl J Med* 1997; 337:581–588.
15. Bowen R, Glicklich A, Kahn M, Rasmussen S, Wadden TA, Bilstad J et al. Cardiac valvulopathy associated with exposure to fenfluramine or dexfenfluramine: U.S. Department of Health and Human Services Interim Public Health Recommendations. *Morb Mortal Wkly Rep* 1997; 46:1061–1066.
16. Molnár D, Török K, Erhardt E, Jeges S. Safety and efficacy of treatment with an ephedrine/caffeine mixture. The first double-blind placebo-controlled pilot study in adolescents. *Int J Obes* 2000; 24:1573–1578.
17. Food and Drug Administration. Final rule declaring dietary supplements containing ephedrine alkaloids adulterated because they present an unreasonable risk. *Fed Regist.* 2004; 69:6787–6854.
18. McBride BF, Karapanos AK, Krudysz A, Kluger J, Coleman CI, White CM. Electrocardiographic and hemodynamic effects of a multicomponent dietary supplement containing ephedra and caffeine: a randomized controlled trial. *JAMA* 2004; 291:216–221.
19. Sjostrom L, Rissanen A, Andersen T, Boldrin M, Golay A, Koppeschaar HPF, Krempf M, for the European Multicentre Orlistat Study Group. Randomized placebo-controlled trial of orlistat for weight loss and prevention of weight regain in obese patients. *Lancet* 1998; 352:167–172.
20. Davidson MH, Hauptman J, DiGirolamo M, Foreyt JP, Halsted CH, Heber D et al. Weight control and risk factor reduction in obese subjects treated for 2 years with orlistat: a randomized controlled trial. *JAMA* 1999; 281:235–242.

21. Hill JO, Hauptman J, Anderson JW, Fujioka K, O'Neil PM, Smith DK et al. Orlistat, a lipase inhibitor, for weight maintenance after conventional dieting: a 1-year study. *Am J Clin Nutr* 1999; 69:1108–1116.

22. Bray GA, Ryan DH, Heidingsfelder S, Cerise F, Wilson K. A double-blind randomized placebo-controlled trial of sibutramine. *Obes Res* 1997; 4:263–270.

23. Rolls BJ, Shide DJ, Thorwart ML, Ulbrecht JS. Sibutramine reduces food intake in non-dieting women with obesity. *Obes Res* 1997; 6:1–11.

24. Hansen DL, Toubro S, Stock MJ, Macdonald IA, Astrup A. The effect of sibutramine on energy expenditure and appetite during chronic treatment without dietary restriction. *Int J Obes Relat Metab Disord* 1999; 23:1016–1024.

25. Lean MEJ. A review of clinical efficacy. *Int J Obes* 1997; 21:30S–36S.

26. Bristol Myers Squibb Company. Glucophage® Package Insert. Princeton, NJ. Available at: http://www. glucophagexr.com/ (accessed February 2005).

27. Lee A, Morley JE. Metformin decreases food consumption and induces weight loss in subjects with obesity and type II non-insulin-dependent diabetes. *Obes Res* 1998; 6:47–53.

28. Fontbonne A, Charles MA, Juhan-Vague I, Bard JM, Andre P, Isnard F et al. The effect of metformin on the metabolic abnormalities associated with upper-body fat distribution. *Diabetes Care* 1996; 19:920–926.

29. Montague CT, Farooqi IS, Whitehead JP, Soos MA, Rau H, Wareham NJ et al. Congenital leptin deficiency is associated with severe early-onset obesity in humans. *Nature* 1997; 387:903–908.

30. Farooqi IS, Jebb SA, Langmack G, Lawrence E, Cheetham CH, Prentice AM et al. Effects of recombinant leptin therapy in a child with congenital leptin deficiency. *N Engl J Med* 1999; 341(12):879–884.

31. Gibson WT, Farooqi IS, Moreau M, DePaoli AM, Lawrence E, O'Rahilly S, Trussell RA. Congenital leptin deficiency due to homozygosity for the 133G mutation: report of another case and evaluation of response to four years of leptin therapy. *J Clin Endocrinol Metab* 2004; 89(10):4821–4826

32. Heymsfield SB, Greenberg AS, Fujioka K, Dixon RM, Kushner R, Hunt T et al. Recombinant leptin for weight loss in obese and lean adults. *JAMA* 1999; 282(6): 1568–1575.

33. Roche Laboratories, Incorporated. Xenical ® use in pediatric and adolescent patients. Nutley, NJ. Available at: http://www.rocheusa.com/ppi/pdfs/Xenical/090f42548009c9ab.PDF (accessed February 2005).

34. Roche Laboratories, Incorporated. Xenical ® Package Insert. Nutley, NJ. Available at: http://www. rocheusa.com/products/xenical/pi.pdf (accessed February 2005).

35. McDuffie JR, Calis KA, Uwaifo GI, Sebring NG, Fallon EM, Hubbard VS, Yanovski JA. Three-month tolerability of orlistat in adolescents with obesity-related comorbid conditions. *Obes Res* 2002; 10(7):642–650.

36. McDuffie JR, Calis KA, Uwaifo GI, Sebring NG, Fallon EM, Frazer TE et al. Efficacy of orlistat as an adjunct to behavioral treatment in overweight African-American and Caucasian adolescents with obesity-related co-morbid conditions. *J Ped Endocrinol Metab* 2004; 17:307–319.

37. Zhi JZ, Moore R, Kanitra L. The effect of short-term (21-day) orlistat treatment on the physiologic balance of six selected macrominerals and microminerals in obese adolescents. *J Am Coll Nutr* 2003; 22(5):357–362.

38. McDuffie JR, Calis KA, Booth SL, Uwaifo GI, Yanovski JA. Effects of orlistat on fat-soluble vitamins in obese adolescents. *Pharmacotherapy* 2002; 22(7):814–822.

39. Norgren S, Danielsson P, Jurold R, Lötborn M, Marcus C. Orlistat treatment in obese prepubertal children: a pilot study. *Acta Pædiatr* 2003; 92:666–670.

40. Berkowitz RI, Wadden TA, Tershakovee AM, Cronquist JL. Behavior therapy and sibutramine for the treatment of adolescent obesity. *JAMA* 2003; 289(14):1805–1812.

41. Godoy-Matos A, Carraro L, Vieira A, Oliviera J, Guedes EP, Mattos L et al. Treatment of obese adolescents with sibutramine: a randomized, double-blind, controlled study. *J Clin Endocrinol Metabol.* 2004. Available at: http://jcem.endojournals.org/ cgi/rapidpdf/jc.2004-0263v1 (accessed February 2005).

42. Berkowitz RI, Fukjioka K, Hewkin A, Walch J, Peng J, Blakesley V, Renz C. Results of a double-blind, placebo-controlled study to evaluate treatment of obese adolescents with sibutramine — efficacy and safety. North American Association for the Study of Obesity's Annual Meeting, Las Vegas, NV, November 14–18, 2004.

43. Lutjens A, Smit JL. Effect of biguanide treatment in obese children. *Helvetica Paediat Acta* 1977; 31(6):473–480.

44. Freemark M, Bursey D. The effects of metformin on body mass index and glucose tolerance in obese adolescents with fasting hyperinsulinemia and a family history of type 2 diabetes. *Pediatrics* 2001; 107(4):55–61

45. Kay JP, Alemzadeh R, Langley G, D'Angelo L, Smith P, Holshouser S. Beneficial effects of metformin in normoglycemic morbidly obese adolescents. *Metabolism* 2001; 50(12):1457–1461.

46. Yanovski JA. Intensive therapies for pediatric obesity. *Pediat Clin N Am* 2001; 48(4):1041–1053.

47. Berkowitz RI, Lyke JA, Wadden TA. Treatment of child and adolescent obesity. In: Johnston FE, Foster GD, Eds. *Obesity, Growth and Development*. London: Smith-Gordon, 2001:169–184.

48. Yanovski JA, Yanovski SZ. Treatment of pediatric and adolescent obesity. *JAMA* 2003; 289(14):1851–1853.

49. Dietz WH. Pharmacotherapy for childhood obesity? Maybe for some. *Obes Res* 1994; 2(1):54–55.

# Section 10

## Surgery

# 18 Surgical Management of Pediatric Obesity

*Thomas Inge, Meg Zeller, Shelley Kirk, and Stephen Daniels*

## CONTENTS

## INTRODUCTION

Surgery has been used for the treatment of clinically severe obesity for almost a half century in the United States. Bariatric surgery is a valuable and proven therapy for obese adults, and several individual procedures were endorsed in 1991 by a Consensus Development Conference of the National Institutes of Health [1]. Largely because of the clearly demonstrated adverse effects of adult obesity on all-cause mortality [2], bariatric surgery is recommended for those adults with a body mass index [BMI] 40 kg/m$^2$ or above and for those 35 kg/m$^2$ or above with severe medical comorbidities who have failed prior nonsurgical obesity management attempts.

Today, extreme obesity is no longer a disease limited to adults. Pediatric specialists are increasingly confronted with a new set of diagnostic and therapeutic dilemmas in severely and extremely obese children and adolescents. At the time National Institutes of Health bariatric guidelines were established, those patients 18 years of age or younger were not included. Thus, recently a multidisciplinary group of pediatric specialists with national representation convened to develop guidelines for adolescent bariatric surgery based on clinical practice and existing evidence [3]. Issues unique to adolescents include the possibility of adverse effects of bariatric surgery on growth and development, concerns about the ability to completely prepare an adolescent for an intervention that changes eating patterns for life, possible effects on future reproductive outcomes, and possible deficiency syndromes if macro- or micronutrient intake is inadequate following operation [3–5].

## PRIMARY CARE PROVIDER CONSIDERATIONS BEFORE REFERRAL OF SURGICAL CANDIDATES

Guidelines that have been proposed [3] for adolescent bariatric surgery necessarily take into consideration the natural history of pediatric severe obesity and the National Institutes of Health consensus guidelines for performing bariatric surgery in adults. Mortality for obese adults begins to rise fairly abruptly above a BMI of 30 to 35 kg/m$^2$ [2] for both men and women. Although adolescents may ultimately suffer the same or greater mortality risk from extreme obesity, it is

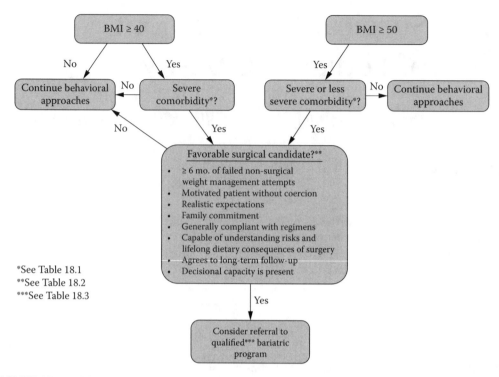

**FIGURE 18.1** Adolescent bariatric management algorithm.

generally held that most teenagers will not suffer a lethal complication of obesity before adulthood. To date, there is no empiric evidence to indicate that different indications for bariatric operation should be used for adolescents compared with adults, though it is rational to be more conservative with adolescents because less is known about the long-term risks and durability of the surgery in youth.

A practical algorithm that can be used to guide initial surgical referral decisions for a clinically severely obese adolescent is shown in Figure 18.1. For adolescents with comorbidities of obesity who have been unsuccessful at attaining a healthier weight during 6 months or more of conventional

---

**TABLE 18.1**
**Comorbidities of Obesity**

**Examples of Severe Comorbidities**

Type 2 diabetes mellitus
Obstructive sleep apnea syndrome
Pseudotumor cerebri

**Examples of Less Severe Comorbidities**

Impaired glucose tolerance
Hyperlipidemia
Hypertension
Venous stasis disease
Nonalcoholic fatty liver disease
Polycystic ovary syndrome
Psychosocial pathology (depression, withdrawal)
Significant impairment in activities of daily living
Gastroesophageal reflux

---

**TABLE 18.2**
**Contraindications for Bariatric Surgery**

Adolescent or family not able to comprehend risks and benefits of the intervention

Adolescent not autonomously motivated to consider operation

Adolescent has unrealistic expectations for results of the surgical intervention

Family/adolescent not able to commit to compliance with postoperative nutritional recommendations and long-term medical and nutritional monitoring

History of noncompliance with treatment regimens or planned health care provider visits

Presence of a medically correctable cause of obesity

Existence of a medical, psychiatric, or cognitive condition that may impair the ability of patient to assent to surgery or adhere to postoperative dietary and medication regimen

Inadequately documented weight loss attempts

Existence of substance abuse in preceding year

Current lactation, pregnancy, or plans for pregnancy in upcoming 2 years

Patient lacks decisional capacity

Inability to provide informed assent (patient) and consent (family)

Adolescent has not attained skeletal maturity (expected adult stature)

dietary and physical activity measures, bariatric surgery may be an option (Table 18.1). It is difficult to precisely define the concept of "failure" of conventional weight management attempts, and failure must be defined on an individual basis, in the context of the weight-management resources that are locally available for the adolescent. Because the number of dedicated adolescent weight-management programs is limited, this approach may be unavailable to the majority of individuals in need of services. The decision to pursue intensive therapies such as surgery necessarily must be made with the agreement of the primary care provider that all reasonable and available nonsurgical weight management attempts have been exhausted. Finally, there are a number of factors that should represent contraindications to pursuit of surgical therapy (Table 18.2).

Adolescents being considered for bariatric surgery should be referred to specialized centers of excellence with a multidisciplinary bariatric team capable of evaluating and managing medical comorbidities of obesity, providing long-term follow-up, and managing the unique challenges posed by the severely obese adolescent (see Table 18.3). Guidelines have been established by the National Institutes of Health [6], the American Society for Bariatric Surgery (http://www.asbs.org) [7], the American College of Surgeons, and the Surgical Review Corporation (http://www.surgicalreview.org) that indicate that such teams should include specialists with expertise in obesity evaluation and management, psychology, nutrition, physical activity, and bariatric surgery. Depending on the individual needs of the adolescent patient, additional expertise in adolescent medicine, endocrinology, pulmonology, gastroenterology, cardiology, orthopedics, and ethics should be readily available. At present, specialized adolescent bariatric programs are being established at a number of academic medical centers in the United States.

The timing for surgical treatment for adolescents is controversial and depends, in most cases, on the compelling health needs of the patient. However, there are certain physiological factors that need to be considered in planning an essentially elective operation. Physiologic maturation is generally complete by sexual maturation (Tanner) stage 3 or 4 [8]. Skeletal maturation (adult stature) is normally attained by the age of 13 to 14 years in girls [9] and 15 to 16 years in boys [10]. Overweight children generally experience accelerated onset of puberty. As a result, they are likely to be taller and have advanced bone age compared with age-matched nonoverweight children. If there is uncertainty about whether adult stature has been attained, skeletal maturation (bone age) can be objectively assessed with a radiograph of the hand and wrist [11]. If an individual has attained 95% or more of adult stature [12], there should be little concern that a bariatric procedure would significantly impair completion of linear growth.

**TABLE 18.3**
**Suggested Institution and Program Qualifications**

1. The program has support for excellence in the care of adolescent bariatric surgical patients at the highest level of administration.
2. The bariatric surgeon meets training criteria recommended by the American Society for Bariatric Surgery (http://www.asbs.org).
3. The bariatric program maintains a "medical director" with expertise in pediatrics who participates in the decision-making process leading to surgery.
4. The program is staffed with a qualified and specially trained allied health worker (e.g., physician's assistant or advanced practice nurse) to act as a bariatric patient care coordinator. This individual's role is dedicated to the close monitoring and continuing education needed in the postoperative care of adolescent bariatric patients.
5. The program maintains a psychologist with expertise in bariatric patient evaluation.
6. The program maintains a dedicated dietician with subspecialty experience or training in bariatric nutritional care.
7. The program maintains a full complement of the various consultative services required for the care of morbidly obese surgical patients including the immediate availability of in-house critical care services.
8. The institution maintains a full line of medical equipment and instruments for the care of bariatric patients throughout the hospital environment (including the clinic area, operating room, intensive care unit, emergency room, and radiologic facilities) suitable for the size and weights seen with extremely obese patients.
   a. The hospital beds, gurneys, operating room tables, clinic exam room and waiting room furniture, scales, wheel chairs, and commodes need to be strong enough and extra wide to accommodate the extremely obese patient and family members.
   b. Patient movement/transfer systems for morbidly obese patients must be in place wherever the morbidly obese receive care.
   c. The computed tomography scanner, fluoroscopy tables, and nuclear medicine equipment must have sufficient capacity to handle morbidly obese patients.
9. The program has a bariatric surgeon who spends a significant portion of his or her efforts in the field of bariatric surgery, who achieves annual continuing medical education in bariatrics, and who has qualified coverage and support for patient care during times of his absence.
10. The program uses clinical pathway orders that facilitate the standardization of perioperative care.
11. The hospital should have a subset of nurses who routinely care for bariatric patients and receive regular bariatric in-service education.
12. The program provides long-term medical follow-up of all patients undergoing bariatric procedures with a monitoring and tracking system for outcomes assessment.

## COMPREHENSIVE TEAM ASSESSMENT OF THE PATIENT REFERRED FOR BARIATRIC SURGERY

Optimal bariatric management (preoperative patient selection and postoperative monitoring) of the adolescent is provided by a team consisting of a pediatrician with weight-management expertise, a psychologist with adolescent expertise, a qualified bariatric surgeon with a special focus in adolescent bariatric practice, a dietician with special focus in bariatric nutrition, and an advanced practice nurse dedicated to care coordination for this special-needs patient group.

Comprehensive assessment of potential bariatric patients by the team begins with a thorough review of the patient's past medical and behavioral history and history of weight-loss attempts provided by the primary care physician. Objective testing, which should be considered during evaluation for bariatric surgery, is shown in Table 18.4. These preliminary studies may indicate the need for consultation by a cardiologist, pulmonologist, endocrinologist, or other specialists. The history will often raise psychosocial concerns that the psychologist will need to be prepared to address.

The psychologist is an integral member of the adolescent bariatric team. The psychologist not only provides considerable input into selection of patients appropriate for surgery but also provides ongoing consultation and management of adherence and psychological issues postsurgery. The

**TABLE 18.4**
**Preoperative Assessment**

| System | Measure |
|---|---|
| Endocrine | Fasting glucose and insulin, hemoglobin A1C, and glucose tolerance testing if indicated by abnormal fasting glucose; thyroid function testing; pregnancy test for females |
| Hepatobiliary/ Nutritional | Liver function tests, albumin, consider ultrasound of gallbladder (if symptoms indicative of cholelithiasis) |
| Cardiovascular | Lipid profile, consider transthoracic echocardiogram |
| Hematologic | Complete blood count |
| Pulmonary | Consider polysomnogram for patients with symptoms of obstructive sleep apnea |
| Skeletal | Bone age assessment should be considered for those patients for whom doubt exists regarding whether adult stature has been obtained |
| Anthropometrics | Height, weight, waist and hip circumferences, and bioelectrical impedance (or DEXA if <300 pounds) |

DEXA = dual-energy x-ray densitometry.

**TABLE 18.5**
**Goals of Psychological Evaluation**

Determine the level of cognitive and psychosocial development, primarily to judge the extent to which the adolescent is capable of participating in the decision to proceed with the intervention

Expose emotional or behavioral problems that may bear on postoperative compliance with nutritional requirements

Identify past/present psychiatric or eating disorders

Define potential supports and barriers to regimen adherence, as well as family readiness for surgery and the required lifestyle changes (particularly if one or both parents are obese)

Assess whether there are reasonable outcome expectations

Assess family unit stability and identify psychological stressors or conflicts within the family

Determine whether the adolescent is autonomously motivated to consider bariatric surgery or whether any element of coercion is present

preoperative psychological evaluation of the prospective adolescent bariatric patient differs considerably from the evaluation of adult candidates. Goals of the evaluation are provided in Table 18.5. Briefly stated, prospective patients are screened for psychopathology, including binge-eating symptoms, as well as cognitive and emotional maturity, history of adherence to medical regimens, and family support. This evaluation is conducted in part with the patient and family together, as well as with the adolescent patient alone. Such a comprehensive family-centered psychosocial assessment provides the bariatric team with the information needed to make decisions about the appropriateness of surgical intervention for each adolescent and to tailor the management to improve adherence with nutritional regimens.

Once the bariatric team's evaluation is complete, decision making regarding a patient's candidacy for surgery must take into account all information obtained. Further input from other involved caregivers (particularly the referring pediatrician) can be important for gauging an adolescent's autonomous motivation for surgery and the patient's prior history of compliance with prescribed regimens and office visits. The multidisciplinary team considering patients for adolescent bariatric surgery acts much like a tumor board or organ transplant team, discussing the advantages and disadvantages of a complex surgical intervention and weighing the myriad psychological, developmental, medical, and social/family factors that may well effect an individual's chances of success with the intervention.

Once the decision has been made to proceed with bariatric surgery, adequate preoperative education of the patient and family is critical. The dietician plays a necessary role, counseling the patient and family about the appropriate postoperative nutritional regimen. Preoperatively, the progression of acceptable food items, emphasis on high-protein foods, appropriate consistency, and meal volumes prescribed during the first week, first month, and subsequent months are discussed to prepare the patient and family for the drastic dietary change. Having the patient and the primary caregivers participate in a "taste-testing" exercise to concretely experience the various high-protein drink products allowed during the first weeks after surgery can help to improve adherence to the advised dietary regimen. The high-protein drinks tasted are ranked according to the patient's preference. Commercially available products and those made from recipes, which allow the patient to design high-protein drinks with flavors of his or her choosing, provide the patient with many options. This feature of the preoperative education was developed to encourage patients to take an active role in their postoperative diet, increase awareness about their food preferences, and help families plan in advance for obtaining the selected food items that will be most acceptable to the patients.

The dietician, along with the advanced practice nurse and surgeons then review required postoperative medication and micronutrient supplementation regimens. Complications and expected side effects specific to the operation are discussed in great detail, and written testing is used to document the patient's mastery of the information presented. Thorough and repeated education of the family and the patient is of paramount importance for adequate preoperative preparation. Most believe that the more informed the patient and the family are, the lower the likelihood of preventable complications.

## POSTOPERATIVE MANAGEMENT

The most common procedure currently used for adolescents is roux-en-Y gastric bypass, although the adjustable gastric band may be a satisfactory option pending approval for this age group by the U.S. Food and Drug Administration. Malabsorptive procedures such as biliopancreatic bypass with or without duodenal switch are currently performed in adults but are probably not suitable for most adolescents. Following surgery, patients are typically cared for in a monitored, nonintensive care unit setting, and maintenance fluids are administered based on lean body weight (typically 40 to 50% of actual weight). Early warning signs of complication include fever, tachycardia, tachypnea, increasing oxygen requirement, oliguria, hiccoughs, regurgitation, worsening abdominal pain, a feeling of anxiety, or acute alteration in mental status. These signs warrant immediate attention and appropriate investigation as they may foreshadow a gastrointestinal leak, pulmonary embolus, bowel obstruction, or afferent loop syndrome (acute dilation and resultant rupture of the bypassed gastric remnant). Routinely, a water-soluble upper gastrointestinal (UGI) contrast study is obtained on postoperative day 1. Special radiologic considerations for adolescent patients undergoing bariatric surgery are outlined elsewhere [13]. After satisfactory passage of contrast is documented, patients are begun on clear liquids and subsequently advanced to a high-protein liquid diet for the first month after surgery.

Postoperative medical surveillance after adolescent bariatric surgery is intensive — weekly for 1 month, then monthly for 6 months, then every third month for the next 18 months. For local patients, this monitoring is best provided by the bariatric program, whereas for distance patients, this care and monitoring is shared with the local pediatrician on an alternate visit basis.

Dietary advancement after surgery is a stepwise process of introducing new items of gradually increasing complexity toward the goal of a well-balanced, small-portion diet, which ensures a daily intake of one-half to 1 g protein per kilogram of ideal weight. This goal is based on the desire to lose fat mass while preserving lean mass postoperatively — a goal that is achievable in our experience [14]. The recommended stages of the dietary protocol for the adolescent patient are presented in Table 18.6. Though general guidelines are given for the timing of each stage, the progression through each of these stages is individualized and dependent on the patient's rate of recovery from the surgery, initial weight status, and tolerance of foods being introduced. To

## TABLE 18.6
## Postoperative Dietary Protocol

| Dietary Stage | Form | Description |
|---|---|---|
| 1 | Liquids | Water and ice chips: duration: 1–2 days; fluid goals:1–2 oz per hour |
| 2 | Liquids | Sugar-free clear liquids; duration: up to 1 week; fluid goals: 4–6 oz per hour; total: 48–64 oz per day |
| 3 | Liquids | High-protein drinks, protein-supplemented pudding, or yogurt; meal pattern: consumed three to four times per day; fluid goal: 90 oz per day; duration: about 3–4 weeks; volume: one-half to two-thirds of a cup per meal; goals/day: protein: 50–60 g, calories: 500–600 kcal |
| 3A | Liquids + solids | Semisolid high-protein foods (e.g., baked fish, tuna salad, chicken salad, cottage cheese, low-fat cheese, shaved turkey, scrambled eggs, egg salad, skim milk); consistency: foods are blenderized, pureed, or chopped into pieces no larger than the size of a pea before eating, and fat-free broth, fat-free mayonnaise, or plain yogurt is added to help moisten foods, as needed, for easier digestion; duration: 2–3 weeks; volume: one-half to two-thirds of a cup per meal; goals/day: protein: 50–60 m, calories: 500–600 kcal |
| 3B | Liquids + solids | Introduction of complex carbohydrate foods (note: foods listed below are added to the meals consisting of a semisolid high-protein food): part I: protein-supplemented blended soups, potato, hot cereal; part II: crackers, toast; goals/day: protein: 50–75 g, calories: 500–600 kcal |
| 3C | Liquids + solids | Introduction of other carbohydrate foods (e.g. vegetables, fruits, low-sugar cold cereal, rice, pasta); new foods: try one-quarter cup per meal, introduce one new food every 2–3 days |
| 4 | Liquids + solids | Follow acceptable food choices from stages 3A, 3B, and 3C: goals/day: protein: 75–100 g, calories: 600–800 kcal, volume: less than or equal to 1 cup per meal; starts approximately 3 months postsurgery |
| 5 | Liquids + solids | Follow acceptable food choices from stages 3A, 3B, 3C, and 4: new foods: red meat, pork, grapes, and raisins; goals/day: protein, 75–100 g, calories: 800–1000 kcal/day, volume: less than or equal to 1 cup/meal; starts approximately: 6 months postsurgery |
| 6 | Liquids + solids | Starts approximately 12 months postsurgery; goals/day: protein: 75–100 g, calories: 1000–1200 kcal/day (may vary according to level of physical activity), volume: less than or equal to 1.5 cups per meal; will continue to avoid foods high in fat and sugar; duration: for life |

determine whether there are any associated adverse reactions to new foods consumed, the foods are introduced individually over a 2- to 3-day period.

The risk of adverse reactions to liquid and solid food items will be minimized if foods high in fat or sugar are avoided and if food volumes are minimized initially. Consumption of sweets or high-fat foods and overeating can result in the dumping syndrome. "Dumping" occurs because after gastric bypass, the gastric phase of digestion is essentially eliminated, and consumed items very quickly pass from the new gastric pouch into the small intestine. This syndrome is associated with abdominal cramping, sweating, a rapid heart rate, vomiting, and diarrhea. To avoid association of such adverse reactions to food items, education must be provided that will encourage use of product nutrition labels to aid in food and drink selection. It is also critical that patients and families learn to identify sources of "hidden" fats (e.g., prepared food from restaurants) and sugars (e.g., condiments such as ketchup) that can cause adverse reactions and ultimately limit the success of the weight-loss operation.

During the first several months following gastric bypass, it is not uncommon to observe caloric intakes in the 300 to 500 kcal/day range. Given the extremely limited intake of solid food (and hence the limited intake of the water content of most solid foods), patients must focus on intake of 90+ ounces of water or nonnutritive liquids per day to avoid dehydration. To ensure that fluid intake does not compromise the patient's capacity to consume necessary solid foods, no liquids are consumed during the half hour before or after a meal or during meals.

Nonsteroidal antiinflammatory medications should be avoided to reduce the risk of intestinal ulceration and bleeding. Ursodiol and ranitidine are prescribed for 6 months, as is the practice for most adult bariatric programs, to reduce the risk of gallstone development and gastrointestinal ulceration. Alcohol should be avoided after gastric bypass, owing to the reduced threshold for intoxication and adverse effects on the function of liver already compromised with steatosis or steatohepatitis [15]. Postoperative vitamin and mineral supplementation consists of two pediatric chewable multivitamins and a calcium supplement, plus an iron supplement for menstruating females. Strong consideration should also be given to additional supplementation of B-complex vitamins beyond what is contained in multivitamin preparations to augment thiamine and folate supplementation because of the risk of beriberi [5] and the possibility of pregnancy in the postoperative period. It is strongly recommended that pregnancy be avoided for the initial 2-year postoperative period, as this is the period of most rapid weight loss. Contraception should be well thought out and deliberate to avoid potential nutritional problems for mother and fetus.

We routinely reemphasize five basic "rules" with each patient encounter: eat protein first, drink 64 to 96 ounces of water or sugar-free liquids daily, no snacking between meals, exercise at least 30 minutes per day, and always remember vitamins and minerals. Behavioral strategies, such as goal setting, self-monitoring, and incentives, can help ensure compliance to the postoperative protocol. Written contracts are used to specify nutrition and physical activity goals and the level of family support that is developmentally appropriate. Daily tracking of the type and amount of food and drink consumed and of vitamin and mineral supplements taken helps patients' dietary regimen adherence. In some cases, incentives can be a useful behavioral tool to help keep adolescents motivated to maintain their new eating habits and to reach increasing activity goals. Available and achievable incentives are selected by the patient and provided by the family and are earned when contracted goals are met over a set period of time.

## FINAL WORDS OF CAUTION

These postoperative guidelines necessitate significant lifestyle changes on the part of the adolescent. It is noteworthy that these changes must occur for a severely obese adolescent who has demonstrated failure at maintaining similar dietary and physical activity changes in the past. Nonadherence to medical regimens is typically worse in the adolescent patient, with medication nonadherence rates of 55% being reported for long-term regimens [16]. Furthermore, these lifestyle changes must occur within an environment that has contributed to the development of the critical weight and health status of the adolescent. Thus, these postoperative nutritional demands need to be considered within the context of a family environment, the parent–adolescent relationship, and other significant interpersonal relationships (peers, siblings) if they are to be successful. Finally, adolescence is a period of rapid change in emotional, cognitive, interpersonal, social, and career/vocational development. The fluidity of this developmental period may present unique challenges for the adolescent bariatric surgery patients that are not seen in the adult patient. All of these factors contribute to the need for caution and closer postoperative monitoring of the adolescent than is seen in adults.

Given that bariatric surgery for the severely obese adolescent patient has not been extensively studied, data describing predictors of positive surgical outcomes are nonexistent. Thus, the development of this area of research is of critical importance to understand the implications of this treatment for long-term psychosocial and physical health. The largest published study in the literature reported 33 adolescents who underwent various forms of gastric restriction and bypass between 1981 and 2001 [17]. Although significant weight reduction and health improvement were seen overall, five patients regained some or all of their body weight 5 to 10 years after surgery. The sole study that has looked at adolescent adherence to the postoperative bariatric regimen indicated that incomplete adherence to dietary, vitamin supplementation, and physical activity recommendations may be as high as 80 to 90% for adolescents [18]. These findings indicate variable adherence patterns following gastric bypass in adolescents that may affect clinically important outcomes.

## SUMMARY

The obesity epidemic in this country has generated a population of adolescents with the premature onset of adult disease. It is clear that bariatric surgery can result in significant weight loss. However, it is not yet clear whether weight loss or comorbidity resolution after adolescent bariatric surgery is sustainable over a lifetime or will have unintended negative consequences. At present, we can only apply rational principles of adolescent medicine and psychology, as well as evidence from adult bariatric surgical studies to guide the application of these procedures to a group of young patients who have serious medical and psychological comorbidities of obesity. Adolescent bariatric surgery programs should have expertise that enables them to assess and meet the unique medical, cognitive, physiological, and psychosocial needs of the adolescent and should be modeled after those adult bariatric programs demonstrating best practices. In the absence of scientifically valid evidence documenting long-term outcomes of bariatric surgery in adolescents, criteria for surgery should be conservative; the surgery should be performed in centers committed to clinical research and capable of long-term, detailed follow-up and outcomes assessment.

## REFERENCES

1. Hubbard, V. S. and W. H. Hall. Gastrointestinal surgery for severe obesity. *Obes. Surg.*, 1991, pp. 257–265.
2. Calle, E. E., M. J. Thun, J. M. Petrelli, C. Rodriguez, and C. W. Heath, Jr. Body-mass index and mortality in a prospective cohort of U.S. adults. *N Engl J Med*, 1999, pp. 1097–1105.
3. Inge, T. H., N. F. Krebs, V. F. Garcia, J. A. Skelton, K. S. Guice, R. S. Strauss et al. Bariatric surgery for severely overweight adolescents: Concerns and recommendations. *Pediatrics*, 2004, pp. 217–223.
4. Garcia, V. F., L. Langford, and T. H. Inge. Application of laparoscopy for bariatric surgery in adolescents. *Curr. Opin. Pediat.*, 2003, pp. 248–255.
5. Towbin, A., T. H. Inge, V. F. Garcia, H. R. Roerig, R. H. Clements, C. M. Harmon, and S. R. Daniels. Beriberi after gastric bypass surgery in adolescence. *J. Pediat.*, 2004, pp. 263–267.
6. Gastrointestinal surgery for severe obesity: National Institutes of Health Consensus Development Conference Statement. *Am. J. Clin. Nutr.*, 1992, pp. 615S–619S.
7. American Society for Bariatric Surgery. Society of American Gastrointestinal Endoscopic Surgeons. Guidelines for laparoscopic and open surgical treatment of morbid obesity. *Obes. Surg.*, 2000, pp. 378–379.
8. Tanner, J. M. *Growth at Adolescence*. Oxford: Blackwell Scientific Publications, 1962.
9. Marshall, W. A. and J. M. Tanner. Variations in pattern of pubertal changes in girls. *Arch. Dis. Child.*, 1969, pp. 291–303.
10. Marshall, W. A. and J. M. Tanner. Variations in the pattern of pubertal changes in boys. *Arch. Dis. Child.*, 1970, pp. 13–23.
11. Greulich, W. and S. I. Pyle. *Radiographic Atlas of Skeletal Development of the Hand and Wrist*. Palo Alto, CA: Stanford University Press, 1983.
12. Tanner, J. M. *Assessment of Skeletal Maturity and Prediction of Adult Height (TW2 method)*. San Diego: Academic Press, 1983.
13. Inge, T. H., L. F. Donnelly, M. Vierra, A. Cohen, S. R. Daniels, and V. F. Garcia. Managing bariatric patients in a children's hospital: radiologic considerations and limitations. *J. Ped. Surg.*, 2004.
14. Inge, T. H., M. L. Lawson, V. F. Garcia, S. Kirk, and S. Daniels. Body composition changes after gastric bypass in morbidly obese adolescents. *Obes. Res.*, 2004, p. A53.
15. Xanthakos, S. M., L. Bucuvalas, J. Daniels, S. Garcia, V. and T. Inge. Histologic spectrum of NASH in morbidly obese adolescents differs from adults. *Obes. Res.*, 2004, p. A211.
16. Rapoff, M. A. *Adherence to Pediatric Medical Regimens*. Dordrecht: Kluwer Academic Publishers, 1999.
17. Sugerman, H. J., E. L. Sugerman, E. J. DeMaria, J. M. Kellum, C. Kennedy, Y. Mowery, and L. G. Wolfe. Bariatric surgery for severely obese adolescents. *J. Gastrointest. Surg.*, 2003, pp. 102–108.
18. Rand, C. S. and A. M. Macgregor. Adolescents having obesity surgery: a 6-year follow-up. *South. Med. J.*, 1994, pp. 1208–1213.

# Section 11

*Interdisciplinary, Interactive, Group Instruction*

# 19 Interdisciplinary, Interactive Group Instruction: Orientation, Evaluation and Monitoring Progress

*Lauren Keely Carlisle and Stewart T. Gordon*

## CONTENTS

## INTRODUCTION

### PROGRAM OVERVIEW

The Interdisciplinary, Interactive Pediatric Weight-Management Program is a comprehensive program designed especially for the needs of the overweight child aged 7 to 17 years. The staff is a team of medical, health, and nutrition professionals whose primary concern is the safety and success of the child in the program.

A pediatrician or family physician serves as the medical director for the program. He or she provides overall medical supervision and guidance. In severely overweight children, calorie restriction is recommended. The very low calorie diet called the protein-modified fast (PMF) is described in detail in Appendix A3. The PMF diet must be closely supervised by a pediatrician or family physician. Health assessments are given quarterly, and results are discussed with parents and mailed to referring family physicians or pediatricians.

A registered dietitian provides nutrition supervision and guidance for the program. He or she conducts weekly educational sessions on nutrition topics and instructs patients in the proper administration of the prescribed diet. Nutrition sessions are conducted in group settings with patients, parents, siblings, and extended family and friends in attendance.

A child development or behavior specialist provides instruction in behavior-modification skills and techniques for the program. He or she conducts weekly educational sessions on the psychosocial aspects of obesity in children. Behavior modification skills are introduced using discussion, modeling, role playing, and guided problem solving. Topics such as self-monitoring, commitment, limit setting, habit formation, goal setting and action plans, decision-making skills, attitudes, and assertiveness training are discussed.

An exercise physiologist provides the exercise supervision and guidance for the program. He or she conducts weekly exercise sessions on various health and fitness topics and leads a weekly exercise class. Each session is a mixture of sharing information on topics such as heart-rate monitoring and injury prevention as well as the actual exercise. In addition, fitness counseling includes motivational techniques to increase daily activity levels and improve body movement awareness based on social cognitive theory [1].

## FAMILY INTERVENTION

Because successful behavior modification depends on what happens in the home, the Pediatric Weight-Management Program makes parents an integral part of the weekly intervention. We have found that the child's successes are determined not only by the child's commitment but also by that of his or her parents as well. At least one parent is required, and siblings and extended family are encouraged to attend the weekly sessions with the overweight child. The parent's participation in the interactive nutrition, behavior, and exercise instruction is strongly promoted.

## FOUR-LEVEL PROGRESSION

The needs of the overweight child depend on his or her level of overweight. There are four distinct levels of the Pediatric Weight-Management Program, each developed specifically for the individual needs of each level of obesity.

### Level I (Red)

This is an inpatient or outpatient level that serves the needs of the child with severe obesity or special medical indications.

### Level II (Yellow)

This level is for children who are diagnosed as overweight. Weekly outpatient sessions address issues of diet, behavior, and fitness.

### Level III (Green)

This level is for the child who is at risk for developing an overweight condition. Weekly outpatient sessions are designed to arrest and reverse the onset of obesity through nutrition education, increased physical activity, exercise training, and behavior modification.

### Level IV (Blue)

This is the maintenance program. Weekly exercise sessions and monthly multitopic meetings reinforce the healthy habits learned in intervention levels I, II, and III. The goal is for a lifetime of healthy eating and activity. This program may also serve as an obesity prevention program for healthy-weight children with primary risk factors.

## ORIENTATION

The following discussion will be delivered by the Medical or Program Director during the first orientation meeting. A parent handout is located in Appendix A1.11.

The founders of the Interdisciplinary, Interactive Pediatric Weight-Management Program are primarily concerned with the prevention and treatment of pediatric obesity. We believe that individualized treatment accompanied by long-term educational follow-up is the most effective approach to this goal. In our clinics, the intervention is closely supervised and the child receives uncompromising care of the highest quality from the pediatric, behavior, exercise, and nutrition specialists. We use a tailored approach in a group setting. The immediate goal is the improvement of the child's physical and emotional well-being. Weight loss and weight maintenance are the attractive side-effects of the overall lifestyle focus of the program.

Overweight children are often labeled by their classmates and even family members as lazy, fat, or stupid, which can lead to a significant erosion of confidence and to depression. By providing a support group structure for overweight children, the Pediatric Weight-Management Program helps to rebuild self-esteem and self-confidence. The children are powerfully motivated by seeing their peers face and overcome similar problems. Almost every child who completes the Pediatric Weight-Management Program enjoys a measurable increase in self-esteem. The program aims to educate children and their families in lifelong healthy behaviors and skills they need to prevent mild overweight from becoming obesity and to maintain healthy weight once achieved. Our long-term program is a family resource for support and reinforcement of the education provided during the treatment intervention.

We believe the success of the Pediatric Weight-Management Program is a result of the "A" Factors:

1. **Availability** of highly committed program professionals: We are deeply concerned with the child's progress, health, and overall emotional well-being.
2. **Accountability** of the child to the program staff: Each week the parents and children report their progress to the staff and are responsible for compliance with the program guidelines. Written records of weight, exercise, and diet are examined by the staff every week, which we believe increases program compliance and success.
3. **Attention** of only the positive kind: When the child does well, she or he receives strong positive reinforcement from the program staff. If the child does not do well, he or she receives encouragement to try harder the next week, but attention is quickly focused to another area of the program.

## EVALUATION

The objective of the medical component of the pediatric weight management program is to ensure that the intervention is safe and effective. This is determined by evaluating the program's effect on physiologic, metabolic, biochemical, and psychosocial parameters. We have shown in several clinical observations that the program promotes enhanced physical fitness [2,3], increased physical activity levels [4], decreased total body weight [5–8], decreased body mass index [2,5,8], decreased body adiposity [5,7,9,10], maintenance of lean body mass [10], maintenance of resting energy expenditure [11], improved lipid profiles [12,13], maintenance of biochemical status [5,14,15], and improved psychosocial parameters [15].

Physical fitness and activity are evaluated by determining heart rate during daily activity, self-reported physical activity (the Godin Leisure Time Exercise Questionnaire and the self-administered physical activity checklist), maximal oxygen uptake ($VO_2$ max), levels of muscular strength and endurance, and levels of flexibility. Weight status and body composition are evaluated by measuring weight, height, body mass index and percentile, waist and hip circumference, dual-energy x-ray absorptiometry, skinfolds measurement, or bioelectrical impedance analysis. Resting energy expenditure may be evaluated by indirect calorimetry. Cardiovascular risk factors are assessed by blood pressure and resting heart rate and blood chemistry (CBC w/diff and CHEM 20 including total cholesterol, triglycerides, and high and low-density lipoprotein). Psychosocial parameters are assessed by the following questionnaires: Piers-Harris Children's Self-Concept Scale, Childhood Depression Inventory, Olsen FACES III test, Culture-Free SEI Form B, Achenbach Child Behavior Checklist (ages 4 to 18), Children's Attributional Style Questionnaire, Student Behavior Checklist, and Family Dynamic Assessment. Maturation is assessed by Tanner staging. Detailed protocols of these measures are found in Appendix A2, and clinical procedures for conducting testing are detailed in Chapter 2 by Sothern.

## MONITORING PROGRESS

Participants are assigned to groups I, II, or III on the basis of their initial body mass index percentile (Appendix A1.10). This level is also used to determine a recommended term of treatment. Children in level 1 are encouraged to attend the program for 1 to 2 years. Those in level II should participate in the program for at least 1 year, and children in level III are given a 6- to 12-month term of treatment.

During the first few months of the program, children and adolescents attend weekly 2-hour comprehensive sessions (Table 19.1). During the medical monitoring period, students who are waiting can be directed to an outdoor park area that includes stationary park equipment and outdoor game supplies such as jump ropes, balls, and hula hoops. This will provide an additional opportunity for the families to engage in physical activity. An indoor nutrition/fitness activity center may also be set up with nutrition books, puzzles, games, and indoor physical activity supplies such as jump ropes, soft balls, mats, music, and videos, in case of inclement weather. This center will also serve as a demonstration area to encourage parents to create environments for play inside and outside of their own homes. Parents are instructed to supervise the children in the center during the free-play sessions.

Weekly sessions begin with a weigh-in and medical monitoring period. This is followed by a group discussion highlighting the patients' accomplishments for the week (Table 19.1). Positive reinforcement is given for trying new vegetables, turning down high-calorie snacks, or participating in physical activity. Behavior modification skills are introduced using discussion, modeling, role playing, and guided problem solving. Topics such as self-monitoring, commitment, limit setting, habit formation, goal setting and action plans, decision-making skills, attitudes, relapse prevention, and assertiveness training are discussed (Table 19.2). Patients with psychological problems are referred to a therapist for additional individual counseling while continuing in the program. Award certificates, inexpensive sports equipment, and other incentive items are given quarterly as positive reinforcement for achieving short-term goals. Special events such as roller-skating parties, park/field days, and holiday parties are organized during the 1-year program to encourage continued participation.

At the beginning of the program, the participants receive books [16], color-coded goal-setting forms, and self-monitoring records specific to their level of overweight. The color-coding of the forms and records is used as positive reinforcement as participants move from one weight level into another.

The maintenance level (blue) will begin after a participant achieves his or her goal weight, which is determined quarterly after each evaluation by the dietician and the physician. Once the

**TABLE 19.1**
**Sample Weekly Clinic Schedule**

| Time, PM | Activity |
| --- | --- |
| 4:30–5:00 | Weigh-in and medical monitoring |
| 5:00–5:15 | Group session — accomplishments |
| 5:15–6:30 | Group activity sessions on nutrition, behavior, and exercise |

**TABLE 19.2**
**Sample Weekly Intervention Schedule**

| Week | Topic | Activity Description | Time, PM |
|---|---|---|---|
| 1 | Nutrition | Diet instruction | 5:00–6:00 |
| | Behavior | Goal-setting and self-monitoring | 6:00–6:20 |
| | Exercise | Safety and exercise/MPEP step | 6:20-6:30 |
| 2 | Nutrition | Questions and answers | 5:00–5:15 |
| | Behavior | Commitment rating | 5:15–5:30 |
| | Exercise | Metabolic systems of the body: aerobic versus anaerobic metabolism — low-impact aerobics to music | 5:30-6:30 |
| 3 | Nutrition | Fun in the kitchen — oven-fried chicken | 5:00–5:30 |
| | Behavior | Benefits and sacrifices: limit setting and rules for eating | 5:30–5:50 |
| | Exercise | Aerobic field sports | 5:50-6:30 |
| 4 | Nutrition | Fun in the kitchen — low-calorie pizza | 5:00–5:30 |
| | Behavior | Habit formation: ABC's of behavior; behavior chain | 5:30–6:00 |
| | Exercise | The MPEP pump — strength training | 6:00-6:30 |
| 5 | Nutrition | Portion control | 5:00–5:30 |
| | Behavior | Individual sessions | 5:30–6:00 |
| | Exercise | Body composition — aerobic circuit | 6:00-6:30 |
| 6 | Nutrition | Restaurant choices | 5:00–5:30 |
| | Behavior | Eating patterns, practical solutions, goal check | 5:30–6:00 |
| | Exercise | The flex test — stretch 'n flex series | 6:00–6:30 |

MPEP = moderate intensity progressive exercise program.

goal weight is achieved, subjects are encouraged to continue to attend weekly 2-hour sessions for the remainder of their recommended term of treatment. The staff will continue to instruct participants concerning nutrition, behavior modification, and exercise (Table 19.2).

## SAMPLE ACTIVITY DESCRIPTIONS

### Group Behavior — Goal Setting

The behavior specialist will discuss with the participants how to set weekly, realistic behavior goals. The participants will be encouraged to record the goals in the program workbook so that the specialist can revisit the goals during the next weekly class. Goals will be set in nutrition and physical activity. For example, a nutrition goal may be to replace two unhealthy snack foods with new vegetables. An exercise goal may be to perform 10 stomach crunches three times during the week or to stretch while watching a favorite television program. Please refer to Chapter 20 and Appendix A3 for more examples of the weekly educational sessions.

### Group Exercise — Aerobic Field Sports

Children will participate in outdoor field games such as softball, volleyball, and soccer. The rules will be altered to encourage movement at all times. For example, aerobic softball requires that all team members walk/run the bases when a run is scored and perform 10 jumping or side jacks when the batter gets a strike. During aerobic volleyball, upbeat dance music is played while the teams hit a beach ball. Whenever the ball hits the ground, the team members must dance for 10 counts in different moves, twist, skip, run in place, and so on while the ball is retrieved for the next serve. In aerobic soccer, there are no boundaries other than those for safety reasons. Therefore, the ball is always in play. Offense and defense players switch places every 10 minutes to enable all members to run up and down the field. Only 5 seconds is allowed to begin play after a goal is achieved. Teams are selected as follows: all children line up behind the instructor, who alternately assigns the children to one of two colors to designate the different teams (e.g., blue and red). This is very time efficient and discourages captains and elimination issues (e.g. being picked last for a team; see also Chapter 20 and Appendix A3).

### Group Nutrition — Portion Control

The dietician will discuss the importance of portion control during a kitchen demonstration. Foods from different nutrient groups will be measured and evaluated for nutrient content, calorie level, and fat content. Parents will participate in the demonstration by measuring the foods (see also Chapter 12 and Appendix A3).

### Procedures for Absentees

Absentees are handled in the following manner: After one absence, children should be telephoned and encouraged to come in the next week. After two absences, they should again be telephoned and reminded that they do not have to report their weight during the meeting. They will be encouraged to provide nutrition and physical activity accomplishments during the following meeting. It is very important at this point that the patient be handled in a positive manner when he or she returns. Instructors should refrain from giving negative attention to their re-gain or lack of compliancy.

After three absences, the patient's physician should be notified and encouraged to telephone the patient. Also, the staff behavioral specialist or psychologist should be notified. After four absences, the family should be scheduled for a group consultation with all of the members of the staff. After this meeting, if attendance does not improve, the patient should be asked to leave the program. A follow-up questionnaire should be completed before their departure that explains their reason for leaving. Every attempt should be made to avoid negative reinforcement of poor attendance or relapse. Words such as "cheating" or "fat" should not be used when interviewing patients. Exercise staff (instructors, interns, and assistants), nutrition staff (dietitians, interns, and assistants), and medical staff (nurses and physician) should confine questions and comments to exercise, nutrition, and medically related issues. Behavior issues should be addressed by the behavioral specialist or psychologist experienced in counseling families.

## SUMMARY

We feel the success of the Pediatric Weight-Management Program's integrated, four-level approach is a result of several factors: the sessions are designed to entertain the children and promote initial success; the program features parent-training methods in short, interactive, educational sessions; in severely overweight children, the diet intervention results in noticeable weight loss that motivates the patient to continue; improved exercise tolerance resulting from the weight loss promotes increased physical activity; and the program team provides consistent feedback. The patients and their families receive results and updates every 3 months. Most important, the program is conducted in groups of families. The child/family group dynamics and peer modeling are primary components of the successful management of obesity in youth.

## REFERENCES

1. Bandura, A. *Social Foundations on Thought and Action: A Social Cognition Theory.* Englewood Cliffs, NJ: Prentice-Hall, Inc., 1986.
2. Sothern, M. S. Exercise as a modality in the treatment of childhood obesity. *Pediatr Clin North Am.* 48:995–1015, 2001.

3. Sothern, M. S., M. Loftin, U. Blecker, and J. N. Udall, Jr. Impact of significant weight loss on maximal oxygen uptake in obese children and adolescents. *J. Investig. Med.* 48:411–416, 2000.

4. Reed, J., C. VanVrancken, M. Loftin, C. Singley, J. Udall, and M. Sothern. Self-reported increases in physical activity in obese youth after a 10 week specialized moderate intensity exercise program. *Obes. Res.* 9:101s, 2001.

5. Sothern, M., J. Udall, R. Suskind, A. Vargas, and U. Blecker. Weight loss and growth velocity in obese children after very low calorie diet, exercise and behavior modification. *Acta Paediatr.* 89:1036–1043, 2000.

6. Sothern, M. S., H. Schumacher, T. K. von Almen, L. K. Carlisle, and J. N. Udall. Committed to kids: an integrated, 4-level team approach to weight management in adolescents. *J. Am. Diet. Assoc.* 102:S81–S85, 2002.

7. Sothern, M. S., J. M. Loftin, J. N. Udall, R. M. Suskind, T. L. Ewing, S. C. Tang, and U. Blecker. Safety, feasibility, and efficacy of a resistance training program in preadolescent obese children. *Am. J. Med. Sci.* 319:370–375, 2000.

8. Sothern, M. S., S. Hunter, R. M. Suskind, R. Brown, J. N. Udall, Jr., and U. Blecker. Motivating the obese child to move: the role of structured exercise in pediatric weight management. *South. Med. J.* 92:577–584, 1999.

9. Sothern, M., J. Loftin, T. Ewing, S. Tang, R. Suskind, and U. Blecker. The inclusion of resistance exercise in a multi-disciplinary obesity treatment program for preadolescent children. *South. Med J.* 92:585–592, 1999.

10. Olivier, L., G. Pinsonat, M. Loftin, C. Van Vrancken, K. Carlisle, S. Gordon et al. The effect of significant weight loss on body composition by DEXA in obese youth. *Int. J. Obes.* 26:S194, 2002.

11. Sothern, M., M. Loftin, R. Suskind, and J. Udall. The impact of significant weight loss on resting energy expenditure in obese youth. *J. Investig. Med.* 47:222–226, 1999.

12. Sothern, M. S., B. Despinasse, R. Brown, R. M. Suskind, J. N. Udall Jr., and U. Blecker. Lipid profiles of obese children and adolescents before and after significant weight loss: differences according to sex. *South. Med. J.* 93:278–282, 2000.

13. Brown, R., M. Sothern, R. Suskind, J. Udall, and U. Blecker. Racial differences in the lipid profiles of obese children and adolescents before and after significant weight loss. *Clin. Pediatr.* (Phila). 39:427–431, 2000.

14. Suskind, R., U. Blecker, J. Udall, T. von Almen, H. Schumacher, L. Carlisle, and M. Sothern. Recent advances in the treatment of childhood obesity. *Pediatr. Diabetes.* 1:23–33, 2000.

15. von Almen, T.K., R. Figueroa-Colon, and R. Suskind. Psychological considerations in the treatment of childhood obesity. In: *The Obese Child.* L. R. Giorgi PL, Catassi C, Eds. Basel: Karger Press, 1991.

16. Sothern, M., T. K. von Almen, and H. Schumacher. *Trim Kids: The Proven Plan That Has Helped Thousands of Children Achieve a Healthier Weight.* New York: Harper Collins Publishers, 2001.

# 20 Interdisciplinary, Interactive, Group Instruction

*T. Kristian von Almen, Melinda S. Sothern, and Heidi Schumacher*

## CONTENTS

## BEHAVIORAL THERAPY: GROUP COUNSELING SESSIONS, FOLLOW-UP, AND RELAPSE PREVENTION

### INTRODUCTION

Learning theorists such as Ivan Pavlov [1] Albert Bandura [2–4], and B. F. Skinner [5–8] have provided the foundation for the behavioral techniques and applied strategies used in weight loss programs for children and their families. In addition, developmental theorists such as Jean Piaget [9,10] have added substantially to our understanding of the cognitive capabilities of children and adolescents. Last, the transtheoretical approach, initially used in the treatment of smoking and alcohol cessation [11–14], has been adapted for use in a variety of health promotion settings [15–17]. The essence of these theories will be presented when appropriate; for a detailed description of the research and writing underlying these theories, please refer to the references cited.

This chapter presents behavioral techniques or strategies, adapted for the treatment of childhood obesity, which are used by health care professionals to help children and families achieve healthier lifestyle habits. The appendices contain many of the behavior-oriented tools developed for the Committed to Kids Weight Loss Program [18–21] at the Louisiana State University Health Sciences Center over the last 20 years. The Popular Press book, *Trim Kids* [21], written for parents of overweight children, provides a discussion of these behavioral strategies and contains related forms. *Trim Kids* is currently used by a variety of healthcare professionals and programs treating childhood overweight and obesity.

Twenty years of researching and treating overweight children, teens, and families highlights the ambivalence and reluctance of this population to seek treatment. Many patients are also nervous to join or share themselves in a group setting. As such, an important issue in treating childhood obesity relates to the interpersonal bond established between the health care professional or interventionist and the family. It is essential that therapists are viewed as professional and knowledgeable as well as available, as the amount and degree of patient change and long-term success is frequently related to the interpersonal relationship between the health care professional and family. Rapport begins at the initial meeting between an interventionist and familyand is established early in therapy. One easy way of establishing rapport with patients is by asking questions, preferably open ended, that relate to their lives or what is important to them. For example, the health professional may ask, "Who is your favorite actor, actress, or sports star?" "Who is your best friend?" "What do you want to be when you grow up?" "How do you feel about your weight?" "Do you want to be healthier?" "Why?" "Why not?" "What do you think you can do to be healthier?" For this reason, an initial group check-in form (Appendix A3.11) are used during the first multidisciplinary outpatient group session in the Committed to Kids program.

These initial, nonthreatening interactions, which focus on patient-related concerns, are a good way to break the ice, begin establishing rapport, and facilitate group bonding and dynamics. In addition, information gathered at this time gives the health care professional a better understanding of what the patients view as important and what they feel they can and cannot change. Such factors are extremely important and are detailed in social action theory [22] and motivational interviewing techniques [23,24], the latter of which focuses attention on client-specific expectations, strivings, and problem-solving strategies. Motivational interviewing incorporates the FRAMES model (feedback, responsibility, advise, menu, empathy, self-efficacy) into therapy and provides health care professionals with guidelines related to patient interviewing techniques. The Committed to Kids program [18–21] relies heavily on the A-Factor (availability, accountability, attention), which is designed to provide an overall supportive, positive attitude and approach for behavior change in the clinic setting. Participant accountability is reinforced by using a weekly check-in form [21] (Appendix A3.12), which allows participants to discuss accomplishments and difficulties encountered as they progress through the program.

Many programs have found that it is beneficial to assess child and parent readiness to change [11–14] or commitment to weight loss efforts [19,21–24] before the initiation of the actual weight loss intervention. The Committed to Kids program, for instance, has parents and children fill out a committment rating scale [21] (Appendix A3.13). Interventionists ask parents and children the following questions during their intake visit: "On a scale from 1 to 100, how important is this weight-loss program to you?" and "How committed are you to trying to change your high-calorie, sedentary behaviors to healthier habits?" A realistic amount of skepticism is expected, but children or parents who rate their initial commitment to following the weight loss program extremely low or who report significant resistance to changing habits should be questioned about the appropriateness of entering into such a program. Supportively confronting the individual (e.g., "It sounds like you or your child is not ready to change your lifestyle," or "When you're ready to help yourself or your child in this program, we'll be here," or "We find it best not to attempt to treat children and families who would rather not be here or who are extremely resistant to making healthy lifestyle changes") is the therapist's best response in this situation. The Committed to Kids program also asks children and parents to fill out the benefits and sacrifices form (Appendix A3.14) which illuminates the participants' preconceived positive and negative expectations of the program.

Most successful weight loss interventions for children (7 to 17 years of age) and their families focus on many relevant factors, including the child's developmental, cognitive, and social–emotional levels; parental values and behaviors; peer values and behaviors; and the behaviors and values of significant others in the child's environment. For instance, children must be able to distinguish low-caloric density foods from those with a high caloric density in various food groups to adhere to a healthy diet. Children must also be able to distinguish activities that are high versus low in terms of energy expenditure to adhere to a healthy activity regimen. Cognitively, children of this age level are capable of such tasks. Piaget would categorize 8- to 10-year-old children's cognitive abilities in the concrete operational stage. Children at this stage of development are capable of performing logical, reversible mental operations on objects. Children of this age are also capable of serially and conceptually arranging objects or concepts into preexisting categories (assimilation) or into newly developed categories (accommodation). Thus, children of this age are able to make the distinction between high- and low-caloric density foods as well as high- and low-energy expenditure activities that are required for them to eat healthfully and be appropriately active.

Most behaviorally based weight loss interventions use a token economy of some sort in their program. The potency of such positive reward systems has been well documented. Epstein et al. [25] and Stark et al. [26], among others, have demonstrated the effectiveness of a token economy in children of this age and younger. Both groups of authors used a token economy to encourage nutritionally balanced eating in 5- to 6-year-old obese children. The result was a significant increase in the children's consumption of nutritious snacks. In addition, Epstein [27] reported a 40% increase in caloric expenditure in 5- to 8-year-old females who were reinforced for active movements. Thus, it has been well documented that children will respond positively to a token economy system advocating healthier eating and activity behaviors.

We have found it essential to provide behavior education for parents and children. This gives all persons involved a common language and reference as well as insight into their behavior, and what motivates and maintains it. For instance, we discuss habit formation with participants, explaining it as "The ABCs of Behavior Change" (Appendix A3.15). It is best to begin by reviewing a nonthreatening or impersonal scenario such as the one provided in the appendix. The antecedents (what comes before the actual behavior, such as feeling sad, smelling food, being bored), behaviors (the behavior the participant engages in, such as eating high-calorie food, being sedentary), and consequences (what comes after the behavior, such as feeling guilty, happy, or sad) of the scenario should be discussed and linked to the maintenance of behavior patterns. Next, participants' "individualized" scenarios should be discussed. Suggestions can be provided or generated by the individual, family, and group concerning how to change overweight habits to healthier ones.

Attention, positive or negative, is known to drive and maintain human behavior. It is, therefore, important for interventionists and parents to focus on positive behaviors (those compatible with weight loss) while ignoring negative behaviors (those incompatible with weight loss) during interactions. Health professionals should frequently model such responses for parents and encourage them to make similar responses to their children. For instance, a therapist may say "Great, you took the stairs rather than the elevator to class all week and lost 2 pounds — that's exciting" or "Fantastic, you had dessert only twice this week and lost 3 pounds." In addition, the Committed to Kids Program [18–21] uses a four-level treatment approach (based on initial and follow-up measures — at 3, 6, 9, and 12 months — of body mass index [BMI] and fitness level). This allows health professionals another opportunity to positively reinforce children as they progress through the program or graduate from one level to the next.

Parents and interventionists are strongly discouraged from focusing negative attention on unhealthy behaviors or noncompliance. Negative reinforcement occurs when negative parental attention (reprimands, humiliation) follows an undesirable child behavior (e.g., parent yells at child when he is caught at the refrigerator between meals or when the child wants to "lounge" all weekend long and does not want to engage in his prescribed exercise program). The child's undesired behavior typically increases in frequency or intensity (e.g., child is more likely to go to refrigerator between meals or is more likely not to do prescribed exercise) as a result of this negative attention. Health professionals must discourage parents from engaging in negative reinforcement with their child or teen because of its adverse effects. Nagging or "guilt trips" are also strongly discouraged as these responses are a form of negative reinforcement that frequently backfires and fosters counterproductive feelings and behaviors. As such, parents should be encouraged to ignore, redirect, or provide appropriate consequences for their children's unhealthy behaviors or habits.

There are two ways of incorporating behavior change into one's lifestyle. The first, the "all or none" approach, appears fairly attractive to some families but is discouraged by most health professionals. For example, when parents and children discover the high-calorie nature of fast food, chips, or soda, a frequent response is that they will "never eat these foods again." This strategy is bound to fail because these foods are highly available and typically preferred by overweight children and their families. A preferred method is the gradual or "shaping" approach to changing behaviors. For instance, a family may decide that they will eat fast food on Friday evening, thus limiting this high-calorie behavior to once a week instead of three or more times per week. After several weeks of success at eating fast food only on Friday, families should be encouraged to try eating fast food every other week on a Friday evening. We call this approach "having your cake and eating it too — only less often." This approach allows persons to engage in preferred behaviors more responsibly, thus gaining control over high-calorie behaviors, increasing self-efficacy, and facilitating long-term maintenance of weight-loss efforts and habits. However, our clinical experience indicates that the "all-or-none" approach can work for some families some of the time. For instance, a family that "doesn't really care about or really isn't into" condiments such as salad dressing or mayonnaise would have no trouble avoiding or replacing those items with healthier options, whereas a family who enjoys these condiments may be more likely to need a gradual, coaxing approach to change from high-fat to low-fat or non-fat varieties.

## SETTING LIMITS

Parents of overweight children frequently experience great difficulty setting appropriate activity or dietary limits with their children. For instance, very few of our significantly overweight children engage in regular physical activity or eat a variety of vegetables (though most eat "starchy" vegetables such as corn, potatoes, or peas). Parental expectations are very important, as they can positively or negatively affect the child's perceptions of himself as well as the child's actual behavior. For example, Waxman and Stunkard [28] found that parents of overweight children believe their children require more calories per day and expect less activity from their obese child. The authors reported that overweight children were less active when at home. No difference was found in their activity level outside the home or at school, however, when compared with a control population of normal-weight children. Therefore, for any weight loss intervention to work with children, parents must view it as appropriate and important for their children to follow. As such, it is necessary to empower parents with the skills necessary to set enforceable limits they are comfortable with for their children. One way to accomplish this is to challenge unhealthy behavior patterns such as inactivity and the eating of only selected foods at meals. For instance, parents are encouraged to enforce a "three-bite rule" at all meals for all family members (other programs use the "be polite, take a bite" strategy). Family members are also encouraged to "grade the new foods." Foods receiving an A through C can be eaten regularly, whereas those receiving a D or F should not be forced on the family. Encourage families to try these non-preferred foods at a much later date or prepared in a much different fashion (e.g., raw versus cooked). Parents are also encouraged to enforce the "30-minute rule," where children are to be active for 30 minutes when returning home from school, rather than watching television or doing homework. Those family members who adhere to the new family rule or limits are rewarded after each meal or 30-minute burst of activity (e.g., a quarter in their bank or bedtime extended by 30 minutes). Rewards should be provided less frequently once family members adopt the rule (e.g., after 1 week of adherence, the family member gets to choose a fun family weekend event, inexpensive toy, or to have a friend stay the night). Nonadherence should be ignored or simply shrugged off by the parent. An appropriate parent response to nonadherence at lunch may be, "You can always earn a quarter after you try three bites of all foods at dinner tonight, or after riding your bike for 30 minutes tomorrow after school."

Children and families are bound to have difficulty with as well as challenge new house rules or limits so that they can again eat only preferred foods or be inactive. Interventionists must challenge parents and children by highlighting the importance of long-term lifestyle changes in foods eaten and activity undertaken for successful long-term weight loss and maintenance. Health professionals should counteract this inevitability by praising both parents and children on doing well at a task that has been difficult but essential for maintenance of weight loss. Such an approach models the use of positives for parents and allows them to feel the effects first-hand. Parents who repeatedly experience difficulty setting or maintaining new limits may be supportively confronted (preferably in a parent-alone group) with, "So, who is the parent and who makes rules in your house?" or "It sounds like you're trying to change something about your family that you're not really comfortable with or serious about; maybe you should try something else, or a different strategy."

Bandura's social learning theory [3] emphasizes the importance of significant others' (models such as parents, teachers, or heroes) behavior on human behavior. In summary, we are likely to emulate or model the behavior of significant others in our environment. Children do not model the "advice" but, rather, the actual behavior. As such, parents who enter their child in a weight-loss program should not then purchase or consume high-calorie foods (such as ice cream, cookies, chips) while restricting them from the enrolled child. Similarly, health professionals treating these families would be wise to alter their own behavior and not consume high-calorie foods such as soda or be inactive during sessions. Imagine the embarrassment a professional would experience if an overweight family observed him or her purchasing high-calorie foods at the market or consuming a "super-sized" fast food meal. Likewise, overweight children whose parents are inactive, eat high-calorie food, or provide this food for normal-weight siblings often report feeling angry and discriminated against or unloved. These children are frequently the ones who sneak or purchase high-calorie food when no one is around — and, in fact, do so to spite their parents. Parents and health professionals must seek alternative ways to meet children's needs and not expose these overweight children to such behavior. For instance, if they must, parents may be encouraged to go to lunch and consume a high-calorie dessert outside the child's presence. Later, the parent may be advised to incorporate the child into this "weekly or bi-monthly treat." The parent or child might even be advised to try splitting his favorite dessert or entree.

A review of the literature examining parental involvement yields conflicting results concerning whether adolescents treated alone or with parents present respond better to weight loss treatment [29–32]. We have found it best to encourage lifestyle changes in the parents, siblings, and extended families of both children and adolescents, regardless of their ages. This allows the entire family to adopt a healthier lifestyle while supporting the child during the change process. This approach also avoids discrimination toward the overweight child. One way to accomplish this is by having families set a weekly goal in addition to having the overweight child set a weekly goal.

## SELF-MONITORING OF FOOD AND ACTIVITY

Self-monitoring is an excellent way of assisting participants in understanding, controlling, and changing unhealthy behavior patterns (Appendix A3.10). Although genetic factors contribute to disease entities such as obesity, health professionals must impress on participants the importance of changing both food- and activity-related behaviors to achieve and maintain weight loss. Each day, participants record food eaten and activities or exercise during the initial phase (3 months) and are asked to keep these records during the maintenance phase only when experiencing difficulty or weight regain. It is important that participants record as precisely as possible, which aids interventionists in counseling and in tailoring the program to the individual and family. As such, the day, time, and amount and type of food or activity, as well as the feelings associated with eating and activity, are included on the record form and should each be filled in as completely as possible. Depending on the child's developmental level and ability to write, parents may be encouraged to assist the child in keeping food and activity records. Parents should be discouraged from keeping records for their children. Food and activity records should be reviewed each week by the dietician and exercise physiologist. Children keeping records are praised, whereas those who fail to keep records are ignored (not praised or positively reinforced) and are supportively confronted if the trend continues.

## CUE ELIMINATION

Ivan Pavlov demonstrated that dogs salivated to the sound of a bell that was consistently rung before their feedings [1]. This same phenomenon holds true for humans. The technique of cue elimination may be used by parents and children and involves physically eliminating the high-calorie or sedentary cues from one's environment. For instance, if parents do not purchase chips or cookies, these are unavailable to be seen or eaten. Quite literally, the chips and cookies are "out of sight" and "out of mind." Children may be tempted by the sight or smell of a bakery or fast food restaurant on their way home from school. Simply by taking an alternate route home, the child eliminates the cue and the subsequent temptation to give in to it. Another example of this phenomenon is television commercials full of high-calorie advertisements, which are very tempting. A family who mutes television commercials and does a quick chore, gets active, or walks from room to room during commercials removes this tempting cue and, it is hoped, the high-calorie behaviors associated with it.

## STIMULUS CONTROL

This technique could also be called "downsizing." Parents should be encouraged to buy "single servings" rather than "jumbo packages" of tempting or high-calorie foods. Organized parents can also break a "jumbo package" into single servings. This technique may fail when a parent discovers that their overweight child has consumed several "single servings" at one time. A parent in this position should be encouraged to discuss the need to adhere to a single serving of the high-calorie food per day. We have found in our clinical experience that most children and families discover one or more "temptation foods" that they have difficulty consuming responsibly. If necessary, the parent should be encouraged to no longer purchase the tempting, high-calorie food and instead consume it only on special occasions when dining out or at the malls, where a single serving may be purchased and eaten, or shared.

## GOAL SETTING: SHORT-TERM, LONG-TERM, AND WEEKLY

Most behaviorally based lifestyle interventions use goal setting with children and families in an attempt to modify high-calorie, sedentary behaviors into healthier behaviors. This technique reinforces a gradual approach to changing behavior. A short-term (3 months) and long-term (6 to 12 months) goal should be set by participants before starting a weight-loss program (Appendices A3.16 and A3.17. This allows parents and children to discuss personalized views and endpoints of their lifestyle change efforts. Examples of short-term goals may be to maintain current weight, lose 5 to 10 pounds, or walk a half mile without resting. Long-term goals may include walking a 5K race, eating three to five fruits and vegetables a day, or reaching an "ideal" body weight. Participants must be discouraged from setting unrealistic, unattainable short- or long-term goals.

Weekly goals are also set that concentrate on changing specific eating and activity behaviors each day or several times during the week. Health professionals should review cognitive restructuring techniques with children and families to facilitate attainment of goals that are set (Appendix A3.18). For example, a family may be encouraged to drink reduced-fat (2%) milk rather than whole (4%) milk for several weeks, followed by another change weeks later to skim milk. Allow families to take an intermediate or smaller step toward goals when necessary (e.g., a family might switch from 4% to 3% to 2% to 1% milk if the 4% to 2% milk switch was too difficult and unattainable). A family might also set a goal to ride their bikes for 20 minutes, 4 days per week. An intermediate step would be to have the family walk or ride bikes for 20 minutes on 3 days. Goals must be small steps, easy to accomplish, and very specific to ensure an easy transition and understanding of what is to be done. We encourage both family- and child-oriented goals. A child's goal may be to drink water, or some other calorie-free beverage 2 days a week (rather than the juice or soda typically consumed). After several weeks of accomplishing this goal, the child may then be encouraged to drink water 3 days per week. Small incentives or rewards are very helpful and even essential in ensuring the attainment of goals. For example, a pat on the back as well as a trip to the park or skating rink, or an inexpensive toy or other incentive should accompany reaching one's goal for the week. Incentives should vary (they can be social or material) and be used less frequently as time goes on and behaviors become established. Healthy professionals should strongly discourage, even disallow, using high-calorie food choices as rewards.

## GOAL ASSESSMENT

The Committed to Kids program asks children and parents to review their previously set goals after 6 weeks of attendance (Appendix A3.19). This allows participants to discuss those goals that have been both easy and difficult for them to accomplish and maintain. It also allows health care professionals to reinforce the importance of maintaining previously set goals and to assist families in problem solving or individualizing their goals and the program.

## BEHAVIORAL SUBSTITUTION OR REPLACEMENT

Behavioral substitution or replacement is similar to goal setting and involves substituting the eating of high-calorie foods or engaging in sedentary behaviors with the eating of low-calorie foods or engaging in more active behaviors (Appendix A3.20). For example, a child may choose to eat frozen yogurt rather than ice cream. Similarly, watching television after school may be replaced with riding a bike or walking the dog around the neighborhood. This technique works best when parents actively participate with their child as well as frequently praise the child for engaging in the new or substituted behavior (e.g., "Great, Johnny, you rode your bike for over an hour after school today instead of watching TV. I'm very proud of you."). This praise, again, may be diminished over time as the new behavior develops into a new habit. Health professionals should consistently praise both children and families for these changes and attempt to help problem-solve difficult or failed substitutions and replacements. For instance, a therapist could respond, "Maybe it would be easier for your family to have fruit rather than cookies as a snack twice this week" because four times a week was initially too difficult.

## RELAPSE PREVENTION

Research with individuals who have successfully changed and those who have maintained addictive habits such as smoking and drinking revealed that all persons, successful and unsuccessful, experience difficulty within 6 months of the initial change program, and most slip or lapse into prior, aberrant behavior patterns [33]. Further, it appears that it is the person's response to this initial lapse that dictates whether he or she will relapse and resort to prior behaviors or will renew their efforts and engage in health-related behaviors. A review of Marlatt and Gordon's cognitive-behavioral model of the abstinence violation effect highlights participant and family cognitions (primarily their attributions) and situational factors that precede and follow their relapse [33]. These researchers report that successful recovery from relapse is most likely when participants blame the relapse on external, unstable, and specific high-risk factors (e.g., "I always eat fries at fast-food spots" or "It's hard to resist a hot dog at the ballpark"). Unsuccessful relapse recovery is likely when participants blame the relapse on internal, stable factors ("I'm weak when it comes to desserts; I just can't say no" or "I always mess up; I'm a failure"). Discuss the Relapse Roadmap with participants and families (Appendix A3.21). Health professionals should highlight the individuals' and families' potential sources of relapse as well as their typical responses. A discussion of healthy, acceptable, family or child alternatives should follow. Interventionists should also clarify "slips" as a lapse (once a week), relapse (two to three times a week), or a collapse (four or more times a week) for participants. Lapses or "treats" should be allowed — and even encouraged on occasion — to avoid feelings of deprivation and increase feelings of self-control.

Relapses and collapses should be discussed, problem solved, discouraged, and supportively confronted if they continue. As such, we engage in discussions concerning these issues shortly after the intense 3-month portion of our weight-loss program to educate children and families to processes and pitfalls typically encountered by others in health-change programs. We hope that such discussion allows participants to more successfully change behaviors for the long term and not give up or "collapse" in the face of a single or isolated slip or lapse. Some health care professionals promote "planned lapses," where participants are encouraged to lapse and later discuss their feelings, potential solutions, and outcomes to such events.

## APPLIED ACTIVITIES AND EXPERIENCES

The Committed to Kids program also covers rules for eating (Appendix A3.22), which is another way for health professionals to help parents set limits or establish new house rules. Behaviors for controlling eating habits and alternative behaviors to eating [21] (Appendix A3.23) are also reviewed. The societal triggers form [21] (Appendix A3.24) illuminates the persons, places, times, and events that either assist or sabotage participants' weight-loss efforts. Addressing temptations with positive self statements (Appendix A3.25) is also reviewed and discussed during the initial and maintenance phases of the program. Additional ideas for role plays and discussion are also provided (Appendix A3.26), as is a Weight-O-Rama game (Appendix A3.27) that is played with children and families at the end of the initial 3-month phase of treatment. Last, the Committed to Kids program incorporates a variety of fun and applied experiences into sessions for the children and families during the maintenance phase. For instance, trips to the grocery store or local parks, recreation activities (such as skating, water slides, picnics, and theme parks), or community events are conducted. These applied sessions allow children and families to practice healthy behaviors in the "real world" while in the presence of supportive interventionists.

## FAMILY PHYSICAL ACTIVITY AND FITNESS EDUCATION SESSIONS

### INTRODUCTION

With specialized populations such as overweight children and adolescents, clinicians and educators are at a great disadvantage when attempting to prescribe appropriate activities and deliver educational interventions. By implementing specialized programs that address these issues, successful prevention and treatment of obesity may be possible. Clinical treatment intervention programs designed to promote behavior change should contain activities structured to the specific physical, emotional, and cognitive needs of the participants.

Both structured exercise and lifestyle physical activity programs are shown to promote improvements in weight status in short-term [34–39] and long-term [34,40,41] multidisciplinary weight-management programs. Younger children, who are naturally active, should be given the opportunity to engage in enjoyable, intermittent exercise of varied intensities and durations, with less emphasis on the improvement of aerobic capacity [21,42,43]. However, older children require more structured programs that include specific recommendations for aerobic, muscular strength and endurance, and flexibility exercises. Research indicates that standard exercise prescription methods may not be applicable in children of different overweight conditions based on the submaximal and maximal response to graded exercise tolerance tests [44–46]. Pediatric weight management programs should, thus, include specialized recommendations specific to the physiologic needs of children of varied weight levels. Alternative modalities of exercise may be considered initially for severely overweight individuals unable to sustain weight-bearing exercise. Intensity, duration, and frequency of exercise should be prescribed in relation to the age, medical history, and weight status of the child. Recommendations should include gradual increases in exercise and daily physical activity, along with consistent behavior modification that includes nutrition and fitness education [47–49]. In all cases, exercises for overweight children should follow the guidelines of the American College of Sports Medicine [50–55].

## PEDIATRIC OBESITY AND EXERCISE PERFORMANCE

Physical activities for overweight individuals should be appropriate to their specific physiologic needs. Overweight children and adolescents are physiologically and emotionally different from their normal-weight counterparts. In a recent study, Schwimmer and colleagues [56] demonstrated that severely overweight children were five times more likely than healthy children to have impaired physical functioning. The BMI $z$ score among severely overweight children was inversely correlated with physical functioning. In addition, similar findings were reported by Doll and colleagues [57], who observed that physical functioning decreased with increasing weight among adults. Moreover, the authors concluded that the diminished ability to move with increasing weight leads to a decrease in caloric expenditure, with a further mismatch in energy balance leading to additional weight gain — or a vicious cycle [57].

Researchers at the Louisiana State University Health Sciences Center (LSUHSC) in New Orleans determined that children with greater obesity levels respond differently to weight-bearing activity (walking) than do nonoverweight children [58]. The overweight and severely overweight children consistently displayed greater physiologic and metabolic responses for a given level of intensity than did the at-risk and normal-weight youth [58]. In a subsequent study, maximal exercise effort ($VO_2$ max) was obtained in 11 overweight children before participation in a pediatric weight management program and again after 10 weeks, using cycle ergometry and indirect calorimetry [46]. There was a significant average weight loss of 8.1 kg ($P < .0001$), and the average height increased significantly from 157.0 ± 9.0 cm at baseline to 158.1 ± 9.0 cm at 10 weeks ($P < .005$). The mean BMI decreased significantly from 34.1 ± 4.8 to 29.4 ± 5.8 ($P < .001$). During the 10-week period, all of the children achieved a lower category of obesity (i.e., from severely overweight [>99th percentile BMI] to overweight [>95th to 99th percentile BMI], from overweight to at risk for overweight [>85th to 95th percentile BMI], and from at risk for overweight to normal weight [<85th percentile BMI]). The increase in relative $VO_2$ max mL/kg per minute from baseline (19.2 ± 3.0 mL/kg per minute) to 10 weeks (22.5 ± 5.8 mL/kg per minute) was significant ($P < .001$). However, when expressed in absolute values (liters/minute), the baseline measure (1.54 ± 0.26 L/min) did not differ significantly from the 10-week measure (1.54 ± 0.29 L/min), indicating that the improved exercise performance was caused by a reduction in weight status. The results of these studies illustrate that the effect of obesity level on physiologic function during weight-bearing activity in overweight children is relative to the intensity of the exercise, and that during weight-bearing activity of increasing intensities, the disparity between the different levels of obesity may be increased. In addition, short-term weight loss improves exercise tolerance in overweight youth.

Increasing levels of obesity may decrease exercise performance because less mechanical work is performed to overcome friction between the thighs, arms, and torso of the overweight individual when walking and pulmonary function may be impaired because overweight individuals must move a heavier body mass forward. Thus, in overweight children, an increased cardiac output and respiratory effort are required to maintain a similar level of work to accommodate the excess load. Finally, during weight-bearing exercise, such as walking, the skeletal musculature is responsible for supporting and moving the entire body mass forward. The increased recruitment of muscle to compensate for the additional fat weight load thereby results in an increased uptake in oxygen. When overweight children exercise at submaximal workloads, excessive body weight induces an excess load that increases the energy required to maintain the same level of exertion as nonoverweight children [59,60].

This is important information that can be used to set appropriate, specific exercise guidelines for overweight children. Neiman [61] was the first to suggest that individuals with varied levels of obesity should receive specialized programs specific to their weight status. The level approach has been successfully implemented in cardiac rehabilitation programs where clinicians implement specific exercise guidelines for each stage of recovery following heart surgery [62]. In addition, the program provides the patient with repeated short-term opportunities to succeed and be promoted to increasing levels of competency.

## EXERCISE INSTRUCTION IN INTERACTIVE, INTERDISCIPLINARY CLINICAL SETTINGS

Researchers at the LSUHSC and Pennington Biomedical Research Center have evaluated a program that provides quality medical, nutritional, psychosocial, and exercise intervention for at risk and obese children along with their families in a weekly outpatient clinical setting [18,21,49,63–65]. The program is unique because of its integrated, four-level approach that encourages short-term (12-week) goal-setting, quarterly feedback, and motivational techniques to improve health behaviors (Table 20.1) [1,63–66].

The interdisciplinary, four-level exercise program is an individualized approach to the prevention and treatment of obesity conducted in a family group setting. Weight loss is just a by-product of the overall focus of the program that is to assist the patient and his or her family in making healthy lifestyle changes, thus promoting positive alterations in body weight. The group family

**TABLE 20.1**
**Initial Physical Activity Strategies by Medical History, Age, and Weight Condition [18,21,63][a]**

| Level | Age, Years | Physical Activity Approach |
|---|---|---|
| Normal Wt ≥1 obese parent | ≤6 | Family counseling, fitness education, free play, reduction of television watching, parent training |
| >85th BMI | 7–18 | Structured weight-bearing activities, free play, reduction of television watching, parent training |
| >95th BMI | 7–18 | Alternate non-weight-bearing activities, free play, reduction of television watching, parent training |
| >99th BMI | 7–18 | Non-weight-bearing activities, free play, reduction of television watching, parent training[b] |

[a] Approach should be adjusted every 3–6 months depending upon child's progress.
[b] Close medical supervision required.

setting has the added benefit of encouraging parent and peer modeling and support among the participants. Unlike the typical physical education class or youth recreational program in which the overweight child often feels inhibited, in the interdisciplinary, four-level exercise setting, all of the students and family members feel comfortable around peers who possess similar levels of physical conditioning. The appropriate exercise intensity and skill level of the activities guarantee initial success to all participants.

The structured exercise protocol and physical activity education includes a moderate-intensity progressive exercise program (MPEP) for children with increasing levels of obesity [18,21,52,63,65]. The model is based on a treatment approach suggested by Neiman and is similar to the medical cardiac rehabilitation model [61,62]. The intervention methods use social cognitive theory [66] and self-efficacy beliefs [64], which motivate children and adolescents to change their behavior by providing mastery experiences, physiological feedback, knowledge transfer, and real or imagined role models (see Chapter 14 for more information).

The exercise recommendations are specific to the different levels of obesity (i.e., initially the severely overweight children have shorter beginning durations and frequencies than the overweight children or those at risk for developing overweight conditions (at-risk)). Initially, at-risk children are advised to exercise more than overweight and severely overweight children. Severely overweight children initially are also prescribed less challenging activities. In addition, because excess fat weight places an increased burden on an individual's cardiorespiratory and musculoskeletal systems, the recommended exercise activities for the overweight and severely overweight adolescents are "arm specific" and less weight bearing. Students are allowed to choose the type of aerobic activity from an extensive list provided in the program book [21].

The approach includes not only guidelines for exercise frequency, duration, and intensity (see Chapter 14) but also a series of 52 weekly dynamic and interactive group sessions that promote increased physical activity and improved body movement awareness [21,45,63–65]. The program also includes specific recommendations for type or modality of exercise based on the individual overweight level and physiologic function (Tables 20.2 to 20.4) [21,52,58,60,63]. This specialized program is designed to ensure that the recommended physical activities may be successfully performed by individuals with various overweight conditions. In addition, the educational content is organized in a developmentally appropriate manner that is easily comprehended by students of all ages. Therefore, the program is designed to better serve the emotional and cognitive, as well as physiologic, needs of overweight individuals. By providing activities that illicit initial success, it is proposed that the program will improve mastery concepts, thereby increasing self-efficacy beliefs [64,66].

During the 1-year program, participants and their families attend weekly 2-hour comprehensive sessions. During these sessions, patients receive medical supervision, nutrition instruction, physical

**TABLE 20.2**
**Children at Risk for Overweight Conditions (>85th BMI), 7–18 Years of Age**

Limit access to television/video/computer
Recommended Aerobic Activities [21,63]: weight-bearing such as brisk walking, treadmill, field sports, inline skating, roller skating, hiking, racket ball, tennis, martial arts, skiing, jump rope, indoor/outdoor tag games.
Parent training and fitness education
Pacing skills

*Note:* Guidelines should be readjusted every 10–15 weeks based on evaluation results.

**TABLE 20.3**
**Overweight Children (>95th percentile BMI), 7–18 Years of Age**

Limit access to television/video/computer
Recommended Aerobic Activities [21,63]: alternate non-weight-bearing such as swimming, cycling, arm ergometer (crank), recline bike, with strength/aerobic circuit training, arm-specific aerobic dancing, and interval walking[a]
Parent training and fitness education

*Note:* Guidelines should be readjusted every 10–15 weeks based on evaluation results.

[a] Walking with frequent rests, as necessary. Gradually work up to longer walking periods and fewer rest stops.

**TABLE 20.4**
**Severely Overweight Children (>99th percentile BMI), 7–18 Years of Age**

Limit access to television/video/computer
Recommended aerobic activities [21,63]: non-weight-bearing only such as swimming, recline bike, arm ergometer, seated (chair) aerobics, and seated or lying circuit training
Parent training and fitness education
Other emotional and dietary concerns must be addressed during treatment

*Note:* Guidelines should be readjusted every 10–15 weeks based on evaluation results

activity education, exercise activities, and behavior modification. Exercise instruction is conducted at each visit by a clinical exercise physiologist and includes fitness counseling.

Each session is a mixture of sharing information on topics such as heart-rate monitoring and injury prevention, as well as the actual exercise [21,63]. In addition, fitness counseling includes motivational techniques to increase daily activity levels and improve body movement awareness based on social cognitive theory [3,66].

The exercise activities correspond with the group's physiological condition of obesity and ability to comprehend, synthesize, and apply health and fitness information to daily-life situations. The structured exercise component (MPEP) includes three types of exercise: cardiorespiratory endurance or aerobic exercise, muscular strength and endurance exercise, and muscular flexibility exercise. The muscular strength and endurance and the flexibility exercises are illustrated in detail in the program book [21] and are also demonstrated in the exercise DVD (Appendix A3.1.1).

The exercise DVD (Appendix A3.1.1) contains 5 minutes of slow movement to music as a warm-up (Appendix A3.3). Thirty to 45 minutes of moderate-intensity, low-impact aerobic dancing follows the warm-up. A 20-minute strength training session begins after a 5-minute period of slow movement (cool down [Appendix A3.3]). Eight to 12 strength exercises are performed to music, using hand and leg weights (Table 20.5). The routine is balanced focusing on all of the major muscle groups. The students perform one set of 10 to 12 repetitions of slow movement (2 to 4 seconds to lift or pull [concentric], 2 to 4 seconds to lower or release [eccentric]) for each of the strength exercises. Careful attention is given to proper technique, full extension of the joints, and full contraction of the muscles. The exercise DVD (Appendix A3.1.1) ends with 5 minutes of flexibility exercises designed to balance the physique and enhance posture (Table 20.6).

Students are explained how to use the exercise DVD (Appendix A3.1.1) and how to record their activities on the Aerobic Activity and Food Checklist (Appendix A3.10). The checklist, which lists the frequency, duration, and type of exercise, is kept by each student and is checked weekly by the exercise physiologist. Students are also instructed on how to obtain heart rates and rates of perceived exertion [67] during exercise sessions to ensure compliance with the moderate exercise intensity (45 to 55% $VO_2$ max or 55 to 65% maximal heart rate). Incentives, in the form of awards, are given for consistent reporting of exercise patterns and for overall compliance with the weight-management program. The program is also prescribed for use at home, and children are encouraged to select a variety of aerobic activities that they enjoy [21,46,49,68].

The primary objective of the four-level exercise program is to motivate students to adopt specific behaviors associated with long-term emotional, physical, and psychological health (i.e., the reduction

### TABLE 20.5
### Strength Exercises [21,52,65]

| Exercise | Muscle Groups |
| --- | --- |
| Leg extension | Quadriceps |
| Leg curl | Hamstrings |
| Rowing | Upper back |
| Overhead press | Shoulders |
| Biceps curl | Biceps |
| Triceps extension | Triceps |
| Pelvic tilt | Gluteals, hips |
| Dumbbell press | Chest |
| Low back extenson | Low back |
| Crunch | Abdominals |
| Squat | Gluteals, quadriceps |
| Standing calf | Calf |

### TABLE 20.6
### Flexibility Exercises [18,21,63]

| Exercise | Muscle Groups |
| --- | --- |
| Shoulder stretch | Shoulder |
| Chest stretch | Chest |
| Upper back stretch | Upper back |
| Single rear shoulder stretch | Shoulder |
| Lying quad stretch | Quadriceps |
| Seated hamstring stretch | Hamstrings |
| Modified butterfly stretch | Hips, hamstrings |
| Butterfly stretch | Hips, hamstrings |
| Straddle stretch | Hips, hamstrings, quadriceps |
| Calf stretch | Calf |

of overall body weight, the improvement of eating patterns, and the increase in the daily energy expenditure). Students learn to identify safe and effective methods for achieving and maintaining weight loss. They acquire knowledge of the basic principles of good nutrition and healthy eating patterns. They become aware of their eating behaviors and activity patterns and learn alternate behaviors to promote long-term health. In terms of fitness, students gain the body movement awareness necessary to adopt activity patterns that will promote long-term health.

The exercise program has been evaluated in several investigations [18,46,48,49,52,64,65,69]. The comprehensive, integrated, four-level approach is successful because of several factors: first, the program features entertaining nutrition and exercise education for children, as well as parent-training methods in short, interactive sessions; second, the improved exercise tolerance resulting from the weight loss promotes increased physical activity; and third, the program team provides consistent feedback. The patients and their families receive results and updates every 3 months. Most important, the program is conducted in groups of families, and the parents' participation in exercise class is strongly encouraged.

The program also encourages participation in a graded exercise test before the beginning of the intervention program, at the end of the 6-month weight-loss intervention, and annually thereafter. The results of the test are used to individualize the exercise recommendations and provide positive feedback to encourage continued participation. Although the four-level recommendations are appropriate for most overweight youth, the results of the exercise test provide additional information that will assist in determining the most appropriate initial modality, intensity, duration, and frequency of exercise. In addition, the results of the test will help to determine compliance with the proposed exercise recommendations.

Moderate progressive exercise sessions at weekly 2-hour sessions include warm-up and cool-down exercises, low-impact aerobics, brisk walking, cycling, strength training, proper exercise techniques, and team sports (Tables 20.2 to 20.4).

The specific guidelines for levels 1, 2, and 3 are as follows.

## CARDIORESPIRATORY ENDURANCE OR AEROBIC EXERCISES

The children will be allowed to choose the type of aerobic activity. A list of appropriate activities is included in the program book [21]. However, children are advised to adhere to the following guidelines:

Intensity: 45 to 55% $VO_2$ max (approximately 55 to 65% of heart rate maximum)
Frequency: One to two times per week in week 1, gradually increasing to five to six times per week in weeks 12 to 30 (see Chapter 14)
Duration: 20 to 30 minutes per session in week 1, gradually increasing to 45 to 60 minutes in weeks 12 to 30 (see Chapter 14)

## MUSCULAR STRENGTH AND ENDURANCE EXERCISES

Intensity: 60 to 80% of one repetition maximum.
Frequency: One time per week in week 1, gradually increasing to two times per week in weeks 12 to 30 (see Chapter 14)

Resistance training may be used safely to enhance the efforts to prevent and reverse childhood obesity and other chronic pediatric diseases in clinic-based interventions [44,55,70,71]. Strength exercises, specifically designed for overweight children, are performed in one set of 8 to 12 repetitions (Table 20.5). The movement time is 2 to 4 seconds concentric and 2 to 4 seconds eccentric through a full range of motion. Children under 14 years of age begin at the lowest intensity. Proper technique is emphasized. Participants increase load (weight or resistance) only when the 12th repetition is performed with ease and in perfect form.

## MUSCULAR FLEXIBILITY EXERCISES

A balanced routine of 10 static stretches specifically designed for overweight children will be performed five times a week (Table 20.6). Dynamic stretches are included in the warm-up and cool-down periods of the aerobic exercise sessions.

Family intervention is an integral component of the interdisciplinary, four-level exercise program. In other studies, family-based programs in which parents were trained to reinforce their children's physical activity have been shown to increase both activity and fitness levels in overweight children and adolescents [41,72–76]. Healthy-weight, as well as overweight, parents, siblings, and extended family are encouraged to participate in the many varied activities offered during the exercise portion of the weekly meetings. Likewise, parents' participation at home with their children during exercise sessions improves compliance and overall success.

## SUMMARY

The interdisciplinary, four-level exercise program is based on the individual needs of children in different ranges of obesity. In each level, the activities described have been chosen because they are safe and effective for the child with a particular overweight physical condition. Also, because these are physically inactive youth, the duration and frequency increase gradually, about 10% per week [77]. Although the learning activities are designed to be somewhat interchangeable, the instructor should not deviate from the recommended movement technique or intensity of an individual exercise. Some activities may be interchanged, but only if their technical aspects and intensities are similar. Instructors may also introduce movement or activities of their own creation, but only if these are similar in technique and intensity to the recommended exercises and are implemented cautiously. Do not compromise safety for the sake of creativity. If you are unsure whether a movement is safe or appropriate for the overweight children in your class, then choose another activity.

The interactive, interdisciplinary environment promotes positive attention, student accountability, and teacher availability. The overweight students learn while they participate in physical activity. They move while they listen. They are provided with specific activities that are challenging but that may always be accomplished. Positive attention reinforces their behavior changes. Teachers and parents become the positive role models for the children in the family. Short-term goals are set and reached. As the overweight individual graduates from one level to another, he or she increases his or her physical activity and, thus, his or her level of fitness. He also increases his knowledge of health and fitness concepts and his ability to manage his weight and medical condition more effectively.

The remainder of this chapter provides a sample interactive, interdisciplinary exercise curriculum for children with varied overweight levels (Table 20.7). A list of suggested activities that can be used as additional exercise sessions in group interactive, interdisciplinary weight management settings may be found in Table 20.8. The skills required for the activities at each level are easily attained to ensure that overweight children will experience mastery, which will motivate them to continue the program. If you notice that during an activity any child is having difficulty, please adjust the activity accordingly.

## LESSON 1: BENEFITS OF EXERCISE, EXERCISE SAFETY, WARMING-UP, EXERCISE PRESCRIPTION, AND INCREASING YOUR DAILY ACTIVITY — THE MPEP-STEP

Materials needed include books (program book [21]), exercise attire, CD player for music, exercise mats, exercise DVD (Appendix A3.1.1), aerobic activity, and food checklist (Appendix A3.10).

**TABLE 20.7**
**Exercise Lesson Plans — Suggested Activities [18,21,63]**

Lesson 1: Benefits of Exercise, Exercise Safety, Warming Up and Increasing Your Daily Activity — The MPEP-STEP
Lesson 2: Exercise Intensity and Pacing Skills (Metabolic Systems), Cooling Down after Exercise
Lesson 3: Aerobic Exercise — Modified Field Sports, The Homework Rule
Lesson 4: Muscular Strength and Endurance: MPEP PUMP, Strength Training Circuit, Creating Indoor Play Areas
Lesson 5: Family Field Sports — Aerobic Volleyball, Creating Outdoor Play Areas
Lesson 6: Flexibility, Flex Test I, and Stretch and Flex Class
Lesson 7: Aerobic Exercise and Cardiopulmonary Endurance, Steady State — Monitoring Heart Rate and Aerobic Circuit
Lesson 8: Exercise Prescriptions: the Fit Kit Walking Program
Lesson 9. Review Muscular Strength and Endurance: Pull Your Own Weight Series
Lesson 10. Park Day — Outdoor Play

**TABLE 20.8**
**Additional Exercise Sessions — Suggested Activities [18,21,63]**

Water Aerobics
Specialty Aerobics (Guest Instructor)
Body Sculpting I: Injury Prevention; Individual Differences (body composition); Exercise Myths [21]
Line Dancing
Rockin' to the Oldies Aerobic Dance [21]
Modified Yoga
Getting the Most Out of Your Workout; 20 Ways to Burn 20 Calories [21]
Super Abdominals [21]
Tennis Lesson and Drills
Cross Training [21]
Band-Aid for Out-of-Shape Muscles [21] (Muscular Strength and Endurance)
Field Day — Annual
Martial Arts: Demonstrations
Team Sports: Basketball
The MPEP Ultimate Workout [21]
Ultimate Frisbee™
Field Trip: Fun Walk/Run Race in the Park
Advanced Resistance Training
Field Trip: Roller Skating — Annual Party
Field Trip: Walk in the Park
Field Trip: Water Slide/Park
Combined Strength and Aerobic Circuit
Beach Party Aerobics with Beach Balls
Balloon games [21] (Balloon Pop; Battle Ball)
Body Sculpting II: Standing Strength Class to Music
Relays: Indoor or Outdoor
Aerobic Musical Chairs [21]
Aerobic Equipment Triathlon
Power Sports: Guest Speaker: Pro Athlete
Tennis Game
Obstacle Course
Holiday Games [21]: Aerobic Easter Egg Hunt Charades; Thanksgiving Family Flag Football; Fourth of July
  Family Field Games
Keeping Fit on Your Trip — Vacation Strategies [21]

Briefly discuss the health benefits of being physically active [21]. Review the safety rules located in Appendix A3.3. Discuss the importance of warming up. Demonstrate warm-up movements to music (Appendix A3.3). Discuss the specific exercise guidelines for each level of overweight (Appendix A3.3), referring parents to the program book [21] and exercise DVD (Appendix A3.1.1). Emphasize the importance of filling out the Aerobic Activity and Food Checklist (Appendix A3.10).

Ask the parents to take a moment to observe their child's demeanor. Notice his or her posture, how quickly or slowly he or she walks, his or her overall physique, and how it makes him or her look. Then ask children to walk around the room so their parents can watch. Most children shuffle slowly with bent heads and shoulders rolled forward. See Appendix A3.3 for verbal cues.

Explain that lots of overweight kids move slowly, with hunched shoulders, appearing as though they do not feel confident. Improving the way your child walks can burn considerably more calories and make him or her look and feel healthier.

Explain to the parent and child that burning calories does not only happen when one is doing hard exercise or playing — calories are burned all the time. Verbal cues located in Appendix A3.3 can help relay this concept and invite the children to quicken their pace.

You will then encourage the children to walk more briskly, with better posture. Tell them that this is called the MPEP-Step ("MPEP" stands for "Moderate Intensity Progressive Exercise Program"). Demonstrate how to do the MPEP-Step, and then ask the children to do it. Remind them that when they walk with their chins up, shoulders back, and in a brisk manner, they appear taller, trimmer, and more in control. Plus, walking with the MPEP-Step burns about 350 to 450 calories per hour. Tell the parents to encourage their child to walk this way every day — no matter where he or she is or what he or she is doing — for the next week. Better yet, tell parents to model this behavior for their child from here on.

## LESSON 2: EXERCISE INTENSITY AND PACING SKILLS (METABOLIC SYSTEMS), COOLING DOWN AFTER EXERCISE

Materials needed include books (program book [21]), exercise attire, portable stereo, exercise mats, exercise DVD (Appendix A3.1.1), and aerobic activity and food checklist (Appendix A3.10)

Children will interact by moving to different types of music at different intensities. During the first 10 minutes of the class, the exercise instructor will demonstrate very simple moves that are easily mastered by the patients. During this time, the concept of low-intensity aerobic exercise will be discussed. Gradually the intensity and speed of the music will increase in an effort to illustrate how the body shifts from aerobic to anaerobic metabolism. The benefits and drawbacks to each will be discussed as the participants dance to the music (Appendix A3.3). The class will end in a cool-down or return to low intensity, followed by stretching exercise. Kids follow the instructor's verbal cues (Appendix A3.3) for the cool-down exercise segment.

## LESSON 3: AEROBIC EXERCISE — MODIFIED FIELD SPORTS, THE HOMEWORK RULE

Materials needed included books (program book [21]), exercise attire, portable stereo, aerobic activity and food checklist (Appendix A3.10), softballs, bats, bases, home plate, field markers (cones), soccer goal, soccer ball, colored flag belts or scarves, football, and whistle,

The students and parents will participate in a soccer game outdoors. The warm-up will include a soccer skill review followed by drills for about 5 minutes. When organizing teams use this method: Tell the students and parents to make a "train" behind you. Then assign every other participant to a different color. For example: red team, blue team, red team. Assign the red team to one side of the field and the blue team to the other.

Periodic breathing and heart-rate checks will illustrate to the kids and parents how soccer raises the metabolic rate, thus encouraging an increase in activity levels and calories burned.

To make the soccer game more aerobic or steady-state, and to increase caloric expenditure, try these modifications: announce to the kids and parents that you are playing by aerobic rules. Allow the ball to go outside of the regular boundaries to keep it in play. Only call the ball out of bounds when it presents a danger to the kids. Otherwise, the ball is always in play. This will increase the amount of total physical activity because overall play will not stop as a result of the referee assigning a player to pass the ball back into play.

If you do call the ball out of bounds, allow 3 seconds only for placing the ball back in play from the sideline or the goal. The team loses the ball if they exceed 3 seconds. In addition, every 5 to 10 minutes alternate the playing assignments from offense to defense. This will allow all students a chance to do both vigorous and moderate activity in small enough doses so that they do not become too fatigued. At the conclusion of the class, the instructor should introduce the Homework Rule (Appendix A3.3). In addition, detailed descriptions of other modified field sports may be found in Appendix A3.3.

## LESSON 4: MUSCULAR STRENGTH AND ENDURANCE: MPEP PUMP, STRENGTH TRAINING CIRCUIT, CREATING INDOOR PLAY AREAS

Materials needed include books (program book [21]), exercise DVD (Appendix A3.1), fat and lean weight models, exercise attire, chairs, exercise mats, aerobic activity and food checklist (Appendix A3.10), station markers, hand weights, exercise resistance band, and a stopwatch.

Discuss the benefits of strength training and factors that affect the results. Proper technique and methods should be emphasized. Dismiss weight-lifting myths, using verbal cues (Appendix A3.C.4.a) for the children. The instructor should pass around models of muscle tissue and fat tissue for the kids to feel and observe using verbal cues in Appendix A3.3. The instructor reviews the technique for the strength exercises. These are illustrated in the program book [21] and in the second half of the exercise DVD (Appendix A3.1.1). The children will then participate in a circuit strength-training session. The strength-training stations will follow the exercises illustrated in the program book [21] and on the Strength and Flexibility Workout Chart [21]. During the circuit, the instructor will discuss facts concerning strength training.

A balanced routine of 8 to 12 muscular strength and endurance exercises (moderate-high intensity, 60 to 80% of one repetition maximum [MPEP pump]), specifically designed for overweight children, should be performed. Children begin performing the exercises as instructed on the exercise DVD without weight or resistance for a 4-week period according to the goals suggested on the exercise record cards. During the fourth week, the exercise physiologist instructs the children on the proper technique during the scheduled weekly session. During the session, parents are enlisted as spotters to ensure safety. The children are then instructed to perform the exercise routine according to the DVD instruction and as indicated on the exercise record cards, twice per week, with at least 1 day of rest between sessions.

The children initially use 1-pound weights in each hand and 1- to 3-pound weights on each ankle to perform the exercises. They initially perform eight repetitions per exercise, with emphasis on proper technique. When eight repetitions are performed in perfect form with ease, the exercises are then increased to nine repetitions. This pattern continues until 12 repetitions can be done in perfect form. The amount of weight to be lifted is then increased to 3 pounds for each hand and 3 to 5 pounds for each ankle, and the repetitions are reduced to eight per exercise. The progression described above is then repeated. Exercises for the upper and middle back muscles use an exercise band. Children use the band with lowest resistance initially and then progress through the same pattern of increased repetitions and intensity. The complete resistance training circuit, consisting of 8 to 12 different exercises, can be easily performed in 20 to 30 minutes.

Parents can be recruited as spotters for the kids, or the kids can be paired as buddies: as one child is executing the exercise the buddy or parent spots, and then they change places. At the completion of the circuit, using verbal cues (Appendix A3.3), the instructor will then review methods to create indoor play areas in the home.

## LESSON 5: FAMILY FIELD SPORTS — AEROBIC VOLLEYBALL, CREATING OUTDOOR PLAY AREAS

Materials needed include books (program book [21]), exercise attire, volleyball net, soft volleyball or beach ball, portable stereo, and aerobic activity and food checklist (Appendix A3.10)

The instructor will gather the children and their family members and set up a volleyball game. Select a game set that includes a soft volleyball or use a beach ball instead. You will need some music to make it complete — along with these few additional guidelines: When the opposing team scores a point, the receiving team has to do 10 aerobic moves to the music such as aerobic dance moves (modified jumping jacks, the twist, the grapevine, and the cha-cha) while the ball is being retrieved. When the serving team gets a "side out" (they lose the point and the serve to the opposing team), they have to do 10 dance movements to the music.

It's also fun to ask those who fumble the ball or foul to walk, jog, or dance around the court. At the end of the volleyball game, the instructor will discuss methods to create outdoor play areas in the home using verbal cues in Appendix A3.3.

## LESSON 6: FLEXIBILITY, FLEX TEST I, AND FLEX AND STRETCH CLASS

Materials needed include books (program book [21]), exercise DVD (Appendix A3.1.1), pen or pencil, exercise attire, chairs, exercise mats, portable stereo, and aerobic activity and food checklist (Appendix A3.10).

The instructor will discuss the importance of flexibility using verbal cues (Appendix A3.3). In pairs, students will be guided through the Flex Test sequence located in the program book [21]. The instructor will emphasize the importance of balance as it relates to flexibility and strength. The instructor will guide the parents and children through an evaluation of different areas of the body. Initially, the parent will observe the child from a side view to determine whether the head and shoulders are aligned with the rest of the body. An appropriate area will be checked in the program book if an imbalance is present. The child will then observe the parent. The instructor will discuss methods to correct the imbalances. He or she will also demonstrate corrective exercises. The parents and children will repeat this process with the other areas of the body (back, knees, etc.). The class will end with a stretching routine to music.

Students will be shown how to keep the knees "soft" (or slightly bent) and not locked or overextended during activities. Corrective exercises, designed to improve the imbalanced areas of the body, will be introduced. The Flex and Stretch series in the program book [21] and exercise DVD (Appendix A3.1.1) will be reviewed to music. A sample stretching exercise is located in Appendix A3.3.

## LESSON 7: AEROBIC EXERCISE AND CARDIOPULMONARY ENDURANCE, STEADY STATE — MONITORING HEART RATE AND AEROBIC CIRCUIT

Materials needed include books (program book [21]), exercise attire, portable stereo, exercise mats, jump rope, aerobic activity and food checklist (Appendix A3.10), station markers, and a stopwatch. Optional equipment includes a treadmill, cycle ergometer, rowing ergometer, rowing machine, or stair climber.

Students will participate in an aerobic station routine. A different aerobic move will be described on a card. Each student will begin at one of the stations. After 2 minutes of movement to music, the instructor will call "rotate" and the students will move in a clockwise fashion to the next station. This continues until all stations have been visited. Alternatively, you may choose to conduct the aerobic circuit using available aerobic exercise equipment. For example: station 1, treadmill; station 2, side jacks; station 3, cycle ergometer; station 4, heel backs with arms up; station 5, rowing ergometer; station 6, twist; station 7, stair climber; and so on. The instructor uses station markers and guides the students from one station to another. Two minutes should be spent at each station, followed by 30 seconds to change stations. The instructor may choose to use music to help motivate the children. Using the verbal cues (Appendix A3.3), the instructor should then discuss heart rate monitoring.

## LESSON 8: EXERCISE PRESCRIPTIONS: THE FIT KIT WALKING PROGRAM

Materials needed include books (program book [21]), exercise attire, exercise DVD (Appendix A3.1.1), pedometers (optional), and aerobic activity and food checklist (Appendix A3.10).

The instructor will discuss the importance of exercise to maintaining weight loss. He or she will review "The Fit Kit Walking Program" located in the program book [21], using verbal cues (Appendix A3.3). The parents and children will be encouraged to begin the program as a family project. The instructor may choose to encourage the families to purchase pedometers so that they may track the distance walked each day and week.

## LESSON 9: REVIEW MUSCULAR STRENGTH AND ENDURANCE: PULL YOUR OWN WEIGHT SERIES

Materials needed include books (program book [21]), exercise attire, portable stereo, exercise mats, exercise DVD (Appendix A3.1.1), and aerobic activity and food checklist (Appendix A3.10).

The instructor will review muscular strength and endurance facts and the exercises listed in the program book [21]. He or she will lead a class in the Pull Your Own Weight Series in the program book [21], using only the child's own body weight. Follow the instructions and follow the verbal cues as listed in Appendix A3.3. Sample exercises are also located in Appendix A3.3.

## LESSON 10: PARK DAY — OUTDOOR PLAY

Materials needed include books (program book [21]), exercise attire, portable stereo, aerobic activity and food checklist (Appendix A3.10), various outdoor game and play equipment, water containers, water, ice, and tables.

Family and friends will be encouraged to join the students in a Park Day/Outdoor Play. One week prior, the instructor will inform the students to bring a bike, roller skates, roller blades, skateboard, and so on to class on this day. The students, family, and friends will be allowed to circle the park in groups using whatever equipment they bring along. Water stations will be set up at one-half to 1-mile intervals.

The instructor may choose to set up volleyball nets, soccer goals, and so on and to bring extra balls along for those children who do not want to walk and do not have bikes, skates, and so forth. Additional ideas for family fitness field trips are listed in Table 20.9.

## NUTRITION EDUCATION SESSIONS

An overview of the interactive, interdisciplinary nutrition education program is provided in Chapter 12 by Schumacher and colleagues. In this chapter, we provide five additional lesson plans that can

---

**TABLE 20.9**
**Additional Suggestions for Nutrition Education Sessions**

Questions and Answers; Write Your Own Sample Meal Plan [21]
Cooking Demonstrations: Fun in the Kitchen — Vegetable Stir-Fry [21]
Individual Sessions
Cooking Demonstrations: Fun in the Kitchen — Healthy Omelets [21]
Class Discussion: Restaurant Choices — Healthy Restaurant Dining [21]
Class Discussion: Low-Fat/Low-Calorie Cooking Guidelines and Substitutions
Food Lab: Starch and Bread Group
Food Lab: Milk/Dairy and Fat Groups
Class Discussion: Write Your Own Restaurant Menu
Class Discussion: Recipe Substitution Exercise [21]
Class Discussion: Supermarket Smarts
Class Discussion/Taste Testing: Lean Meat and Substitute Choices
Class Discussion/Taste Testing: Healthy Snacks
Cooking Demonstrations: Fun in the Kitchen — Yogurt Fruit Dip [21]
Cooking Demonstrations: Fun in the Kitchen — Healthy Holiday Recipes
Understanding Food Labels [21]
Cooking Demonstrations: Fun in the Kitchen: Low-Fat Breakfast Sausage
Balancing Your Way to Good Nutrition: Vitamins and Minerals [21]
Healthy Breakfasts [21]
Food-Label Jeopardy

---

be implemented in a family-based, multidisciplinary weight management setting. A listing of additional suggestions for nutrition education sessions is located in Table 20.9.

## DIET INSTRUCTION

Materials needed include the program book [21], protein-modified fast diet handout (Appendix A3.G), and notepad and pen.

This lesson should be instructed to severely overweight children only with close medical supervision. Review the protein-modified fast diet (Appendix A3.8), discuss vitamin and mineral supplementation, and review the process for filling out the aerobic activity and food checklist (Appendix A3.10).

## FOOD LABS: FRUIT AND VEGETABLE GROUP

Materials needed include the table of food portions and units (Appendix A3.D), food groups/units (Appendix A3.4), recipes (Appendix A3.6), program book [21], fruit juice (apple, orange, grape, cranberry), fresh fruit, dried fruit, measuring cups and spoons, large bowl of lettuce, salad dressing, cooked broccoli, cheese sauce, cooked vegetables, and V-8™ or tomato juice

Instruction: Review fruit and vegetable units (Appendix A3.4)
Activity: Measure items and calculate caloric value; emphasize different caloric values; have class estimate caloric and fat values before weighing; emphasize caloric density
Specific activities:
1. Measure out one exchange/serving of fruit juice into a glass; emphasize the caloric density of fruit juice by calculating the caloric value of a 12-oz glass of grape juice
2. Calculate the caloric value of various fresh fruits
3. Measure out one exchange/serving of dried fruit; emphasize caloric density of dried fruit
4. Measure items and calculate caloric value

Activity: Emphasize different caloric and fat values before and after additions such as salad dressing and cheese sauce.

Specific activities (have participants volunteer to measure items):

1. Measure lettuce and calculate the caloric value. Add one tablespoon of salad dressing (average salad dressing value is 100 calories and 10 g fat per tablespoon) at a time, calculating caloric value after each addition. Emphasize caloric difference between plain lettuce and lettuce with various amounts of salad dressing.

2. Measure and calculate the caloric value of broccoli. Add one tablespoon cheese sauce (average cheese sauce value is 50 calories and 5 g fat per tablespoon) at a time, calculating the caloric value after each addition. Emphasize the caloric difference between plain broccoli and broccoli and various amounts of cheese sauce.

3. Measure and calculate the caloric value of various vegetables including vegetable juice.

## COOKING DEMONSTRATIONS: FUN IN THE KITCHEN — OVEN-FRIED CHICKEN

Materials needed include the recipe located in program book [21]; skinless, boneless chicken breasts; bread crumbs or flour; egg substitute; nonstick cooking spray; baking sheet; and an oven.

Activity: Prepare oven-fried chicken

Specific Instructions: Preheat the oven to 370°F. Dip the chicken breasts in the egg substitute, then into the bread crumbs. Repeat this process for an extra-crispy coating. Spray a baking sheet with the nonstick cooking spray and place the chicken breasts onto the sheet. Bake at 370°F for 45 minutes or until chicken is cooked throughout. Thoroughly wash your hands and all work surfaces with soap after handling raw meat.

Discuss the caloric value and nutrient content of the recipe. Allow children and parents to sample the oven-fried chicken following the exercise session.

## NUTRITION GAMES: FAST-FOOD FOLLIES

Materials needed include grilled chicken sandwich (no mayonnaise or cheese), small fries, diet drink, double-meat sandwich, large fries, regular drink, fried chicken dinner, and biscuit.

Activity: Review Fast-Food List in program book [21]. Have participants volunteer to weigh food. Calculate caloric and fat content of various fast-food meals in class.

Compare best and worst choices (fried chicken dinner vs. grilled chicken dinner and bacon-double cheeseburger with large fries and a regular drink vs. grilled chicken sandwich with small fries and a diet drink)

Measure and weigh items in class.

Have participants touch and feel the grease on the fried items.

Specific Instructions: Average values

Fried chicken: 100 calories and 10 g fat per ounce.

Fried hamburger: 100 calories and 10 g fat per ounce.

Grilled chicken: 55 calories and 3 g fat per ounce.

Cheese on sandwich: 100 calories and 10 g fat per ounce (average)

French fries: 125 calories and 5 g fat per ounce.

Average mayonnaise on sandwich: 1 tablespoon: 135 calories and 15 g fat per ounce

Free toppings: mustard, ketchup, lettuce, tomato, pickles, onions

Hamburger bun: two servings starch/bread, 160 calories and 0 to 2 g fat per whole bun

Biscuit: average 125 calories and 5 g fat per ounce.

## Class Discussion: Understanding Fiber

Materials needed include the handout Filling up with Fiber (Appendix A3.9), program book [21], samples of foods rich in fiber (Table 20.10), notepad and pen, flip chart, erasable markers, or chalk board.

> Activity: Review and discuss the role and benefits of fiber. Using the samples, compare the fiber content of various foods.
>
> Specific Instructions: Dietary fiber is the part of plant food that humans cannot digest or absorb. The recommended daily intake of fiber for children 3 to 18 years old is the child's age in years plus 5 g. For adults it is 20 to 30 g per day.

There are several benefits to increasing the amount of fiber in your diet.

### Benefits of Fiber

Fiber can draw water into the digestive tract to make stools softer and easier to pass. Dietary fiber reduces the risk of certain digestive diseases, such as diverticulosis, hemorrhoids, and irritable bowel syndrome. This is because fiber increases the rate at which food travels through the digestive tract. Dietary fiber can also help in weight loss. Dietary fiber increases the bulk of a meal and promotes a feeling of fullness in the stomach, which in turn may reduce the amount of food eaten. High-fiber foods generally require more chewing and may take longer to eat.

Certain types of dietary fiber lower cholesterol and triglyceride levels in the blood, and dietary fiber may help in the prevention of certain types of cancer. There is evidence that high-fiber foods may help to prevent colon cancer by binding with cancer-causing agents and speeding their progress through the digestive tract.

### Adding Fiber to Your Diet

When you increase the amount of fiber in your diet, you should do so gradually. Your stomach and your intestines need time to get used to this change. Adding fiber too quickly or using too much fiber on a regular basis may cause gas, diarrhea, and bloating. Be sure to drink plenty of water and other liquids as well. Aim for at least 8 glasses of water per day. Assist patients who do not drink water regularly to gradually achieve this goal over several weeks. Table 20.10 details foods that provide fiber and the grams per serving of each.

**TABLE 20.10**
**Best Fiber Sources — Grams of Fiber**

| Food | Fiber, g |
|---|---|
| **Breads** | |
| Whole-wheat, regular, 1 slice | 2–3 |
| Pumpernickel, 1 slice | 2 |
| Rye, 1 slice | 2 |
| Pita, whole wheat, 1 | 5 |
| Whole-wheat, hearty or heavy, 1 slice | 4–6 |
| **Legumes** | |
| Beans, cooked, ½ cup | 8 |
| Lentils, cooked, ½ cup | 4 |
| **Cereals and Other Starches** | |
| Barley, cooked, ½ cup | 3 |
| Cereal, bran, ½–1 cup | 6–15 |
| Oatmeal, cooked, ½ cup | 2 |
| Popcorn, 1 cup | 1 |
| Rice, brown, cooked, ½ cup | 2 |
| **Vegetables** | |
| Asparagus, cooked, ½ cup | 2 |
| Broccoli, cooked, ½ cup | 2 |
| Brussels sprouts, cooked, ½ cup | 3 |
| Cabbage, cooked, ½ cup | 2 |
| Carrots, cooked, ½ cup, or raw, 1 medium | 3 |
| Cauliflower, cooked, ½ cup | 2 |
| Green beans, cooked, ½ cup | 2 |
| Potato (with skin), cooked, 1 medium | 4 |
| Spinach, cooked, ½ cup | 2 |
| **Fruits** | |
| Apple (with skin), 1 medium | 3–4 |
| Apricots, dried, ⅓ cup | 4 |
| Blueberries, 1 cup | 4 |
| Banana, 1 medium | 2 |
| Figs, dried, 2 | 4 |
| Orange, 1 medium | 3 |
| Pear (with skin), 1 medium | 4 |
| Peach (with skin), 1 medium | 2 |
| Prunes, dried, 4 | 2 |
| Raisins, ¼ cup | 2 |
| Strawberries, 1 cup | 4 |

# REFERENCES

1. Pavlov, I. P. *Conditioned Reflexes.* (G. V. Anrep, Trans.). London, Oxford University Press, 1927.
2. Bandura, A. *Principles of Behavior Modification.* New York: Holt, Rinehart and Winston, 1969.
3. Bandura, A. *Social Learning Theory.* Englewood Cliffs, NJ: Prentice-Hall, 1977.
4. Bandura, A. *Social Foundations of Thought and Action.* Englewood Cliffs, NJ: Prentice Hall, 1986.
5. Skinner, B. F. *The Behavior of Organisms*: *An Experimental Analysis.* Acton, MA: Copley, 1938.

6. Skinner, B. F. *Science and Human Behavior*. New York: Macmillan, 1953.
7. Skinner, B. F. The science of learning and the art of teaching. *Harvard Educ Rev.* 24:86–97, 1954.
8. Skinner, B. F. *The Technology of Teaching*. New York: Appleton-Century-Crofts, 1968.
9. Piaget, J. *The Moral Judgment of the Child*. New York: Harcourt, 1932.
10. Piaget, J. Piaget's theory. In: P. H. Mussen, Ed. *Carmichael's Manual of Child Psychology*. New York: Wiley, 1970.
11. Prochaska, J. O., DiClemente, C. C. Stages and processes of self-change of smoking: toward an integrative model of change. *J Consult Clin Psychol.* 51:390–395, 1983.
12. Prochaska, J. O., DiClemente, C. C., Norcross, J. C. In search of how people change. Applications to addictive behaviors. *Am Psychol.* 47:1102–1114, 1992.
13. Prochaska, J. O., DiClemente, C.C. *The Transtheoretical Approach*. New York: Basic Books, 1992, pp. 300–334.
14. Prochaska, J. O., DiClemente, C.C. *Stages of Change in the Modification of Problem Behavior*. Sycamore: Sycamore Publishing Company, 1992, pp. 184–214.
15. Berg-Smith, S. M., V. J. Stevens, K. M. Brown, L. Van Horn, N. Gernhofer, E. Peters et al. A brief motivational intervention to improve dietary adherence in adolescents. The Dietary Intervention Study in Children (DISC) Research Group. *Health Educ. Res.* 14:399–410, 1999.
16. Feldman, R. H., Damron, D., Anliker, J., Ballesteros, R. D., Langenberg, P., DiClemente, C., Havas, S. The effect of the Maryland WIC 5-A-Day promotion program on participants' stages of change for fruit and vegetable consumption. *Health Educ. Behav.* 27:649–663, 2000.
17. Lee, R. E., Nigg, C. R., DiClemente, C. C., Courneya, K. S. Validating motivational readiness for exercise behavior with adolescents. *Res. Q. Exerc. Sport.* 72:401–410, 2001.
18. Sothern, M. S., H. Schumacher, T. K. von Almen, L. K. Carlisle, and J. N. Udall. Committed to kids: an integrated, 4-level team approach to weight management in adolescents. *J. Am. Diet. Assoc.* 102:S81–S85, 2002.
19. von Almen, T. K., Figueroa-Colon, R., Suskind, R. M. Psychological considerations in the treatment of childhood obesity. In: P. L. Giorgi, Suskind, R. M., Catassi, C. Ed., *The Obese Child*. Basel, Switzerland: Karger Press, 1991, pp. 162–171.
20. von Almen, T. K., Figueroa-Colon, R., Suskind, R.M. Psychological considerations in the treatment of childhood obesity. *Pediatr Adolesc Med.* 2, 1992.
21. Sothern, M., von Almen, TK, Schumacher, H. *Trim Kids: The Proven Plan That Has Helped Thousands of Children Achieve a Healthier Weight*. New York: Harper Collins Publishers, 2001
22. Ewart, C. K. Social action theory for a public health psychology. *Am. Psychol.* 46:931–946, 1991.
23. Miller, W. R., Rollnick, S. *Motivational Interviewing: Preparing People to Change Addictive Behavior*. New York: The Guilford Press, 1991.
24. Miller, W. R., Rollnick, S. *Motivational Interviewing: Preparing People for Change*, 2nd ed. New York: The Guilford Press, 2002.
25. Epstein, L., Masek, B., Marshall, W. A nutritionally based school program for control of eating in obese children. *Behav. Ther.* 9:766–788, 1978.
26. Stark, L. J., F. L. Collins, Jr., P. G. Osnes, and T. F. Stokes. Using reinforcement and cueing to increase healthy snack food choices in preschoolers. *J. Appl. Behav. Anal.* 19:367–379, 1986.
27. Epstein, L. H. Adherence to exercise in obese children. *J Cardiac Rehab.* 4:185–195, 1984.
28. Waxman, M., Stunkard, A. J. Caloric intake and expenditure of obese boys. *J. Pediatr.* 96:187–193, 1980.
29. Kingsley, R. G., Shapiro, J. A comparison of three behavioral programs for the control of obesity in children. *Behav. Ther.* 8:30–36, 1977.
30. Epstein, L. H., Wing, R. R., Koeske, R., Andrasik, F., Ossip, D. J. Child and parent weight loss in family-based behavior modification programs. *J. Consult. Clin. Psychol.* 49:674–685, 1981.
31. Brownell, K. D., Kelman, J. H., Stunkard, A. J. Treatment of obese children with and without their mothers: changes in weight and blood pressure. *Pediatrics.* 71:515–523, 1983.
32. Kirschenbaum, D. S., Harries, E. S., Tomarken, A. J. Effects of parental involvement in behavior weight loss therapy for preadolescents. *Behav. Ther.* 15:485–500, 1984.
33. Marlatt, A. G., Gordon, J. R. *Relapse Prevention: Maintenance Strategies in the Treatment of Addictive Behaviors*. New York: The Guilford Press, 1985.
34. Epstein, L., Wing, R., Penner, B. C. et al. Effect of diet and controlled exercise on weight-loss in obese children. *J. Pediatr.* 7:358–361, 1985.

35. Gutin, B., Litaker, M. Islam, S., Manos, T., Smith, C., Treiber, F. Body-composition measurement in 9-11-y-old children by dual-energy X-ray absorptiometry, skinfold-thickness measurements, and bio-impedance analysis. *Am. J. Clin. Nutr.* 63:287–292, 1996.

36. Epstein, L. H., Wing, R., Koeske, R., et. al. A comparison of lifestyle exercise, aerobic exercise and calisthenics on weight loss in obese children. *Behav. Ther.* 15, 1985.

37. Becque, M. D., Katch, V. L., Rocchini, A. P., Marks, C. R., Moorehead, C. Coronary risk incidence of obese adolescents: reduction by exercise plus diet intervention. *Pediatrics.* 81:605–612, 1988.

38. Brown, R., Sothern, M., Suskind, R., Udall, J., Blecker, U. Racial differences in the lipid profiles of obese children and adolescents before and after significant weight loss. *Clin. Pediat.* (Phila). 39:427–431, 2000.

39. Sothern, M., Gordon, S. Prevention of obesity in young children. *Clin. Pediat.* 42:101–111, 2003.

40. Epstein, L. H. Methodological issues and ten-year outcomes for obese children. *Ann N Y Acad Sci.* 699:237–249, 1993.

41. Epstein, L. H., Valoski, A., Wing, R. R., and McCurley, J. Ten-year follow-up of behavioral, family-based treatment for obese children. *JAMA.* 264:2519–2523, 1990.

42. Bailey, R., Olson, J., Pepper, S., Porszasz, J., Barstow, T., Cooper, D. The level and tempo of children's physical activities: an observational study. *Med Sci Sports Exerc.* 27:1033–1041, 1994.

43. DiNubile, N. A. Youth fitness — problems and solutions. *Prev Med.* 22:589–594, 1993.

44. Bar-Or, O., Foreyt, J., Bouchard, C. et al. Physical activity, genetic and nutritional considerations in childhood weight management. *Med Sci Sports Exerc.* 30:2–10, 1998.

45. Bar-Or, O. A., Rowland, W. *Pediatric Exercise Medicine: From Physiologic Principles to Health Care Application.* Champaign, IL: Human Kinetics, 2004

46. Sothern, M. S., Loftin, M., Blecker, U., Udall, Jr., J. N. Impact of significant weight loss on maximal oxygen uptake in obese children and adolescents. *J. Investig. Med.* 48:411–416, 2000.

47. Epstein, L. H., Goldfield, G. S. Physical activity in the treatment of childhood overweight and obesity: current evidence and research issues. *Med. Sci. Sports Exerc.* 31:S553–S559, 1999.

48. Sothern, M. S., Loftin, M., Suskind, R. M., Udall, Jr., J. N., Blecker, U. The impact of significant weight loss on resting energy expenditure in obese youth. *J. Investig. Med.* 47:222–226, 1999.

49. Sothern, M., Udall, Jr., J. N., Suskind, R. M., Vargas, A., Blecker, U. Weight loss and growth velocity in obese children after very low calorie diet, exercise, and behavior modification. *Acta Paediatr.* 89:1036–1043, 2000.

50. Pollock, M., Glasser, G., Butcher, J., Despres, J., Dishman, R. et al. American College of Sports Medicine Position Stand. The recommended quantity and quality of exercise for developing and maintaining cardiorespiratory and muscular fitness, and flexibility in healthy adults, *Med Sci Sports Exerc.,* 975–991, 1998.

51. Sothern, M. S., Loftin, M., Suskind, R. M., Udall, J. N., Blecker, U. The health benefits of physical activity in children and adolescents: implications for chronic disease prevention. *Eur. J. Pediatr.* 158:271–274, 1999.

52. Sothern, M. S., Loftin, J. M., Udall, J. N., Suskind, R. M., Ewing, T. L., Tang, S. C., Blecker, U. Safety, feasibility, and efficacy of a resistance training program in preadolescent obese children. *Am. J. Med. Sci.* 319:370–375, 2000.

53. Hass, C. J., Feigenbaum, M. S., Franklin, B. A. Prescription of resistance training for healthy populations. *Sports Med.* 31:953–964, 2001.

54. Pescatello, L. S., Franklin, B. A., Fagard, R., Farquhar, W. B., Kelley, G. A., Ray, C. A. American College of Sports Medicine position stand. Exercise and hypertension. *Med. Sci. Sports Exerc.* 36:533–553, 2004.

55. Stratton, G., Jones, M., Fox, K. R., Tolfrey, K., Harris, J., Maffulli, N. et al. BASES position statement on guidelines for resistance exercise in young people. *J. Sports Sci.* 22:383–390, 2004.

56. Schwimmer, J. B., Burwinkle, T. M., Varni, J. W. Health-related quality of life of severely obese children and adolescents. *JAMA.* 289:1813–1819, 2003.

57. Doll, H. A., Petersen, S. E., Stewart-Brown, S. L. Obesity and physical and emotional well-being: associations between body mass index, chronic illness, and the physical and mental components of the SF-36 questionnaire. *Obes. Res.* 8:160–170, 2000.

58. Sothern, M., Loftin, M., Suskind, R., Wilson, J., Singley, C., Udall, J., Blecker, U. The impact of level of obesity on physiologic function during rest, submaximal and maximal weight-bearing exercise in obese youth. *Obes. Res.* 5:35S, 1997.

59. Maffeis, C., Schutz, Y., Schena, F., Zaffanello, M., Pinelli, L. Energy expenditure during walking and running in obese and nonobese prepubertal children. *J. Pediatr.* 123:193–199, 1993.

60. Sothern, M. S., Loftin, J., Suskind, R. M., Udall, J. N., Blecker, U. Physiologic function and childhood obesity. *Int. J. Pediatr.* 14:135–139, 1999.

61. Neiman, D. *Fitness and Sports Medicine: An Introduction.* Palo Alto, CA: Bull Publishing Co., 1990

62. Pollock, S. E. Human responses to chronic illness: physiologic and psychosocial adaptation. *Nurs Res.* 35:90–95, 1986.

63. Sothern, M. S. Exercise as a modality in the treatment of childhood obesity. *Pediatr. Clin. N. Am.* 48:995–1015, 2001.

64. Sothern, M. S., Hunter, S., Suskind, R. M., Brown, R., Udall, Jr., J. N., Blecker, U. Motivating the obese child to move: the role of structured exercise in pediatric weight management. *South. Med. J.* 92:577–584, 1999.

65. Sothern, M. S., Loftin, J. M., Udall, J. N., Suskind, R. M., Ewing, T. L., Tang, S. C., Blecker, U. Inclusion of resistance exercise in a multidisciplinary outpatient treatment program for preadolescent obese children. *South. Med. J.* 92:585–592, 1999.

66. Bandura, A. Health promotion by social cognitive means. *Health Educ. Behav.* 31:143–164, 2004.

67. Borg, G. *Borg's Perceived Exertion and Pain Scales.* Champaign, IL: Human Kinetics, 1998

68. Rippe, J. M., Hess, S. The role of physical activity in the prevention and management of obesity. *J. Am. Diet. Assoc.* 98:S31–S38, 1998.

69. Sothern, M. S., Despinasse, B., Brown, R., Suskind, R. M., Udall, Jr., J. N., Blecker, U. Lipid profiles of obese children and adolescents before and after significant weight loss: differences according to sex. *South. Med. J.* 93:278–282, 2000.

70. Metcalf, J. A., Roberts, S. O. Strength training and the immature athlete: an overview. *Pediatr. Nurs.* 19:325–332, 1993.

71. LeMura, L. M., Maziekas, M. T. Factors that alter body fat, body mass, and fat-free mass in pediatric obesity. *Med. Sci. Sports Exerc.* 34:487–496, 2002.

72. Epstein, L. H., Klein, K. R., Wisniewski, L.. Child and parent factors that influence psychological problems in obese children. *Int. J. Eat. Disord.* 15:151–158, 1994.

73. Epstein, L. H., Koeske, R., Wing, R. R., Valoski, A. The effect of family variables on child weight change. *Health Psychol.* 5:1–11, 1986.

74. Epstein, L. H., Valoski, A., Koeske, R., and Wing, R. R. Family-based behavioral weight control in obese young children. *J. Am. Diet. Assoc.* 86:481–484, 1986.

75. Epstein, L. H., Wing, R. R., Koeske, R., Valoski, A. Effect of parent weight on weight loss in obese children. *J. Consult. Clin. Psychol.* 54:400–401, 1986.

76. Batch, J. A., Baur, L. A. Management and prevention of obesity and its complications in children and adolescents. *Med. J. Aust.* 182:130–135, 2005.

77. Strong, W., Malina, R., Blimkie, C., Daniels, S. et al. Evidence based physical activity for school-aged youth. *J. Pediatr.* 146:732–737, 2005.

# APPENDIX 1
## Clinical Management Forms

## A1.1 SAMPLE JOB DESCRIPTION — CLINICAL COORDINATOR

| |
|---|
| Position: Clinic Coordinator |
| Terms of Employment: Unlimited |
| Hours of Employment: 20 hours per week, scheduled as necessary |

### Duties and Responsibilities

**Daily**

Check voice mail and return phone calls from parents and referring physicians or others; mail out information packets to parents and referring physicians; file patient information as necessary

Replace forms in files as necessary

Respond to patient/parent concerns and complaints and refer medical concerns to the physician, nutrition concerns to the dieticians, behavior concerns to the psychologists, and exercise concerns to the exercise physiologist; process all registration, insurance, and public relations/marketing items; document all correspondence and information in patient files

**Weekly**

Make phone calls to absentees from weekly weight clinic; make notes in patient files and report any special circumstances to medical director

Schedule meeting room and set-up

Schedule patients for physician office visits or additional medical testing as required

Maintain office and clinic supplies, order as necessary

Process check requests for supplies as required

Process reimbursement for petty cash (anything under $50.00) supplies as required

Prepare and distribute flyers concerning class events, free information seminars, orientations

**Monthly**

Schedule meeting room for monthly staff meeting, notify staff

Take minutes at monthly staff meeting, distribute to staff

Update class schedule, prepare flyer, and mail out

Prepare monthly attendance report

Prepare and distribute monthly staff "special events" calendar

Prepare patient birthday list for each month

Order clinic supplies as necessary

**Quarterly**

Organize free information sessions and orientations: meeting space, supplies, patient contact, patient class schedule, slide presentation, sign-in sheet, display table, hand-outs, registration packets

Schedule patients for history and physical exams or refer them to appropriate physician office

Mail packets with copies of progress to referring physicians as per procedure guide

Calculate obesity status [1,2] and assign patients to phase I, II, or III as per procedure guide

Prepare orientation packets including consent forms

Prepare patient files with all necessary forms as per procedure guide and sample file

Mail out test preparation letters 2 weeks before evaluation date as per procedure guide

Make reminder phone calls for blood tests, evaluation reminders, and body composition tests

Prepare awards for graduating from one phase to another — for activity, attendance, and weight loss — as per procedure guide

**Ongoing**

Typeset memos, letters, copies, faxes, phone calls, and so on as necessary for good communication among and between staff physicians and parents

Keep up clinical records and files

Prepare, order, or purchase incentive awards as necessary

Perform quality control for patient files

Arrange pre-/postpicture film developing, photo book organization

Keep up program calendar

## A1.2   PEDIATRIC WEIGHT MANAGEMENT CLASS SCHEDULE FORM

|  | Medicine | Nutrition | Behavior | Exercise |
|---|---|---|---|---|
| 4:00–4:30 | Set-up | Set-up | Set-up | Set-up |
| 4:30–4:50 |  |  |  |  |
| 4:50–5:00 | Accomplishments | Accomplishments | Accomplishments | Accomplishments |
| 5:00–5:30 |  |  |  |  |
| 5:30–6:00 |  |  |  |  |
| 6:00–6:30 |  |  |  |  |
| 6:30–7:00 | Clean up | Clean up | Clean up | Clean up |

## A1.3  PHONE SCREENING AND INFORMATION FORM

| Initials: | |
|---|---|
| ☐ Self-pay or Insurance | ☐ Medicaid |
| **Phone Screening and Information Form** | |
| Date: | Time: |
| Patient Name: | ☐ M    ☐ F |
| Age: | DOB:  /  / |
| Height:_____<br>  (approximate, feet/inches) | Weight: _____<br>  (approximate, pounds) |
| Mother: | Father: |
| Address: | |
| Telephone (Home): | Telephone (Work): |
| Price Quoted: | |
| Additional Comments: | |

**Mailing Checklist**

| | |
|---|---|
| ☐ Local Area | ☐ Out of Town |
| ☐ Out of State | ☐ Information Letter |
| ☐ Brochure | ☐ Business Card |
| ☐ Referral Form | ☐ Registration Form |

## A1.4  PHYSICIAN REFERRAL FORM

**<insert name of institution> Pediatric Weight Management Program**

Date: _____  Appointment Date and Time: _____

Patient's Name: _____  Physician: _____

Date of Birth: _____  ☐ Male   ☐ Female

Parent's Names: _____

Address: _____  Home Phone#:_____

_____  Work Phone#: _____

_____  Other Phone#: _____

### Medical History

Past Medical History: _____

_____

_____

Recent Medical History:_____

_____

Primary Physician: _____

Referring Physician: _____

Address: _____  Phone#: _____

_____  Other Phone#: _____

### Billing Information

☐ Private Insurance:_____

☐ HMO: _____

☐ CHAMPUS    ☐ Payment at Service    ☐ Payment Plan:_____

☐ Accept Insurance Only    ☐ Medicaid    ☐ No Coverage

## A1.5   REGISTRATION FORM

---

**<insert name of institution> Weight-Management Program Registration Form**

| | |
|---|---|
| **Patient Information** | **Emergency Contact** |

**Patient Information**

Last Name:_____ Sex: ☐ M ☐ F

First Name:_____ Date of Birth: _____

Middle Name: _____ Religion: _____

Street Address: _____

City:_____State:____ZIP Code_____

Soc.Sec.#:_____

Home Phone: (_____) _____

Patient Admitted Before:    ☐ Yes    ☐ No

**Emergency Contact**

Please give the name of a relative or friend who does not live with you, who can be contacted in case of an emergency:

Name: _____

Relationship to Child: _____

Street Address: _____

City:_____State:____ZIP Code _____

Phone: (_____) _____

---

**Father's Information**

Last Name: _____

First Name:_____Middle: _____

Street Address: _____

City:_____State:____ZIP Code_____

Home Phone: (_____) _____

Soc.Sec.#:_____

Date of Birth: _____

Marital Status: ☐ single ☐ married ☐ divorced ☐ widowed

Occupation:_____Employer: _____

Work Address: _____

City:_____State:____ZIP Code_____

Work Phone: (_____)_____

**Insurance Information**

Insurance Company: _____

Phone # to verify Ins. Coverage: _____

Policy #: _____

Does your insurance need to be pre-certified? ☐ Yes ☐ No

Name of Insured: _____

SECOND POLICY

Insurance Company: _____

Phone # to verify Ins. Coverage: _____

Policy #: _____

Does your insurance need to be pre-certified? ☐ Yes ☐ No

Name of Insured: _____

---

**Mother's Information**

Last Name: _____

First Name:_____Middle: _____

Street Address: _____

City:_____State:____ZIP Code_____

Home Phone: (_____) _____

Soc.Sec.#:_____

Date of Birth: _____

Marital Status: ☐ single ☐ married ☐ divorced ☐ widowed

Occupation:_____Employer: _____

Work Address: _____

City:_____State:____ZIP Code_____

Work Phone: (_____)_____

**Other Information**

MEDICAID: Please present Medicaid Card

Medicaid #: _____

County:_____Name of Worker: _____

Handicapped Children's Program: ☐ Yes ☐ No

County:_____Name of Worker: _____

REFERRAL INFORMATION

Who is the child's pediatrician?_____

Who referred you to this program? _____

Physician's Name:_____

Health-Care Facility:_____

---

**Person Responsible for Bill**

Name: _____

Street Address: _____

City:_____State:____ZIP Code_____

Relationship to Child: _____

**Office Use Only**

Medical Record#:_____Account#: _____

Doctor:_____Service: _____

Date:_____Time:_____

## A1.6   &lt;INSERT NAME OF INSTITUTION&gt;

### Medical History and Physical Examination Form

#### Historical Data

### A. Health History
   1. Participant
   2. Family

Birth Weight_____Age at obesity _____

Family members who are overweight _____

List attempts at weight reduction_____

List any present or past serious illness _____

List any hospitalization_____

*Gynecological History/Sexual History*

1. Menarche

2. Last menstrual period

3. Breast development     Yes_____ No_____

   Age of onset         _____Yrs.

   Pubic hair          Yes_____ No_____

   Age of onset         _____Yrs.

   Birth control        Yes_____ No_____

   Birth control method _____

   Medications:   Yes, Describe_____

              No_____

   Nonprescription Drugs:   Yes, Name and/or describe _____

              No_____

   Allergy:     Yes_____ No_____

      Food:_____

      Medications: _____

      Other: _____

### B. Dietary History
   1. Participant
   2. Family

Problem foods: _____

Problem places:   Relative's homes_____ Friends_____ Television _____

Dietary History: Food preparation: ___% Fried ___% Broiled ___% Boiled ___% Baked ___% Grilled ___% Other

List the common meats eaten in your family _____

Indicate with or without skin _____

Types of fat-cooking:   Vegetable oil_____ Margarine_____ Butter_____ Lard_____ Other_____

**C. Physical Athletic History**
  1. Participant
  2. Family

Athletic activities:   None_____ Walk_____ Ride bike_____ Skating (Ice and/or roller) _____ Swim _____

Run _____ Jump Rope_____ Dance_____ Other_____

The amount of time each session:   3 times/week_____ 2 times/week_____ Other_____ >20 min_____ <20 min_____

**D. Psychosocial History**

  1. Participant

  2. Family

Do friends make fun of your obesity?      Yes_____ No_____

Why do you want to lose weight? _____

What do you plan to gain by losing weight?_____

*Social Habits:*

Smoking or tobacco:      Yes_____ No_____

   How many pack(s) per day?_____

Drinking:      Yes_____ No_____ How long?_____

   Which type:      Beer_____ Wine_____ Liquor_____

**Physical Examination Form**

| Physical Examination | WNL← | PF↑ |
|---|---|---|
| General appearance | | |
| Skin, hair, nails | | |
| Lymph nodes | | |
| Head, face, ears, eyes, nose, throat, mouth | | |
| Neck | | |
| Chest, breast, lungs<br>Tanner stage: | | |
| Heart | | |

| | | |
|---|---|---|
| Abdomen | | |
| Genitalia, anus, rectum<br>Tanner stage: | | |
| Extremities — appearance (if abnormal, describe finding or identify as listed below): | | |
|   Varus (bowlegged) | | |
|   Valgus (knock knee) | | |
|   "Flat" foot | | |
| Rotation | | |
|   Hip | | |
|   Knee | | |
|   Ankle | | |
| Gait | | |
| Additional description of positive findings: | | |

Temperature _____ Pulse _____ Respirations _____ BP_____

Weight_____ Height_____

*Note:* ←WNL = within normal limits              ↑PF = positive finding

Signature _____

**Review of Systems**

Date: _____ Name:_____

HEENT _____

_____

_____

Cardiopulmonary _____

_____

_____

Gastrointestinal _____

_____

_____

Genitourinary _____

_____

_____

Neurological _____

_____

_____

Other _____

_____

_____

## A1.7   <INSERT NAME OF INSTITUTION> CLEARANCE FORM

_____ has met the medical requirements of screening to enter the weight reduction program.

_____ has not met the medical requirements of screening to enter the weight reduction program.

Labs Pending _____

No Labs Pending _____

### *Referrals*

Pulmonary_____

Endocrinology_____

Orthopedics_____

Others _____

### *Follow-up visit recommended*

10 weeks _____

3 months _____

6 months _____

1 year      _____

Other      _____

## A1.8   PROGRAM INFORMATION LETTER

### Pediatric Weight Management

Thank you for your interest in <insert name of institution> Pediatric Weight Management Program.

A new session of <insert name of institution> will begin in <insert date>. In the last 10 years, the <insert name of institution> program has assisted many children to reach their individual weight loss goals. The comprehensive program includes

- Weekly consultations with a registered dietitian, clinical exercise physiologist, and behavioral modification specialist
- Medical supervision by a pediatrician
- Educational tools including exercise/motivational videos and colorful and fun workbooks and handbooks
- Comprehensive health and fitness evaluations every 3 months
- Achievement certificates, awards, diet/exercise record books, and a backpack
- Lipid profile and chemical blood analysis
- Graded exercise test including metabolic analysis
- Body composition analysis by DEXA, including percentage fat, lean body mass, and bone mineral density

Parents, please follow these easy registration steps:

STEP 1    Your child must have a completed medical history and physical examination to enroll in the program. Make an appointment with your child's primary care physician for a history and physical examination and provide the name, address, and telephone number of your physician so we can mail the appropriate forms to his or her office. If you do not have a primary care physician, you can make an appointment with our medical director to obtain a medical history and physical by calling <insert phone number>. Following the exam, a recommended "term of treatment" will be determined by the medical director.

STEP 2    Attend the free information session on <insert> from <insert> until <insert> at the <insert>.

STEP 3    Register for the next session by returning the enclosed registration form and fee in the self-addressed envelope.

STEP 4    Attend the orientation session after receiving clearance from the medical director. You and your child are now on your way to a healthier and happier life.

All children are required to take an exercise test before the start of the session. If your child has not been tested or scheduled, please call the program secretary at <insert> after completing the medical history and physical to schedule an appointment. Exercise testing is done only on <insert> between <insert> at the (MAP INCLUDED IN PACKET).

One week after the orientation meeting, regular classes will begin. Classes will be held on <insert> evenings from <insert> until <insert>. We require at least one parent to attend these sessions with the child. Weekly attendance is essential to the success of your child's weight loss.

The cost of the program is listed below.

Registration:

- Participants are required to pay a <insert> registration fee, which is due before any testing or classes. This fee includes the cost of the initial screening and health assessment.

Program materials:

- A <insert> fee for educational materials is due at the orientation meeting.

Payment schedule:

- <insert> per class attended is billed monthly to the patient thereafter. Each quarter the patient will participate in a progress screening and health assessment; if the patient does not attend at least 10 of 12 classes, he or she will be billed for this assessment.

Rebate:

- The patient will receive a <insert> rebate if he or she attends 48 classes during the 1-year period. Also, if he or she attends the 1-year progress screen and health assessment, a <insert> rebate will be given.

Total cost:

- The total cost of the pediatric weight management program will be <insert> per year of treatment. Patients receive a 20% discount if the full fee is paid in advance.

Payment options:

- Visa and Master Card are accepted. Monthly cash/check payment plans are available but must be approved before program participation. For your convenience, we also have an agreement with <insert> Loan by phone (1-800-<insert>). This option is available pending credit approval.

If there are any questions that have not been covered here, please call. We hope to see you and your child this next session. Thanks!

## A1.9  INITIAL PARENT QUESTIONNAIRE

Child's Name _____ Date _____

Address _____ Telephone _____

Parents' Names

_____

_____

**General**

1. Why do you want your child to lose weight at this time?

_____

_____

2. Name and address of child's physician

_____

_____

3. Please describe your child's weight during the past 6 months:

   ☐ It has decreased.

   ☐ It has been the same.

   ☐ It has increased.

4. Please describe previous attempts your child has made to lose weight, including at what age:

| Age | Weight lost | How long weight loss maintained | Weight-loss method |
|-----|-------------|--------------------------------|--------------------|
|     |             |                                |                    |
|     |             |                                |                    |
|     |             |                                |                    |
|     |             |                                |                    |
|     |             |                                |                    |

5. Why do you think your child is overweight? (Check all reasons that apply.)

   ☐ Overeats at meals

   ☐ Snacks

   ☐ Low activity level

**Weight and Medical History**

6. Birth weight _____ Age at onset of obesity _____

7. ☐ Breast-fed   or   ☐ bottle-fed

Infant feeding problems:

_____

_____

8. Overweight from 2 years of age              ☐ Yes   ☐ No

9. Teased by other children because of weight   ☐ Yes   ☐ No

10. Previous medical problems:

_____

_____

_____

11. Hospitalizations:

_____

_____

12. Medications:

_____

_____

_____

**Family Medical and Weight History**

13. Grandparents' weights:
Maternal Grandmother _____ Maternal Grandfather _____
Paternal Grandmother _____ Paternal Grandfather _____

14. Parents' weights:
Mother _____ Father _____

15. Siblings' weights:
Sisters _____
Brothers _____

16. Aunts: Number overweight _____

17. Uncles: Number overweight _____

**Medical:**

18. Mother: Other health problems (describe)

_____

_____

_____

19. Father: Other health problems (describe)

_____

_____

20. Has anyone in your family had diabetes, hypertension, or thyroid disease?

_____

_____

_____

**Social History**

21. In what grade is your child? _____ Name of school_____

22. Does your child like school?                  ☐ Yes  ☐ No

23. Does your child have friends at school?        ☐ Yes  ☐ No

24. What are your child's school grades?
   ☐ Above average (As and Bs)
   ☐ Average (Cs)
   ☐ Below average (Ds and Fs)

25. Your child's favorite subjects:

_____

_____

26. How does your child spend most of his or her free time?
   ☐ TV
   ☐ With friends
   ☐ Phone
   ☐ Other

27. Does your child have friends in the neighborhood?   ☐ Yes  ☐ No

28. Please describe any difficulties you have in managing your child at home:

_____

29. What are the attitudes of the following people about your child's weight?

|  | Disapprove (child's fault) | Indifferent (doesn't care) | Sympathetic (wants to help) |
|---|---|---|---|
| Father |  |  |  |
| Mother |  |  |  |
| Siblings |  |  |  |
| Friends |  |  |  |

30. How does your child get along with you?

   ☐ Good   ☐ Average   ☐ Poor

31. How does your child get along with your spouse?

   ☐ Good   ☐ Average   ☐ Poor

32. How does your child get along with his or her siblings?

   ☐ Good   ☐ Average   ☐ Poor

33. How do you get along with your spouse?

   ☐ Good   ☐ Average   ☐ Poor

34. Do you encourage your child to be

   ☐ Active   ☐ Inactive

35. Has your child ever received psychological or other counseling in the past?      ☐ Yes   ☐ No

If your child has received counseling, specify what kind, length of treatment, and place, and give a brief description of the results:

_____

_____

_____

36. How does your child feel about himself (self-image)?

   ☐ Relatively happy, except for weight

   ☐ Fair

   ☐ Dislikes self intensely, including other aspects in addition to weight

**Eating Habits**

37. Is your child a compulsive eater?

   ☐ Yes   ☐ No

38. Does your child eat in binges?

   ☐ Yes   ☐ No   ☐ Sometimes

39. Does your child hide food?

   ☐ Yes   ☐ No   ☐ Sometimes

40. Does your child eat when depressed or anxious?

   ☐ Yes   ☐ No   ☐ Sometimes

41. Does your child crave sweets?

   ☐ Yes   ☐ No   ☐ Sometimes

42. Does your child eat food as a reward?

   ☐ Yes   ☐ No   ☐ Sometimes

43. Does your child eat food as a punishment?

   ☐ Yes   ☐ No   ☐ Sometimes

44. Does your child eat at regular times?

   ☐ Yes   ☐ No   ☐ Sometimes

45. Eating patterns: Times per week meal is eaten:

| Breakfast | 0 | 1 | 2 | 3 | 4 | 5 | 6 | 7 |
|-----------|---|---|---|---|---|---|---|---|
| Lunch | 0 | 1 | 2 | 3 | 4 | 5 | 6 | 7 |
| Dinner | 0 | 1 | 2 | 3 | 4 | 5 | 6 | 7 |

46. Does your child eat second helpings?

   ☐ Yes   ☐ No   ☐ Sometimes

47. Snacking patterns: Times per week:

| Mid-morning | 0 | 1 | 2 | 3 | 4 | 5 | 6 | 7 |
|-------------|---|---|---|---|---|---|---|---|
| After school | 0 | 1 | 2 | 3 | 4 | 5 | 6 | 7 |
| After dinner | 0 | 1 | 2 | 3 | 4 | 5 | 6 | 7 |

48. Types of snacks:

   ☐ Chips          ☐ Frozen dessert

   ☐ Cakes, cookies  ☐ Leftovers

   ☐ Pickles        ☐ Fruit

   ☐ Candy          ☐ Sandwiches

   ☐ Other: _____

   _____

   _____

49. Does your child eat dessert?

   ☐ Usually   ☐ Occasionally   ☐ Seldom

50. What size portions does your child eat?

   ☐ Small   ☐ Medium   ☐ Large

51. How fast does your child eat?

   ☐ Slowly   ☐ Average   ☐ Quickly

52. What beverages does your child drink?

   _____

   _____

53. What are your child's favorite foods?

   _____

   _____

54. Which foods does your child dislike?

   _____

   _____

55. Are there any problem foods?

   _____

   _____

56. What time of the day is a problem for your child overeating?

   _____

57. Does your child eat too many starches?

   ☐ Yes   ☐ No   ☐ Sometimes

58. Does your child eat too much meat and fat?

   ☐ Yes   ☐ No   ☐ Sometimes

59. What about the eating habits of other family members?

Mother:

_____

Father:

_____

Siblings:

_____

60. Does your child take any vitamin or mineral supplements?

☐ Yes        Kind _____

☐ No

61. What is the motivation to lose weight?

Child:

_____

Siblings:

_____

Mother:

_____

Father:

_____

62. Does your child eat any foods (such as cakes, pies, ice cream) directly from the package?

☐ Yes   ☐ No   ☐ Sometimes

63. Does your child usually clean the plate?

☐ Yes   ☐ No   ☐ Sometimes

64. When your child finishes the food on the plate and there is more food available on the table, what does he or she usually do?

☐ Does not take any more

☐ Takes a little more

☐ Takes a lot more

65. When is your child most likely to overeat? (Check all that apply.)

☐ When he/she serves him/herself

☐ When food is served by others

☐ When parents or family urge him/her to eat more

☐ When friends urge him/her to eat more

☐ When others (not family) are present

66. When is your child more likely to eat more food than usual?

☐ When eating alone

☐ When eating in a group

67. Does your child eat more food on certain days of the week?

☐ Eats more on the weekends

☐ Eats more on the weekdays

☐ No difference between the weekends and weekdays

**Exercise Habits**

68. Does your child have a physical education class at school?

☐ Yes        Times per week _____

☐ No

69. Does your child participate in extra athletic activities?

☐ Yes        Kind _____

☐ No

70. Does your child participate in home exercise activities?

| Activity | Times per week |
|----------|----------------|
|          |                |
|          |                |

71. Does your child watch television excessively or engage in other sedentary activities?

☐ Yes        Estimated percent of free time_____

☐ No

72. What is your child's attitude about exercise?

☐ Positive

☐ Negative

☐ Moderate

**Family Exercise Activities**

73. Is father

☐ Active        Activities: _____

☐ Inactive

74. Is mother

☐ Active        Activities: _____

☐ Inactive

75. Are siblings

☐ Active        Activities: _____

☐ Inactive

*Activity Patterns*

76. How many hours per day does your child perform the following activities?

| | |
|---|---|
| Watching television | hours |
| Playing actively (e.g., running, jumping) | hours |
| Playing quietly | hours |
| Completing homework | hours |
| Sleeping | hours |

77. What does your child do for physical exercise, and how often does he or she do it?

_____

_____

_____

## A1.10   FOR BODY MASS INDEX (BMI) AND CDC PERCENTILES

http://www.cdc.gov/growthcharts/

# A1.11  ORIENTATION HANDOUT

&lt;insert name&gt; Pediatric Weight-Management Clinic

Dear Parents,

Welcome! You've just taken an important step toward helping your child to become healthier and happier. These are some commonly asked questions and concerns about our program:

### 1. What Can I Expect from the Program?

*Patient Care:* You can expect the highest quality in pediatric health care from our staff of medical, nutrition, behavior, and exercise specialists. The program is an individualized approach to prevention and treatment of obesity conducted in a group setting. Our main goal is the improvement of your child's physical and emotional health and well-being. Weight loss is just a by-product of the overall focus of the program, which is to assist you and your family in making healthy lifestyle changes. A healthy lifestyle will promote maintenance of appropriate body weight and long-term success.

*Education and Guidance:* During the initial weeks of the program you can expect to see all three instructors and the physician weekly. Likewise, all four topics (Medicine, Nutrition, Behavior Modification, and Exercise) will be presented each week. This is a very intense phase, with a great deal of emphasis on diet and changing activity patterns.

*Reinforcement and Maintenance:* During the long-term phase of the program you and your child will join other families who have been in the program previously. Some children will continue to lose weight during this phase and some will only be concerned with maintenance of weight loss. This depends on your child's level of obesity at the beginning of the program. You can expect to see one to two instructors each week. The topics will alternate and will serve as reinforcement (gentle reminders) of material covered in the first few weeks. This is the most important phase of the program, where either long-term success or relapse (weight regain) occurs.

*Evaluation and Success:* Approximately every 3 months we reevaluate your child to account for normal growth and development. Your child receives a new goal weight and we make careful note of his or her progress. We strongly suggest that even after the program is completed, patients continue to attend at least two or three of these evaluations each year. There is no additional charge for this service.

*Promptness:* You can expect that service will begin promptly at &lt;insert time&gt; with weigh-in; also that classes will end between &lt;insert time&gt; and &lt;insert time&gt; each week. You can expect that at least &lt;insert time&gt; minutes of exercise of varying types will be available each week, weather and room availability permitting.

### 2. What Is Expected from My Family and Me?

*Attendance:* Weekly attendance is absolutely essential to success in the first few weeks of the program. Thereafter, although we strongly encourage weekly attendance, individual families usually decide what is the best situation for their own needs. Some children will need weekly check-ins; others will do just fine attending every 2 to 3 weeks.

*Remember:* We have found that attendance corresponds highly with long-term success.

*Accurate Record Keeping:* You and you child are expected to keep certain records. Your child will be rewarded with stickers and positive attention when he or she turns in completed records each week. You should assist your child in keeping these records accurately.

*Compliance:* The program works only if you follow the plan carefully. Weight loss varies, depending upon how overweight your child is at the beginning. We know that if your child is not losing weight, then he or she is not following the plan.

*Parent and Family Support and Participation:* This is absolutely essential! At least one parent must attend clinic sessions weekly with the child. The more the merrier: siblings and extended family are also encouraged to attend. Parents, as well as children, should come dressed to participate in exercise activities each week. We strongly discourage parents from just observing their children exercise and not joining in on the fun!

### 3. Just What Exactly Does My Fee Cover?

The breakdown of charges is:

- Medical history and physical
- Lab work × 3 (CBC w/dif, SMA20, and lipid profile)
- Nutritional Instruction, Behavior Counseling, and Exercise Prescription (50 classes, 4 evaluations)

The majority of the expense to administer this program to your child accrues in the first 3 months. Therefore, please note that your responsibility for payment will not be dismissed if you discontinue the program prematurely.

*4. Why Does This Program Work, Where Others Fail?*

We like to say it is because of something we call the A-Factor:

- Availability of highly qualified staff of experts — This is not just a job to us: we are deeply concerned with your child's progress, health, and overall emotional well-being. We are the A-Team, so to speak.

- Accountability to the program staff — Each week you and your child report your progress and are responsible for remaining within the designated program guidelines. The staff checks the weight, medical, nutrition, and exercise records each week. This greatly improves program compliance and success.

- Attention — the positive kind only — If your child does well he or she receives tons of positive reinforcement. If not, we encourage your child to try harder next week — but attention is quickly focused to another area of the program.

*5. If I Am Having Individual Problems with the Program, What Do I Do?*

Call the office, and leave a message for one of the three staff members. If it is a medical problem, ask the secretary to contact the pediatrician; if it is a question about the diet or nutrition, ask for the dietitian; if it is exercise related, ask for the exercise physiologist; and if it concerns behavioral problems, ask for the behavior specialist. If you have a general concern about the program, such as insurance, financial, or time conflicts, speak to the weight-management program secretary.

## Philosophy

The founders of the <insert program> are primarily concerned with the prevention and treatment of pediatric obesity. We believe that aggressive treatment accompanied by long-term educational follow-up is the most effective approach to this goal. In our clinics the intervention is closely supervised, and the child receives uncompromising care of the highest quality from the pediatric, behavior, exercise, and nutrition specialists. We use an individual approach in a group setting. The immediate goal is the improvement of the child's physical and emotional well-being. Weight loss and weight maintenance are the attractive side-effects of the overall lifestyle focus of the <insert program>.

## A1.12  ORIENTATION CHECKLIST

**Pediatric Weight-Management Program Orientation Checklist**

Don't forget to

    Hand out patient materials

    Instruct participants on how to fill in food diaries

    Hand out meeting schedule

    Hand out test preparation letters

    Hand out laboratory testing forms

    Other: _____

    _____

    _____

## A1.13   CLASS SCHEDULE: <INSET NAME OF INSTITUTION> PEDIATRIC WEIGHT MANAGEMENT

| Week | Day | Date | Time | Activity | Location |
|------|-----|------|------|----------|----------|
| 0 | | | 6:00 PM | Free info session | Auditorium |
| 0 | | | 6:00–7:00 | Orientation | Classroom |
| 1 | | | 4:30–5:30 PM | Group discussion | Classroom |
| | | | 5:30–6:20 PM | Nutrition Session | Kitchen |
| | | | 6:20–6:30 PM | Exercise | Classroom |
| 2 | | | 4:30–5:30 PM | Group discussion | Classroom |
| | | | 5:30–6:30 PM | Aerobic Class | Auditorium |
| 3 | | | 4:30–5:20 PM | Group Discussion | Classroom |
| | | | 5:20–5:50 PM | Exercise | Cardiac Rehab CTR. |
| | | | 5:50–6:30 PM | Behavior | Classroom |
| | | | | Nutrition | Kitchen |
| 4 | | | 4:30–5:20 PM | Group Discussion | Classroom |
| | | | 5:20–5:50 PM | Exercise | Strength rehab |
| | | | 5:50–6:30 PM | Behavior | Classroom |
| | | | | Nutrition | Kitchen |
| 5 | | | 4:30–5:20 PM | Group Discussion | Classroom |
| | | | 5:20–6:30 PM | Individual Consultations | Classroom |
| 6 | | | 4:30–5:20 PM | Group Discussion | Classroom |
| | | | 5:20–5:50 PM | Exercise | Stretch rehab |
| | | | 5:50–6:30 PM | Behavior | Classroom |
| | | | | Nutrition | Kitchen |
| 7 | | | 4:30–6:00 | Park Day | Off-site |
| | | | 6:00–6:30 PM | Weigh-in/monitor | Classroom |
| 8 | | | 4:30–5:20 PM | Group Discussion | Classroom |
| | | | 5:20–5:50 PM | Exercise | Cardiac Rehab CTR. |
| | | | 5:50–6:30 PM | Behavior | Classroom |
| | | | | Nutrition | Kitchen |
| 9 | | | 4:30–5:20 PM | Group Discussion | Classroom |
| | | | 5:20–5:50 PM | Behavior | Classroom |
| | | | | Nutrition | Kitchen |
| | | | 5:50–6:30 PM | Exercise | Outdoors |
| | | | 6:30–7:30 PM | Free Info Session | Auditorium |
| 10 | | | 4:30–5:15 PM | Water Exercise | Pool |
| | | | 5:30–6:00 PM | Group Discussion | Classroom |
| | | | 6:00–6:30 PM | Behavior | Classroom |
| | | | | Nutrition | Kitchen |
| 11 | | | 4:30–6:30 PM | Evaluations | Clinic |
| 12 | | | 4:30–6:30 PM | Awards | Classroom |

## A1.14  WEEKLY CLINIC CHECKLIST

Don't forget to

    Check and collect food diaries

    Check and collect exercise cards

    Collect goal sheets

    Fill in symptom sheets

    Hand out stickers, awards, or incentives

    Hand out exercise DVDs (Class 1) and exercise bands (Dyna-Bands™) (Class 4)

    Check attendance and forward to coordinator for reminder phone calls

    Other _____

        _____

        _____

## A1.15   WEIGHT RECORD AND VITAL SIGNS

| Patient Name: | | | | | | | | |
|---|---|---|---|---|---|---|---|---|
| Date | Week | Height (cm) | Weight (kg) | Weight (lbs) | Weekly Loss/Gain | Loss to Date | BP | RHR* |
| | | | | | | | | |
| | | | | | | | | |
| | | | | | | | | |
| | | | | | | | | |
| | | | | | | | | |
| | | | | | | | | |
| | | | | | | | | |
| | | | | | | | | |
| | | | | | | | | |
| | | | | | | | | |
| | | | | | | | | |
| | | | | | | | | |
| | | | | | | | | |
| | | | | | | | | |
| | | | | | | | | |
| | | | | | | | | |
| | | | | | | | | |
| | | | | | | | | |
| | | | | | | | | |
| | | | | | | | | |
| | | | | | | | | |
| | | | | | | | | |

* Resting heart rate

## A1.16   TEST PREPARATION LETTER

**<insert name of institution>**

Dear Parent,

Your child is required to have a blood test prior to_____.

He/she will not be allowed to begin the program until this test has been completed.

The laboratory is located at_____.

Their hours of operation are _____ .

To make an appointment call _____ .

Instructions prior to test:

Fasting is required (no food) 12 hours beforehand. We suggest scheduling an early morning appointment so that the fasting may be done overnight. Drinking water is fine.

Should you have any further questions regarding this test please contact the weight management program office at

_____.


Thank You.

Sincerely,

Program Director

## A1.17   EVALUATION CHECKLIST

Patient name: _____

Date:_____

Measurements

- □ Height
- □ Weight
- □ Blood pressure
- □ Resting heart rate
- □ Bioelectrical impedance analysis (BIA)
- □ Skinfolds
- □ Circumferences

□ Photograph

□ Questionnaires and forms

□ Physical activity record

Psychosocial questionnaires

- □ Child
- □ Parent

□ Laboratory forms (blood work: baseline, 10 weeks, 1 year)

□ Consent form

## A1.18 EVALUATION STATION CHECKLIST

1. Behavior Specialist — Patient check-in/check-out, psychosocial questionnaires

2. Physician or Nurse — Weight, height, blood pressure, resting heart rate

3. Exercise Physiologist — Bioelectric impedance analyzer

4. Dietitian — Skinfold measurement, circumferences, growth chart, goal weight review

5. Physician — Answer questions before patients and parents leave

## A1.19   EVALUATION FORM: <INSERT NAME OF INSTITUTION> PEDIATRIC WEIGHT MANAGEMENT PROGRAM

Location: _____

| Weight Management Quarterly Evaluation Form | | | |
|---|---|---|---|
| Name | Sex | DOB | Date of exam |
| Group | Race | Age | Visit |

| Measure | 1 | 2 | 3 | Average | Examiner |
|---|---|---|---|---|---|
| Weight (kg) | | | | | |
| Height (cm) | | | | | |
| Body mass index | | % | | Level of obesity | |
| Midarm circumference (cm) | | | | | |
| Waist circumference (cm) | | | | | |
| Hip circumference (cm) | | | | | |
| Midthigh circumference (mm) | | | | | |
| Triceps circumference (mm) | | | | | |
| Subscapular circumference (mm) | | | | | |
| Medial calf circumference (mm) | | | | | |
| Head circumference (cm) | | | | | |

| BIA resistance | | Resting heart rate (bpm) | | |
|---|---|---|---|---|
| Blood pressure (mmHg) | | | | |
| Number of classes attended | | Number of classes conducted | | Picture (circle one) | Yes | No |

## A1.20  EVALUATION RESULTS FORM

**<insert name of institution> Pediatric Weight Management Program**

**Evaluation Results**

Name:_____　　　　Age:_____

Today's Date:_____　　Level:_____

Group:_____

Your child's weight is _____ lbs.

Your child's height is _____ ft. _____ in.

Your child's Body Mass Index is _____. This value is based on the Pediatric Growth Charts.

Your child is in level _____ of the program.

Based on your child's present height, his/her goal weight is _____. This value will increase as your child grows.

Your child is made up of a range of _____ to _____% body fat. The healthy range for girls ages 7 to 17 is 20–25%, and for boys it is 12–18%. The upper range is based on a measure called BIA, which stands for Bioelectrical Impedence Analysis. The BIA is a machine that predicts fat percentages by using a very low electrical current. The lower range is based on a measure of skinfolds, or fat right under the skin. This means that your child has _____lbs of fat and ____ lbs of muscle, bone, and water combined.

Your child's cholesterol level is _____. The healthy level for children is <170.

Your child's triglyceride level is _____. The healthy triglyceride range for children 7 to 17 years is 10–140.

Your child's LDL (the "bad" cholesterol — Low Density Lipoprotein) is _____. The healthy range for children ages 7 to 17 is <110.

Your child's HDL (the "good" cholesterol — High Density Lipoprotein) is _____. The HDL healthy range for children ages 7 to 17 is >35.

Your child's circumference measurements are_____ in. (waist) and_____ in. (hips).

## A1.21   FITNESS EVALUATION

| Exercise/Fitness Evaluation | | | |
|---|---|---|---|
| Date: _____ | | | |
| Name: _____ | | | |
| DOB: | Age: | Sex: | Tanner Stage: |
| Group: | Site: | Tested by: | |

**Cardiorespiratory Condition**

| Resting Heart Rate<br><br>(RHR, bpm): | Resting Blood Pressure<br><br>(RBP, mm Hg): |
|---|---|
| Maximum Estimated Heart Rate<br><br>(HR, bpm: 220 – age): | |
| Target Heart Rate (THR):<br>220 – age(_____)  RHR(_____) × (_____) – % + RHR(_____) =<br>*Levels I, II, III = 55, 60, or 65%; Level IV = 65, 70, or 75% | |

| Aerobic Capacity | |
|---|---|
| Seat height: | Predicted max heart rate (bpm): |
| 80% predicted max HR (bpm): | Seconds, 30 beats: |
| **Workloads** | **Heart Rates** |
| 1st workload: | 2nd min: |
| kg | 3rd min: |
| watts | 4th min: |
| 2nd workload: | 2nd min: |
| kg | 3rd min: |
| watts | 4th min: |
| 3rd workload: | 2nd min: |
| kg | 3rd min: |
| watts | 4th min: |
| 4th workload: | 2nd min: |
| kg | 3rd min: |
| watts | 4th min: |
| Activity code:         Estimated $VO_2$:         Sub max $VO_2$: | |
| **Flexibility Muscular** | **Strength and Endurance** |
| Trunk flexion: | Overhead press: |
| in | lb |
| cm | reps |

| Refer to FLEX CHECK results | Bench press: |
|---|---|
| | lb |
| | reps |
| | Leg extension: |
| | lb |
| | reps |

| Body Composition | | |
|---|---|---|
| Weight (kg): | Height (cm): | Body mass index: |
| Percentage fat: | | Fat body weight: |
| Goal weight: | | Lean body weight: |

## A1.22  QUARTERLY EVALUATION RESULTS FORM: <INSERT NAME OF INSTITUTION> PEDIATRIC WEIGHT MANAGEMENT PROGRAM

| Quarterly Evaluation Results ||
| --- | --- |
| Name: | Age: |
| Today's Date: | Level: |
| Group: | Quarterly evaluation: |
| ***3 months ago...*** | ***now...*** |
| Your child's weight was _____lbs. | Your child's weight is now _____lbs.<br>Your child lost _____lbs. in the last ___ months! |
| Your child's height was ____ft. ____in. | Your child's height is now ____ft.____in. Your child grew ____in. in the last ___ months! |
| Your child's body mass index was _____. | Your child's body mass index is now _____. |
| Your child was in level ____, the ____color. | Your child graduated to level ____, the ____ color. |
| Based on your child's past height, his/her goal weight was _____lbs. | Your child's new goal weight is _____lbs. This will increase as your child grows. |
| Your child's percentage body fat range was ___–___%. The upper range is based on a measure called BIA, which stands for Bioelectrical Impedence Analysis. The lower range is based on a measure of skinfolds, or fat right under the skin. | Your child's % body fat range is ____–____%. Your child reduced percentage body fat by ____%. |
| Based on the BIA measure, your child had _____lbs of fat, and _____lbs of muscle, bone, and water. | Your child has _____lbs of fat, and _____lbs of muscle, bone, and water. He/she lost ____lbs of fat. |
| Your child's cholesterol level was ____. | Your child's cholesterol level is _____. The normal level for children is <170. |
| Your child's cholesterol level was ____. | Your child's triglyceride level is _____. The normal range for children 7 to 17 is 10–40. |
| Your child's LDL level was _____. This is the "bad" cholesterol! (Low-Density Lipoprotein) | Your child's LDL level is _____. The normal range for children 7 to 17 is <110. |
| Your child's HDL level was _____. This is the "good" cholesterol! (High-Density Lipoprotein) | Your child's HDL level is _____. The normal range for children 7 to 17 years of age is >35. |
| Your child's waist and hip measures were _____in. (waist) _____in. (hip) | Your child's waist and hip measure are _____in. (waist) _____in. (hip)<br>He/she lost ___in. in the waist and ___in. in the hip. |

## A1.23 SAMPLE SPREADSHEET

| Name | Age | Sex | Date of Birth | Weight | Height | Body Mass Index | Body Mass Index Percentile | Level of Obesity |
|------|-----|-----|---------------|--------|--------|-----------------|----------------------------|------------------|
|      |     |     |               |        |        |                 |                            |                  |
|      |     |     |               |        |        |                 |                            |                  |
|      |     |     |               |        |        |                 |                            |                  |
|      |     |     |               |        |        |                 |                            |                  |
|      |     |     |               |        |        |                 |                            |                  |
|      |     |     |               |        |        |                 |                            |                  |
|      |     |     |               |        |        |                 |                            |                  |
|      |     |     |               |        |        |                 |                            |                  |
|      |     |     |               |        |        |                 |                            |                  |
|      |     |     |               |        |        |                 |                            |                  |

| Midarm Circumference (cm) | Waist Circumference (cm) | Hip Circumference (cm) | Midthigh (mm) | Medial Calf (mm) | Head (cm) |
|---------------------------|--------------------------|------------------------|---------------|------------------|-----------|
|                           |                          |                        |               |                  |           |
|                           |                          |                        |               |                  |           |
|                           |                          |                        |               |                  |           |
|                           |                          |                        |               |                  |           |
|                           |                          |                        |               |                  |           |
|                           |                          |                        |               |                  |           |
|                           |                          |                        |               |                  |           |
|                           |                          |                        |               |                  |           |
|                           |                          |                        |               |                  |           |

| Triceps (mm) | Subscapular (mm) | Skinfold Percentage Fat <insert formula> | BIA Percentage Fat | Blood Pressure (mmHg) | Resting Heart Rate (bpm) |
|--------------|------------------|------------------------------------------|--------------------|-----------------------|--------------------------|
|              |                  |                                          |                    |                       |                          |
|              |                  |                                          |                    |                       |                          |
|              |                  |                                          |                    |                       |                          |
|              |                  |                                          |                    |                       |                          |
|              |                  |                                          |                    |                       |                          |
|              |                  |                                          |                    |                       |                          |
|              |                  |                                          |                    |                       |                          |

# APPENDIX 2
## Testing/Measurement Protocols

## A2.1 MEASUREMENTS

### A2.1.1 HEIGHT MEASUREMENT

A calibrated Dyfed stadiometer (e.g., Holtain Ltd., U.K.) should be used to obtain the height in centimeters of each patient. The patient will remove his or her shoes and step onto the floor platform facing in an outward direction with the heels together. The scapula and buttocks will remain in contact with the back of the stadiometer during the measure. The head will be positioned in a horizontal plane. The clinician will move the headboard onto the most superior aspect of the study participant's head. This procedure will be repeated two additional times. The average height to the nearest tenth of a centimeter (0.1 cm) should be calculated on a data statistical form.

### A2.1.2 MEASUREMENT OF WEIGHT

An electronically calibrated scale (e.g., Indiana Scales, Terre Haute, IN) should be used to obtain the weight in kilograms of each patient. The patient will remove his or her shoes and step on the scale. The patient will remain as still as possible. The patient's weight in kilograms will be recorded once the digital reading is constant. The patient will remain on the scale until the weight is recorded. The process will be repeated two additional times. The average weight in kilograms of each measure will be calculated and recorded on the data statistical form.

## ARKANSAS CLINICIAN'S GUIDE TO WEIGHT PROBLEMS IN CHILDREN AND ADOLESCENTS

### Step 1:  Calculate BMI

**BMI is the relationship of weight to height.**

$$BMI = \frac{weight\ (kg)}{height\ (m)\ x\ height\ (m)} \quad OR \quad \frac{weight\ (lb)\ x\ 703}{height\ (in)\ x\ height\ (in)}$$

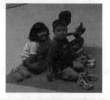

**For example, Gary's BMI = his weight (37 pounds) x 703 divided by his height (41 in) squared or 37 x 703/1681.  Gary's BMI is 15.5**

### Step 2:  Calculate BMI Percentile

To be sensitive to the issue of a child's self-esteem, the term obesity is no longer used.  Remember that the BMI is only a screen for overweight.  Clinical correlation is necessary because adiposity is the actual health risk.  For example, kids who are very muscular may have an elevated BMI but may still have low body fat.  If necessary, contact a dietitian or exercise physiologist who is experienced in measuring body fat.

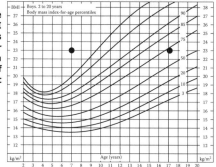

| |
| Underweight = < 5th Percentile |
| Risk of Overweight = 85th to 94th percentile |
| Overweight = ≥ 95th percentile |

Because the BMI of children varies with age and gender, it is necessary to use standardized curves to determine if a child is overweight or not.  As you can see on the chart above, a boy of 7 who has a BMI of 23 is overweight whereas another boy at age 17 with the same BMI is not.

### Step 3:  Choose a course of action

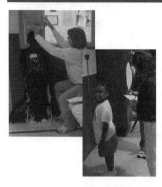

**Underweight**: Screen for chronic diseases, malnutrition, eating disorders and genetic causes (e.g., thin parents).

**Normal Weight:** Assess lifestyle and promote healthy habits including 1) a diet low in sugar, saturated and trans fats and high in fruits, vegetables and calcium; 2) at least 30 minutes of physical activity each day; and 3) limiting TV, video game and computer time to 2 hours a day.

**Risk of Overweight:** Patients with a personal or family history of co-morbidities need full evaluation for overweight. If no history of co-morbidities, encourage healthy lifestyle as above and follow up in 1 year to recheck BMI.

**Overweight:** Needs full evaluation and treatment for overweight.

*Developed by Arkansas Chapters of the American Academy of Pediatrics and the American Academy of Family Practice, UAMS Preventive Nutrition Project, Arkansas Foundation for Medical Care. UAMS College of Public Health. UAMS Department of Pediatrics. Arkansas Department of Health. April 2004*

# ARKANSAS CLINICIAN'S GUIDE TO WEIGHT PROBLEMS
# IN CHILDREN AND ADOLESCENTS

## Full Evaluation for Overweight

### Assess overweight

Age first noted
Perceived causes by child and parent
Prior weight loss attempts
Time in sedentary activities (TV, video games, computer)
Time in physical activity (sports, walking, outdoor play)
Body image, family stress and any depressive symptoms

### Assess Co-Morbidities

Family History: Obesity, Diabetes, Hyperlipidemia, HTN, MI, Stroke
PMH: chronic diseases
ROS: sleep apnea, worsening asthma, exercise intolerance, reflux, limb pain, emotional difficulties, menstrual irregularities

### Assess diet

Milk/dairy (should be 3-5 servings a day of skim or 1%)
Fruits and vegetables (should be 5-9 servings a day)
Intake of soft drinks and fruit and sugar drinks
Fast food consumption
Food behavior (large portions, skipping meals, eating while watching TV, high calorie snacking, binge eating)

### Patient Examination

Body habitus, BP (age appropriate), chest, extremities, acanthosis nigricans, thyromegaly, striae

### Labs:

Cholesterol panel
Consider fasting glucose if FHx of type 2 diabetes or signs of insulin resistance
Other lab based on individual findings

## Treat Overweight: Based on Readiness to Change

| STAGE OF CHANGE | READINESS TO CHANGE | ACTION |
|---|---|---|
| Pre-Contemplation | Not currently interested in changing | Give personalized reasons why change would be valuable; reassess at each visit. |
| Contemplation | Interested in changing within next 6 months but not now | For both contemplation and preparation, ask for start dates for change. Set goals with family and pick goals that can be successfully achieved. |
| Preparation | Willing to initiate change in next 30 days | |
| Action | Already making changes | Give encouragement for small changes. Suggest alternative strategies if weight gain continues. |
| Maintenance | Successful at change and trying to maintain | Continue periodic follow-up visits every 2-3 months as in any chronic disease. |

## Clinical Pearls

- **First goal is no further weight gain. Children may "grow into" their weight as their height increases.**
- **Increase fruits and vegetables, use skim or 1% milk. Decrease sugared drinks, candy, junk and fast foods.**
- **Turn off the TV while eating. Remove unhealthy snacks from view. Put out fruits and vegetables. Regular meal times including breakfast. Child's fist-size portions only. Limit snacking to healthy foods.**
- **Encourage anything that increases breathing and heart rates (brisk walking, bicycling, dancing, other sports). Work up to one hour a day. Set limits on TV, video, and computer time (2 hrs/day total).**
- **Self-monitoring is one of the most helpful tools. Have them record physical activity and diet, weigh every 2-4 weeks. Review records when patient comes back and give praise and/or problem solve.**
- **Parents should act as role models, play with children, and eat meals together at the table at home.**

**If child continues to have inappropriate weight gain, reassess for compliance or the presence of emotional problems. Consider referral for problems beyond your scope of management such as co-morbidities, possible abuse or severe psychopathology.**

## Community Involvement

**To prevent obesity, local school policies on nutrition and physical activity should be improved. Clinicians can and should help guide their local school district's health policy committee.**

## Resources

For resources, referral and other information, or a free CME program, go to the Arkansas Center for Health Improvement website at http://www.achi.net/

## A2.1.3  CIRCUMFERENCE MEASUREMENTS:

An additional method of assessing body composition is the measurement of girth of various body sections [4]. From the sum of the measurements, percentage body fat is determined from equations, tables, or nomograms.

Equipment needed: Metal or fiberglass measuring tape with metric scale.

Several various sections of the body are measured based on gender. The standard areas measured in males are the shoulders, chest, waist, biceps, thigh, and calf. In females, the standard areas are shoulders, bust, waist, abdomen, hips, thigh, calf, and biceps. Regardless of sites to be measured, the general rules are as follows:

1. Both the clinician and subject are in a standing position.
2. Unless noted otherwise, clinician is positioned in front of subject.
3. When applying tape to site, no air space should be between the subjects' skin and the tape. Conversely, the tape should not be pulled tightly.
4. The tape should always be positioned in a horizontal plane to the subject.
5. The tape should be read to the closest 0.25 inch.
6. Clinician should have strong knowledge of anatomy to locate areas to be measured.

The sites mentioned above are located and measured as follows.

For male subjects:
  Shoulders: Subject stands erect with weight evenly distributed between both feet. Shoulders should be back and arms should hang freely at sides. The clinician positions tape over the largest area of the deltoids below the acromion.
  Chest: Subject will stand erect with feet shoulder-width apart. The subject abducts arms slightly so that the tape can be positioned around chest. The clinician locates the fourth costosternal joint, and the measurement is taken at this level.
  Waist: Subject will be undressed or wearing light clothing for this measurement. The subject will stand erect with abdomen relaxed, arms at sides, and feet together. The measurement will be taken at the narrowest part of the torso, above the level of the navel.
  Biceps: Subject stands erect with arms relaxed at sides. Clinician locates the most muscular aspect of the biceps, tape is positioned, and measurement is taken.
  Thigh (midthigh): For most accurate results, clinician will measure the midpoint between the inguinal crease and the proximal border of the patella. This measurement is made when the subject's knee is flexed to 90 degrees. This site is marked and the tape is placed here once the subject returns to an erect, standing position.
  Calf: Subject stands with weight evenly distributed on both feet. Clinician locates maximum circumference of the gastrocnemius (calf) muscle, positions tape, and takes measurement.

For female subjects:
  Shoulders: see male
  Bust: Subject stands erect with arms relaxed at sides. Measurement is made across the chest, at the nipple line.
  Waist: see male
  Abdomen: Subject stands with arms by the sides and feet together. The clinician places tape at the level of the greatest anterior extension of the abdomen. The level will usually be at the navel.

Hips: Subject stands erect with arms at sides and feet together. The tape is positioned at the maximum circumference of the buttocks.

Thigh: see male

Calf: see male

Biceps: see male

## A2.1.4   MEASUREMENT OF RESTING BLOOD PRESSURE

A Dynamap system will be used. Two readings will be taken and averaged. If the two values differ by more than 5 mm Hg, an additional reading will be obtained. A small cuff will be used for the children. The study participant will abstain from eating and heavy exercise for at least 2 hours before the test. Study participants will also be instructed not to ingest caffeine within 30 minutes of blood pressure measurements. The study participant will be comfortably seated, with the arm slightly flexed, palm up, and the entire forearm supported at heart level on a smooth surface.

## A2.1.5   MEASUREMENT OF RESTING HEART RATE

A stethoscope and watch with second hand or digital readout in seconds will be used. The study participant will sit quietly for at least 5 minutes before the test. The heart rate will be taken by auscultation. The stethoscope will be placed to the left of the sternum just above the level of the nipple. The heart beats will be counted for 30 seconds and then multiplied by 2. This will give total beats per minute. An average of three separate readings will be noted.

## A2.2 LABORATORY BLOOD WORK

Biochemical markers, total cholesterol, triglycerides, high-density lipoproteins, and low-density lipoproteins will be examined in a certified laboratory. Study participants will be required to fast for 12 hours before the test.

Blood collection and processing: Venous blood will be collected in the morning after a 12-hour fast with the study participant seated. Blood will be collected in tubes containing 1.5 mg/mL ethylenediaminetetraacetic acid (EDTA) for procedures requiring plasma, in tubes with no additives for serum measures, and in citrate tubes for homeostasis endpoints.

Chemistry and lipid measures: All routine chemistry and lipid analyses will be performed on a Beckman Synchron CX5 automated chemistry analyzer, and the low-density lipoprotein cholesterol is calculated using the Friedewald equation. The coefficient of variation for these assays is less than 2%, and the <insert> laboratory participates in the Centers for Disease Control and Prevention ongoing lipid standardization program. Blind duplicate blood samples will be collected and analyzed in 10% of the study participants tested to verify laboratory values.

## A2.3  BODY COMPOSITION ANALYSIS

Skinfold analysis:

Skinfold analysis measures the thickness of a double fold of skin and subcutaneous adipose tissue at various body locations [5]. The use of skinfold calipers is the most commonly used method for determining obesity. The advantages of this method is its relative simplicity, quickness, and nonevasive nature. In addition, very little space is needed. Various equations have been developed in the prediction of body composition (see chapter 4 for reference) [4,6–13]. A two-site formula developed by Slaughter et al. [14] includes specific equations for overweight youth.

Equipment needed:

Skinfold caliper

Tape measure

Black felt pen

General rules for taking skinfolds are as follows:

1. All measurements should be taken on the right side of the body for uniformity with most U.S. research efforts.
2. Sites to be measured should be marked for best accuracy until clinician is sufficiently skilled.
3. Clinician should feel the sites to familiarize him/herself with the subject and area.
4. Subject should not have exercised immediately before measurement because shifts in body fluid to skin will inflate normal skinfold values.
5. Clinician should take a minimum of three measurements at each site, spacing each measure at least 15 seconds apart.
6. Calipers should be accurately calibrated before measurement.
7. Caliper dial should be read approximately 4 seconds after pressure from hand on caliper jaw has been released.
8. Thumb and index finger pressure should be maintained throughout each measurement.

Several sites have been designated and standardized for use by clinicians. For purposes of this investigation, two sites — triceps and subscapular — will be used. These sites are illustrated as follows:

- Instructions for skinfold measurements at these sites are as follows:
    - Measurement of skinfolds: A skinfold caliper (Harpenden), tape measure and black felt pen will be used to measure triceps and subscapular skinfolds thickness. All measurements will be taken on the right side of the body. All sites will be marked with a black felt pen for accuracy after the anatomic location of the measurement has been verified by a trained technician. The subject will refrain from exercise at least 2 hours before the test. A minimum of three measurements will be taken at each site at least 15 seconds apart. The calipers will be calibrated after before each measurement. The caliper dial will be read approximately 4 seconds after pressure from the hand on the caliper is released.
    - Triceps skinfold: A vertical skinfold on the posterior midline of the upper arm will be examined. With the subject's right elbow flexed at 90 degrees, the clinician will measure the distance between the lateral projection of the acromion process of the scapula and the inferior border the olecranon process of the elbow. The site will then be marked with the black felt pen at the midpoint on the lateral side of the arm. With the subject's arm relaxed at his or her side, the clinician will stand behind he subject and grasp skinfold side with the thumb and index finger approximately one-half inch above the mark. The calipers will then be applied at the mark.

- Subscapular skinfold: A diagonal skinfold will be obtained just below the lowest angle of the scapula. The clinician will feel for the bottom of the scapula to locate the site. The site will be marked and the skinfold will be grasped with thumb and index finger about one-half inch above the mark. The skinfold will then be taken on a 45-degree diagonal line toward the right side of the subject's body.
- Body fat
  - Body impedance has been validated as a measure of body fat and lean body mass. For example: The Tanita Body Composition Analyzer (model TBF-310) measures body weight and body impedance simultaneously by standing barefoot on the scale. Sanitation will be maintained by cleaning the Tanita pads on which the children will stand with alcohol before each measurement. Body fat and lean body mass are automatically recorded using a laptop computer. These variables will be expressed as a percent of total body weight for statistical analyses. The Tanita Body Composition Analyzer has been found to be accurate within 5% of body fat estimation by DEXA and is very reliable, with less than 1% variation within itself.
- Measurement of differential photon absorption using dual-energy x-ray absorptiometry
  - Dual-energy x-ray absorptiometry (DEXA) will be used to determine percentage of fat, lean body mass, and bone mineral density in the program participants. DEXA uses an x-ray source to generate photons to scan study participants. Bone-mineral content measurements previously calibrated against secondary standards with ashed bone sections are used to help calculate fat-free mass (FFM). Percentage of fat and fat-free body can be predicted with accuracy by observing the ratio of absorbency of the different-energy-level photons, which are linearly related to the percentage of fat in the soft tissues of the body. The coefficient of variation of fat-free tissue measurement has been calculated at 2%, which is comparable to that obtained by hydrodensitometry [15–17].
  - The participants will receive total DEXA body scans (e.g., Hologics QRX 2000). This machine has been cleared by the U.S. Food and Drug Administration as a market device used for scanning the anterior/posterior and lateral spine, femur, total body, and forearm to determine bone mineral density. The speed of the scan will be determined by the size of the study participant. Larger study participants will be programmed in the slow speed mode; smaller study participants in the fast speed mode. The study participants will be instructed to remove all metal and jewelry as well as their shoes before they are correctly positioned on the scan table, lying down on their back with their arms to their side. The DEXA will measure x-rays as they are transmitted through the study participant's body. The study participant will be exposed to ionizing radiation, but there is no discomfort during the measurement. When using the DEXA, the dose of radiation is 0.02 to 0.03 mR for each total body scan (Hologics). This exposure is less than the 125 mR/yr, which is the amount individuals receive from nonmedical background radiation (lunar). The low dose of radiation will not adversely affect the bone or surrounding tissue. There are no side effects to using the DEXA, except in pregnant or nursing mothers. As the effects of ionizing radiation to unborn or nursing infants are unknown, females of child-bearing age should participate in a urine pregnancy test prior to testing. Women who are nursing infants should not participate in DEXA testing. The entire process causes very little discomfort and is a totally noninvasive step-by-step process.

## A2.4 MEASURES OF PHYSICAL ACTIVITY LEVEL AND FITNESS

### A2.4.1 SAMPLES OF SELF-REPORT QUESTIONNAIRES

#### Physical Activity

Godin–Shephard Leisure Time Physical Activity Questionnaire [18]. The Godin–Shephard is a four-item self-reported recall of usual physical activities during a typical week. Children are asked to write how many times per week they engage in vigorous-, moderate-, and light-intensity activity for 15 minutes or more. Examples of the types of activity are provided. A total score is derived by multiplying the frequency of each category by a standard metabolic equivalent (Vigorous × 9, Moderate × 5, Light × 3). Children are also asked to report how many times they engage in activity long enough to make them sweat. Adequate reliability and validity have been reported [19] with children as young as in the fourth grade.

#### Sedentary Behavior

Children will be asked to report the number of hours they spend in sedentary pursuits both before and after school. The sedentary activities assessed will include television, video, computer, reading, homework, and telephone. The list of sedentary activities will be taken from the Self-Administered Physical Activity Checklist [20]. Sedentary behavior from this measure is correlated with body mass index percentile in previous research [21].

#### Dieting Social Support

The Children's Dietary Social Support Scale (DSS) [22] is a seven-item measure of perceived social support for healthy dietary choices. The scale assesses support from family, friends, and teachers in a yes–no format. The measure has been shown to relate to behavioral intentions and behavior change [23,24]. The reliability and validity of the measure has been established, and normative data are available [22–24].

#### Physical Activity Social Support

The Physical Activity Social Support Scale (PASS) [23,24] is an 18-item measure that assesses perceived support for physical activity. Support from family, teachers, and friends is assessed in a yes–no format, and positive and negative social support subscales are derived.

### A2.4.2 DETAILED EXERCISE TESTING PROTOCOLS

#### The Physical Work Capacity Test

The physical work capacity test (PWC) is a multi-stage cycle ergometry test. Subjects pedal for three 2-minute stages at progressively increasing workloads. The PWC protocol uses a 5-minute warm-up at 25 watts before maximal testing. The pedal rate should be held constant at 60 rpm throughout testing. The test should begin unloaded at 60 rpm for 2 minutes. After the 2 minutes, workload should increase by 29 watts (0.5 kg) every 2 minutes until 118 watts. From that point, power output should increase by 15 watts (0.25 kg) until volitional termination or a drop in pedal rate of 5 rpm. Heart rates up to 160 bpm are used to extrapolate to the power output at a heart rate of 170 bpm [25].

#### LOFTIN–SOTHERN TEST

The Loftin–Sothern [26] treadmill protocol is a modified Balke [27] protocol that includes a baseline standing measure and three submaximal, steady-state stages. The test was designed to observe baseline, submaximal, and maximal differences in specific metabolic and physiologic parameters between nonobese and obese children during weight-bearing exercise (walking).

Pretest:        Resting in a seated position for 30 minutes.

                Fasting for 4 hours before the time of the test.

                No vigorous activity for 48 hours before the test.

Baseline:       Expired gases are collected with a metabolic measurement cart for 10 minutes while subject is standing, unsupported.

Submaximal:     Expired gases are collected with a metabolic measurement cart during treadmill walking as follows:

                2.5 mph for 5 minutes at 0% grade.

                3.0 mph for 5 minutes at 0% grade.

                3.5 mph for 5 minutes at 0% grade.

Maximal:        3.5 mph until test completion. Grade is increased 2% every 2 minutes until test completion.

## A2.5  PSYCHOLOGICAL TESTING

| Test | Year | Location |
|------|------|----------|
| Child Behavior Checklist: Achenback™ [28,29] | 1991 | University of Vermont<br>1 S. Prospect Street<br>Burlington, VT 05401 |
| Children's Depression Inventory: Kovacs M [30] | 1981 | The Psychological Corporation<br>555 Academic Court<br>San Antonio, TX 78204-2498 |
| FACES III: Olson DH, Portner J, Lavee Y [31] | 1985 | Family Social Science<br>290 McNeal Hall<br>University of Minnesota<br>St. Paul, MN 55108 |
| The Piers-Harris Children's Self-Concept Scale: Piers EV, Harris DB [32–34] | 1969 | Western Psychological Services<br>12031 Wilshire Boulevard<br>Los Angeles, CA 90025-1251 |

## A2.6   TANNER STAGING

Sexual maturity rating will be determined by a physician (trained in pediatric medicine) using methods from Faulkner and Tanner [35] on all study participants.

# APPENDIX 3
## Sample Intervention Materials

## A3.1   RESOURCES

### A3.1.1   Resources for Pediatric Weight Management Educational Materials, Sample Handouts, and Self-Monitoring Forms

---

**Resource**

**Committed to Kids/Trim Kids affiliates:**

Birmingham, Alabama:
  Children's Hospital of Alabama
  1600 Seventh Street South
  Birmingham, Alabama 35233

Denver, Colorado:
  University of Colorado Health Sciences Center
  Department of Pediatrics
  4200 East 9th Avenue
  Box C 225
  Denver, Colorado 80262
  Phone: (303) 315-7037

  The Good LIFE Clinic
  The Children's Hospital – B218
  Department of Pediatrics
  1056 East 19th Avenue
  Denver, Colorado 80218
  Phone: (303) 864-5370

Fort Lauderdale, Florida:
  US BARIATRIC-KIDS
  4800 Northeast 20th Terrace
  Ft. Lauderdale, Florida. 33308
  Phone: (954) 351-7770 x 129
  E-mail: kids@usbariatric.com

Jupiter, Florida:
  Committed To Kids
  Jupiter Institute of the Healing Arts
  175 Toney Penna Drive #101
  Jupiter, Florida 33458
  Phone: (561) 746-1205

Chicago, Illinois:
  Finch University of Health Sciences
  The Chicago Medical School
  3333 Green Bay Road
  North Chicago, Illinois 60064
  Phone: (847) 578-8497

Pikeville, Kentucky:
  Pediatric Clinic
  261-277 Town Mountain Rd
  Pikeville, Kentucky 41501
  Phone: (606) 437-3500 x3805

Baton Rouge, Louisiana:
  Committed to Kids
  Pennington Biomedical Research Center
  6400 Perkins Road
  Baton Rouge, Louisiana 70808
  Phone: (225) 763-2677

New Orleans, Louisiana:
  Louisiana State University Health
  Sciences Center
  Department of Pediatrics
  1542 Tulane Ave.
  New Orleans, Louisiana 70112
  Phone: (504) 556-9822

Holland, Michigan:
  926 South Washington
  Holland, Michigan 49423
  Phone: (616) 494-4065

Gulfport, Mississippi:
  3300 15th Street
  Gulfport, Mississippi 39501
  Phone: (504) 646-1017

St. Louis, Missouri:
  Committed to Kids, St. Louis
  220 VonBeheren
  Chesterfield, Missouri 63005
  Phone: (636) 530-9880

Buffalo, New York:
  Kazabee, Inc.
  PO Box 391
  Buffalo, New York 14226
  Phone: (716) 906-1443
  Web site: http://www.kazabee.com

Columbus, Ohio:
  Matrix — Committed to Kids
  2 Easton Oval, Suite 450
  Columbus, Ohio 43219
  Phone: (614) 475-9500

Salem, Oregon:
  Committed To Kids
  Salem Hospital's Rehabilitation Center
  2561 Center Street N.E.
  Salem, Oregon 97309-5014
  Phone: (503) 561-6990

Corpus Christi, Texas:
  Driscoll Children's Hospital
  3533 South Alemeda Street
  Corpus Christi, Texas 78411
  Phone: (361) 694-4864
  Fax: (361) 694-4832

Fort Worth, Texas:
  709 West Leuda Street
  Fort Worth, Texas 76104
  Phone: (817) 336-7275

McAllen, Texas:
  Committed To Kids, McAllen
  220 South Bicentennial Blvd, Suite A
  McAllen, Texas 78501
  Phone: (956) 668-1060
  E-mail: ChildWellnessRGV@aol.com

Bellevue, Washington:
  Pro Sports Club, 20/20 Lifestyles
  4455 148th Avenue N.E.
  Bellevue, Washington 98007
  Phone: (425) 861-6218
  Fax: (425) 861-6277
  Web site: www.proclub.com/kids/committedToKids.asp

**Other pediatric weight management treatment centers:**

Fit Matters, Larabida Children's Hospital
  http://www.larabida.org

Shapedown
  http://www.shapedown.com

The Hip Hop Clinic at St. Francis Hospital
  http://www.stfrancishospitals.org

| Resource | Contact Information |
| --- | --- |
| Committed to Kids/Trim Kids | www.trimkids.com |
| Trim Kids at eDiets.com | www.eDiets.com/familyandfriends |
| Trim Kids DVD at eDiets.com | www.eDiets.com (store) |
| Healthy Families | http://healthyfamily02@yahoo.com |
| Healthy You | http://www.chkd.org/health_library/ |
| OWL: Optimal Weight for Life Program | http://www.childrenshospital.org/OWL |
| Stanford Pediatric Weight Program | http://pediatricweightcontrol.stanford.edu |
| Winning Ways for Kids | http://www.gundluth.org/nutrition |
| Client-centered approach to nutrition education for the prevention of overweight with children | http://www.dhss.state.mo.us/missourinutrition/resource |
| Families in Balance | http://www.boswellcenter.com |
| Get Kids in Action | http://www.getkidsinaction.org |
| Kids Weight Down | http://www.maimonidesmed.org/clinicalservices/ |
| Positive Choice | http://www.positivechoice.org |
| The Body Shop | http://www.humc.net |
| ICAN — Intensive Counseling Activity and Nutrition | http://www.cardinalhill.org |
| REACH 2010 Project (Oklahoma Native American) | http://www.health.state.ok.us |
| St. Joseph's Mercy Center for Health Management in Macomb | http://www.macombweb.trinity-health.org |
| Teen Choices and Challenges | http://www.teenchoicesandchallenges.com |

## A3.1.2 PROGRAMS AVAILABLE FOR INCREASING PHYSICAL ACTIVITY AND PROMOTING HEALTHY NUTRITION

Active Living Partners: Physical Activity and Health Information News (2003)
Human Kinetics Publishers, Inc.
P.O. Box 5076
Champaign, Illinois 61825-5076
1-800-747-4457
Fax: 217-351-1549
Web site: www.humankinetics.com

American Alliance for Health, Physical Education, Recreation, and Dance
1900 Association Drive
Reston, Virginia 20191-1599
1-800-213-7193 or 703-476-3400
fax 703-476-8316
Web site: http://www.aahperd.org

American College of Sports Medicine
P.O. Box 1440
Indianapolis, Indiana 46206-1440

American Heart Association
7320 Greenville Avenue
Dallas, Texas 75231
1-800-640-4640
Fax: 1-800-242-8721
Web site: http://www.amhrt.org

The American Volkssport Association
1001 Pat Booker Road, Suite 101
Universal City, Texas 78148
210-659-2112 or 1-800-830-WALK

Centers for Disease Control and Prevention, National Center for Chronic Disease, Prevention and
   Health Promotion, Division of Nutrition and Physical Activity
4770 Buford Highway
Atlanta, Georgia 30341
1-888-CDC-4NRG
1-888-232-4674
Web site: http://www.cdc.gov

Child and Adolescent Trial for Cardiovascular Health (CATCH)
The set has a School Nutrition Program Guide, a Guidebook and PE Activity Box, and four different
   curriculums and three video tapes for third, fourth, and 5th graders.
National Heart, Lung and Blood Institute Information Center
P.O. Box 30105
Bethesda, Maryland 20824-0105
301-251-1222

Guidelines for School and Community Programs to Promote Lifelong Physical Activity Among
   Young People
U.S. Dept. of Health and Human Services
Centers for Disease Control and Prevention
*MMWR* 1997: Vol. 46 No. RR-6; Atlanta, Georgia

HeartPower
Resource kit for teachers pre-kindergarten through 8th grade.
American Heart Association, Alaska Region
1057 W. Fireweed, Suite 206
Anchorage, Alaska 99505
1-888-276-0858

How to Promote Physical Activity in Your Community: A Project to Promote Partnering on Physical
  Activity
December 1997, Booklet, ASTDHPPHE
1015 Fifteenth St. NW Suite 410
Washington, D.C. 20005

JumpSTART Program
JumpSTART is a school-based program that offers elementary teachers activities to incorporate
  into existing curricula for grades 3–5. It has a Letter of Introduction and a Teacher's Guide. It
  also includes materials to encourage parent involvement.
National Heart, Lung and Blood Institute Information Center
P.O. Box 30105
Bethesda, Maryland 20824-0105
301-251-1222
Web site: http://www.epi.hss.state.ak.us

Myths and Conceptions, PEI Active Living Alliance
Prince Edward Island, Canada.
Web site: http://www. edu.pe.ca/activeliving/myths2.htm

National Association for Sport and Physical Education
1900 Association Drive
Reston, Virginia 20191-1599
1-800-213-7193 or 703-476-3410
Fax: 703-476-8316

National Association of Governor's Councils on Physical Fitness and Sports
201 South Capitol Avenue, Suite 560
Indianapolis, Indiana 46225
317-237-5630
Fax: 317-237-5632
Web site: http://www.fitnesslink.com

National Coalition for Promoting Physical Activity (NCPPA)
1900 Association Drive
Reston, Virginia 20191-1599
Web site: http://www.ncppa.org/ncppa

National Heart, Lung and Blood Institute
Information Center
P.O. Box 30105
Bethesda, Maryland 20824-0105
Web site: http://www.nhlbi.nih.gov/nhlbi

National Recreation and Park Association
P.O. Box 6287
Arlington, Virginia 22206
1-800-626-6772
Web site: http://www.nrpa.org

Partnership for a Walkable America
National Safety Council
1121 Spring Lake Drive
Itasca, Illinois 60143-3201
630-285-1121
Web site: http://www.nsc.org/walkable.htm

Physical Activity and Health, A Report of the Surgeon General, Executive Summary. U.S. Dept.
of Health and Human Services, Centers for Disease Control and Prevention, The President's
Council on Physical Fitness and Sports, 1996
Superintendent of Documents
P.O. Box 371954
Pittsburgh, Pennsylvania 15250-7954

President's Council on Physical Fitness and Sports
Box SG
701 Pennsylvania Ave., NW, Suite 250
Washington, D.C. 20004
202-690-9000

President's Council on Physical Fitness and Sports
President's Council on Physical Fitness and Sports Report: Physical Activity and Sports in the
Lives of Girls — Physical and Mental Health Dimensions from an Interdisciplinary Approach.
Washington, D.C.: President's Council on Physical Fitness and Sports, 1997.
Preventing Childhood Obesity: Health in the Balance
National Academies Press
202-334-3313 or 1-800-624-6242
Web site: http://www.nap.edu

Ready. Set. It's Everywhere You Go: CDC's Guide to Promoting Moderate Physical Activity Media Kit
Centers for Disease Control and Prevention
U.S. Dept. of Health and Human Services
4770 Buford Highway
Atlanta, Georgia 30341

SPARK (Sports, Play, and Active Recreation for Kids)
A Physical Education Curriculum for students in grades K-6.
1-800-SPARK-PE

U.S. Department of Health and Human Services [USDHHS]. (1996). Physical activity and health:
A report of the Surgeon General. Atlanta, Georgia: Centers for Disease Control and Prevention.

U.S. Department of Health and Human Services [USDHHS]. (2000). CDC's Guidelines for School
and Community Programs: Promoting Lifelong Physical Activity, An Overview. Centers for
Disease Control and Prevention.

Wellness Council of America
7101 Newport Avenue, Suite 311
Omaha, Nebraska 68152
402-572-3590

## A3.1.3   TAKE CHARGE ON-SITE TRAINING PROGRAM FOR PRIMARY HEALTH CARE PROVIDERS

**Take Charge**

A model program designed to increase physical activity among employees.
National Coalition for Promoting Physical Activity (NCPPA)
1900 Association Drive
Reston, Virginia 20191-1599
Web site: http://www.ncppa.org/ncppa

## A3.2 TRAFFIC LIGHT DIET

http://www.trafficlightdiet.com/

**A3.3    SAMPLE EXERCISE LESSONS (From Sothern, M., von Almen, T. K., and Schumacher, H., *Trimkids,* New York: Harper Collins, 2001.)**

1. Lesson 1: Benefits of exercise, exercise safety, warming-up, exercise prescriptions, increasing your daily activity — The MPEP step
   a. Exercise Benefits and Safety
      Refer to the program book [2] for information on the benefits of exercise. Discuss the following safety tips with the students.
      Stop exercising if you feel any discomfort in a muscle or joint. It's normal to feel a gentle burning sensation, but if the pain is worse than that, stop immediately! You'll need to report it to your teacher, coach, exercise physiologist, or doctor the next time you see him or her.
      Do the exercise exactly as instructed. The exercises in the program book have been designed especially for you, and you shouldn't change them.
      Always warm up before and cool down after each exercise session.

   b. Techniques for Warming Up
      Verbal cues: Before you do any type of exercise, you'll need to warm up for at least 5 minutes before each session. Warming up is simple: move each part of your body in a slow, controlled manner. When you slowly move an arm, a leg, or a shoulder, your heart sends blood to that body part, delivering fuel to the muscles and tissues that are in motion. Moving your arms and legs helps the heart pump blood throughout your entire body, preparing your body for more movement. Try the suggestions below, or make up your own!
      Some warm-up suggestions:
      March in place for 3–5 minutes
      Do arm circles forward, then back, 20 times
      Do 10 modified jumping jacks or "side jacks": instead of jumping, alternate placing each heel out to the side on the floor while the arms go above the head
      Tap each foot 20 times, then rise on your toes 10 times.

   c. Exercise Prescriptions: Designing a Formal Exercise Routine
      We have discovered that just telling families to be more physically active is just not enough. Most overweight kids need weekly structured exercise goals. As they do in casual fun and play, allow your patients to choose the exercise activities they most enjoy to make up their formal exercise routine.
      Every child who participates in the program will engage in a tailor-made exercise program. In the beginning, we make absolutely sure that the goals each child establishes are easy to accomplish. It's that initial success that motivates the child to keep going, and each child has his or her own level of ability, which parents and children must respect.
      Severely overweight children will have a more difficult time exercising than will moderately or mildly overweight kids. As a consequence, they should start out doing less, at a slower pace, and fewer times per week. It is perfectly all right to begin with 1 or 2 days a week of approximately 20 minutes of exercise and to increase the amount of activity weekly as pounds are shed. In addition, your patient doesn't have to do all 20 minutes at one time. Ten minutes in the morning and 10 in the afternoon or evening will still burn the same number of calories.
      It's best for seriously obese children to start out doing exercises that support their extra body weight, such as swimming or riding a bike. Moderately overweight children should begin with non-weight-bearing exercise first and gradually alternate with

weight-bearing activities. They can participate in walking or playing tag, for example, or basketball, as long as they take frequent rests when necessary. Again, they can gradually work up to longer walks and fewer rest stops. Mildly overweight children can safely participate in most activities, but even that little bit of extra weight may slow them down somewhat, so pacing is important. Gradually work up to higher speeds, harder movements, and longer duration.

Encourage the parents to consider enrolling their child for one or two afternoons a week in some kind of structured dance, martial arts (such as karate), gymnastics (only for chubby or mildly overweight children), or a similar activity. This will help foster friendships with other children who are active, and it will give you a break from having to supervise his or her entire exercise program. Make sure parents speak to the coach or teacher beforehand to discuss their child's special needs.

Describe the four color-coded levels to your patient and family; identify which one he or she is in, and explain that there is a different exercise and eating program for each color. Let him or her know that when he or she reaches his or her first weight-loss goals, he or she will graduate to the next color level, and that the objective is to attain his or her long-term goal weight and be a lifelong member in the Blue Level.

Weekly exercise activities:

Each week, you will find two types of activities:

• The Weekly Aerobic Activity
• The Weekly Strength and Flex Exercises

Each activity includes recommendations as to how often, and for how long, your patients should perform it. These are meant to be realistic goals — they are also the minimal goals. If your patients want to do more — great! Usually if you give them less, they'll do more. Then you can really praise them for going over and above. This really helps them achieve "mastery" — a feeling that they have accomplished something special.

Read through the following information with your patients and their families to understand the exercise strategy:

The Moderate-Intensity Progressive Exercise Program is designed especially for overweight kids. Remember that moderate — not fast or hard — exercise is the best for losing weight. You can do moderate exercise for hours without getting too tired, which burns the most calories and fat. After about 30 minutes of moderate exercise, your ability to burn fat increases, so the longer you exercise at a moderate pace, the more fat you'll burn.

This program uses moderate workout levels for aerobic, strengthening, endurance, and flexibility exercises. Each color-coded level has its own regimen. It is called progressive because it gradually increases in duration and frequency over time during the 12 weeks.

Duration means the amount of time you spend exercising at each session.

Frequency refers to the number of exercise sessions you do in a given week.

Intensity means how hard and fast you exercise. The intensity of your workout can change according to the speed, grade (steepness), muscles you use, and the force or resistance that you apply.

Vigorous Intensity = >55–70% maximal oxygen uptake ($VO_2$ max) or >65–80% maximal heart rate (MAXHR)

Moderate Intensity = 45–55% $VO_2$ max or 55–65% MAXHR

Low Intensity = <45% $VO_2$ max or <55% MAXHR

The maximal oxygen uptake refers to the total amount of oxygen that an individual will consume when exercising at maximum effort. Called $VO_2$ max for short, it is well accepted as the best indicator of aerobic fitness.

Here is a Sample Week 1 Aerobic Activity: Recommended Goals (refer to the program book for the remaining weeks' goals):

Red Level: the exercise goal this week is 2 days per week for 20 minutes each day.

Yellow Level: the exercise goal this week is 2 days per week for 25–30 minutes each day.

Green Level: the exercise goal this week is 3 days per week for 35–40 minutes each day.

Blue Level: the exercise goal this week is 3 days per week for 30–60 minutes each day.

Encourage your patients to write their goals in the Aerobic Activity and Food Checklist (Appendix A3.10). This is the minimum amount of aerobic exercise that they should perform this week. In the spaces indicated, encourage them to list the activities accomplished this week and how long they were done. If they know their heart rates, it should be written in the space provided.

Check to make sure your patients are performing the activities for the length of time and the number of days per week suggested for each color level. They should do them at a moderate or medium pace and be able to talk without strain while exercising. If breathing becomes rapid or labored, instruct them to slow down. Have them check their heart rates to determine whether 55–65% of maximum age-predicted heart rate has been attained. The program exercise DVD (see Appendix A3.1.1) illustrates how to take a heart rate.

Encourage your patients to do as much playing as possible. Let them know that playing burns even more calories than structured exercise. Resist the urge to push, thinking more will be better. If they can do it, great. But if you assign them less, they may do more.

d. Increasing Your Daily Activity — The MPEP Step

Verbal cues: Think about large people. Do they move fast? Usually not, and that may be one reason why they are large. When you move slowly, you don't burn many calories. You also don't use many muscles, and those you do use aren't used effectively. Now, think of people who walk briskly. They're usually trimmer and appear more energetic. They automatically burn more calories simply because they move faster and cover more ground in less time. It is amazing how simply walking faster, taking longer strides, and holding your chin up a little higher can make you look and feel lighter and more effective. And that feels good!

We want you to burn as many calories as you can as often as you can. To do that, you'll have to work your body more effectively on a regular basis. Now, when you hear the term "work," it will refer to how much energy you expend to burn calories. One way to work more effectively is to walk more briskly, covering as much ground as possible. By walking faster, you automatically increase your daily activity, which will help you lose and keep the weight off.

The following is a description of a role play session as presented in Chapter 20, Lesson 1. The conversation among the insructor, patients, and parents that should be conducted during the lesson is detailed in the program book as follows:

"Does this look familiar?" Dr. Melinda asks as she drops her head, rolls her shoulders and inches slowly forward. "Who do I look like? Do I look very tall? How tall do I look?"

One of the kids snickers, "Four feet tall!" Everyone chuckles, including Dr. Melinda.

"Do I look important and like I know where I'm going? Can you even see my face? When your head is down and your shoulders are hunched forward, no one can see your pretty face! You appear shorter and more overweight."

Then, Dr. Melinda lifts her head and holds her shoulders back. She walks forward briskly, smiling widely. "Now who do I look like?" she asks. "A supermodel, right?" Again, the kids laugh. "Maybe not, but I do look taller and more important, don't I? Actually, I look about six inches taller just because I lifted my head. And because of that, I also look about 30 pounds lighter."

Melissa was a participant in our program and lost 2 pounds in the first week just by walking with the MPEP-STEP. She also reported that others reacted differently toward her, she accomplished more, and she felt much more energetic.

2. Lesson 2: Exercise Intensity and Pacing Skills (Metabolic Systems), Cooling Down after Exercise
   a. Exercise Intensity and Pacing Skills (Metabolic Systems):
   The Body's Metabolic Engine [2]
   Verbal cues: For overweight and even slightly chubby kids, activity may be less frequent because they cannot keep up with the demands of certain sports, dance, or group games. In addition, their metabolic systems — the engines of their bodies — are different. Using a car as a metaphor, we can say that chubby and overweight children run out of gas sooner because the excess weight makes the engine run harder to move the car forward. A small car can go farther than a large truck on the same amount of gas.

   Regardless of weight, your body has three types of engines (or metabolisms), much like a car has three different gears: one for fast take-offs, one for start-and-stop driving, and one for highway driving.

   Medium-slow: This engine enables movement for long stretches of time. This is the engine that is fired up for aerobic exercises. It uses a combination of oxygen, fat stored in the body, and sugar (or carbohydrates) for fuel. After about 20 minutes of activity at the same speed, your body begins to use more of the stored fat for fuel. If you have not eaten for several hours, it will gobble up even more of that stored fat. The longer you maintain the medium-slow speed, the more calories and fat you will burn.

   Because overweight children have more stored fat than others, they can exercise in the medium-slow engine for hours without running out of gas as long as their pace stays low and consistent. But they must keep it slow and steady for a long period of time. It's all right to use the fast engine for a moment as long as it is brief and they return to the easier pace.

   Fast: This engine taps into the body's anaerobic capabilities. "Anaerobic" means "without air" — this engine depends not on oxygen, but primarily on sugar stored in the muscles (glycogen) for its fuel source. You kick-start this engine whenever the speed of your activity increases to a higher level.

   Your chubby child can use the fast engine until the workload becomes too difficult. At this point a substance called lactic acid will build in his muscles, making his muscles burn and feel tired. His breathing rate will also increase because he is trying to take in more oxygen so he can shift gears and begin using the medium-slow engine again. Unfortunately, because the fast engine is anaerobic, trying to take in more oxygen by breathing faster will not help. Your child's body will not allow him to shift to the medium-slow, aerobic engine unless he slows down.

   The fast engine has a very small fuel tank. It only takes between 3 and 5 minutes for your child to run out of gas. Unless activity is reduced to a speed or level to allow the child to shift to the medium-slow engine again, your child will be physically unable to continue.

The fast engine is great for short periods of exercise that promote strength and power. Sprinting is one example. So are stomach crunches.

Super Fast: Skilled and powerful athletes such as Olympic weight-lifters, jumpers, or sprinters use the super-fast engine. It relies on chemicals made from fuel stored directly in muscle fibers and immediately ready for use. The tank of the super-fast engine is even smaller than the fast engine. When children turn on that engine, they will run out of gas in only 10 seconds!

Your body uses different fuel systems for different levels or "intensities" of work:

| Very Fast | Fast | Medium to Slow |
| --- | --- | --- |
| 0–10 seconds then you run out of ATP | 10 seconds–5 minutes then you run out of glycogen and muscles fill with lactic acid | After 5 minutes and for hours and hours after (if you do not go too fast), you breathe out $CO_2$ |

- ATP stands for adenosintriphosphate, a long word for the chemical fuel made from sugar.
- Glycogen is another long word for sugar made from the food we eat.
- Aerobic. The sugar and oxygen we breathe combine with stored fat to give us the "gas" to go.
- Lactic acid — this is what makes your muscles burn and feel tired.
- $CO_2$ stands for carbon dioxide — the air we breathe out or exhale when we do aerobic exercise.

You can increase the size of the tanks in each of these engines by engaging in regular exercise training, and increasing how often (frequency) and how long (duration) you spend being physically active during any given week. Doing this will allow you to exercise for longer periods in all of the metabolic engines.

Don't rush the process! The heavier your child is, the longer it will take for her to comfortably use and improve her engines. Chubby children take at least 3 months to experience a noticeable change, and at least 6 months to reach their full potential for improvement. Heavier kids will take longer.

Verbal cues to parents: Finally, listen to your child. When she is exercising and says that she is tired, that means she is tired! If she says she is hurting, that means she is hurting! Allow her to slow down or stop to catch her breath. Then, gently prod her back into moving at a pace that is more comfortable. You may think she is faking her discomfort, but she is probably not. If you get irritated with her limitations, remember: her excess weight is physically disabling, she needs encouragement, not criticism.

b. Techniques for Cooling Down

Verbal cues: 5–10 minutes before you complete your exercise — whether it's riding your bike, jogging, swimming, walking, or dancing — you need to start cooling down. Do this gradually until you are maintaining a slow, easy pace. Continue at this pace for the last 10 minutes or so of your workout.

Cooling down is important because your body needs time to return to its normal heart rate and breathing pattern. Otherwise, the blood traveling to your exercising muscles will pool, or remain in the muscles. This can make you feel dizzy or nauseous, and you may experience painful muscle cramps.

Cooling down is just like warming up. You simply move your arms and legs slowly after exercising, and your blood leaves the muscles and returns to the heart and lungs. Your legs even have a built-in pump to help with that process, but you have to keep them moving for the pump to work.

Slowing down before stopping your exercise also helps bring your temperature back to its normal range. That's why it's called cooling down!

No matter what exercise you are doing, always slow the pace for the last 5–10 minutes.

3. Lesson 3: Aerobic Exercise — Modified Field Sports; The Homework Rule
   a. Modified Field Sports
   Family Flag Football
   The parents and children will participate in a flag football game (no tackling and use the flag belts if available). If you don't have flag belts, purchase inexpensive table napkins in two different colors. Divide the patients and family members into two teams and ask all of them to tuck one of the colored napkins into their waistband. Play the game of football with these aerobic rules: Allow 20 seconds only to pre-pare for the kick-off. Allow only 10 seconds for the huddle. The ball must be snapped for the next play no more than 10 seconds after it is down. Switch player position: If you are quarterback and your son is running back, switch every 15 minutes. These rules keep the game moving and the calories burning.
   Special Instructions: The parents may serve as goal posts by holding their arms in a "letter L" position facing inward to each other. The instructor will need to have a parent serve as quarterback to help explain the rules of the game to the inexpe-rienced younger children.

   Aerobic Softball
   The group will participate in aerobic softball as follows: The game follows regula-tion rules; however, the participants are instructed that when the opposing team scores a point, they must walk/run the bases; likewise, when the team up to bat gets an out, they must walk/run the bases. You may also add 10 modified jumping jacks for each strike or error in the field, to keep the kids even more active. Peri-odically check breathing and heart rate to illustrate how aerobic softball is just as vigorous as structured exercise.

   b. The Homework Rule: Play Now! Homework Later!
   Don't Do Your Homework — Yet! In 1987, W.B. Strong recommended that children should not be allowed to do homework directly after school [26]. Children have already been confined during the long, often tedious, day in an activity-restricted environment, and need a break to enjoy physical activities and to let off steam.
   The following handout can be given to the children to encourage them to take an activ-ity break upon their return home from school.

---

The MPEP After-School Plan
"Hit those books! No television until all of the homework is done!"
Is this what Mom or Dad says the minute you get home from school?
But it's really hard to start your homework right away, because you feel tired from working and studying at school all day. Do you think it's your body that is tired, or is it just your brain?
Try this instead:
As soon as you get home from school, go to the refrigerator and get a big glass of ice water. Maybe you're tired because you are thirsty ("dehydrated" means you don't have enough water in your body).

Then you should go outside if the weather is nice, and walk, or ride your bike, or skate, or walk the dog. You could play ball, or play tag, or jump rope. If the weather is bad, find a large area inside, and turn on some music and dance. Why don't you get your TrimKids exercise video or workbook and do some exercises? Maybe there is an exercise program on television.

You should try to do at least 30 minutes of any kind of "moving around" before you start your homework (45 to 60 minutes is even better). This will give your brain a chance to rest from the long school day.

Remember, when you get home, your brain is tired, but your body isn't. Work the muscles that have been sitting at a desk all day! Then do your homework after you exercise. You may still have time before dinner for one television show.

Verbal cues to parents: When children get home after a day at school, their brains are tired, but not their bodies. They have already been confined during the long, often-tedious, day in a relatively sedentary environment. They need a break to enjoy physical activities and let off steam.

From now on, hand your child a big glass of ice water, then tell him to go outside and walk, ride a bike, skate, play ball, jump rope, or play tag. If the weather is bad, tell him to do some dancing, go to his imagination station, or play a round of indoor basketball. Make sure he does between 30 and 60 minutes of moving around before he or she starts his homework.

4. Lesson 4: Muscular Strength and Endurance: MPEP pump; Strength Training Circuit; Creating Indoor Play Areas
   a. Muscular Strength and Endurance: MPEP pump

Verbal cues for parents: Aerobic exercise is great for healthy hearts and lungs. But if your child engages in only aerobic exercise, she will be missing two critical components: strength and flexibility. What good is a car with a great engine but that has no tires, hood, top, or doors? Muscles provide the framework for your child's engine and must be strong to protect him or her from injury. A bone is only as strong as the muscle attached to it.

Muscles must be exercised with some kind of weight at least once or twice a week to keep them tight or toned. This happens through the force or resistance of strength training. Children can strengthen their muscles through lifting weights (soup cans will do), or by simply lifting a limb or part of their own body (as in modified push ups). Strength training will become a regular part of their routine in the Trim Kids Program.

Strengthening exercises result in toned muscles. Toned muscles are metabolically active tissues: they burn more calories than fat even when the child is not moving. In fact, a toned muscle burns 33 calories per hour to maintain itself, compared with fat tissue, which burns only two to three calories per hour. Strong muscles are a lot like furnaces. The stronger the muscle, the more intensely the furnace burns. This furnace is called the metabolic rate.

Your pediatrician can guide you to identify the kinds of strengthening activities that are safe for your overweight child. His growing bones and developing joints may be at risk for injury if he asks too much of his body by strenuous lifting, pushing, jarring, or pulling. Even jumping could cause harm. Severely overweight children should only participate in strength exercises that offer good support for their joints. The exercises in the Trim Kids Program were designed especially for overweight children.

On getting your pediatrician's approval and making sure the equipment is in good repair, encourage your child to strengthen her muscles by

- climbing trees
- swinging on monkey bars
- jumping on trampolines with safety nets
- swinging on swing sets
- skipping rope
- playing hopscotch
- climbing in and out of a swimming pool
- participating in gymnastics
- dancing
- learning a martial art

Strength training has many other health benefits: it may prevent bone fractures and arthritis, as well as diseases such as osteoporosis, diabetes, and heart disease. It will make your child look better: strong muscles under his or her skin will make him or her look toned and fit.

Verbal cues: Muscles have very little brains — they remember only after being shown many times. They will stay tight without your telling them to, if you exercise them with weight at least twice a week.

The most important thing is that a muscle that you have exercised becomes a trained muscle. Trained muscles burn calories even when you are not exercising them. Fat tissue just hangs around.

An Introduction to Resistance Weight Training

Resistance weight training includes weight training, strength training, circuit weight training, isometrics, and isokinetics, which involve exercising the muscles against moderate to heavy loads, generally with few repetitions. Its use results in varying degrees of muscle size increase (hypertrophy), increased lean body mass, and increased strength and power.

For years, resistance weight training evoked a negative image and was avoided by athletic and medical professionals alike. This has changed with recent research in this still controversial field of training. Guidelines for resistance training are listed in the program book [2].

Force and Weight Aspects

Individuals should begin the program at 60% or less of their maximum strength threshold. This weight should be maintained until 8 to 12 repetitions can be performed at specified velocities and in perfect form (technique). At this time an increase in weight of 5 to 10% is recommended.

Speed of Movement (Velocity)

A 2- to 4-second count for both the lifting or pulling and lowering or releasing phases with constant movement throughout is recommended. The movement should be performed with no rest and with a slight hold at the highest-force resistance. The velocity can be increased slightly when using free weights, and a hold is not necessary.

Frequency

Untrained children should begin the program at a frequency of once per week, with twice per week the maximum. Trained children can begin the program at a frequency of twice per week, with a minimum of once per week to prevent a loss in strength and muscle size. A minimum of 1 day between workouts is necessary to guarantee enough rest to promote strength gains. Two to 3 days of rest between workouts is advisable for individuals working at peak workloads. This will help to prevent overwork and injury. It is inadvisable to work out with weights more frequently than three times per week.

Duration

A period of 1.5 to 2 minutes per station is suggested. Each station should consist of one or two sets of 8 to 12 repetitions performed as specified. This will induce a balanced workout of muscular strength, muscular endurance, and slight $VO_2$ improvement provided there is a minimum rest period with no more than 30 seconds between stations (a 15-second rest is recommended).

Technique

Body alignment should follow American College of Sports Medicine (ACSM) guidelines with positioning for maximum isolation of designated muscles or muscle groups. The general technique for all exercises is as follows:

- Movement should occur only in the joint adjacent to the muscles being contracted. All other body parts should be stationary and relaxed.
- As the movement begins, the individual should focus on the muscles being worked and fully contract (squeeze and shorten) the muscle into the holding point. When extending the weights, a maximum range of motion should be achieved.
- There should be a light grip on the handles unless specifically working the forearm. This prevents an unnecessary elevation in blood pressure.
- Technique specific to each exercise should be illustrated by a weight-lifting instructor or trainer.
- Breathing should be continuous and at a normal rate throughout with no specific inhalation or exhalation phase. To aid in concentration, a quiet, nondistracting atmosphere is recommended. Warm-up should consist of approximately 5 minutes of low-impact jogging moves, range of motion without weight, and gentle stretching. Cool down should be a similar process with more intense stretching.

Safety

At least one spotter is required on all free-weight stations. A spotter is encouraged on all stations to aid the subject, especially through the latter repetitions of maximum force.

Injury Prevention

It is suggested that exercises be performed as specified only. It is advisable that a spotter be used to correct faulty technique as muscles reach fatigue.

Muscle Soreness

Slight muscle soreness and tightness are normal 1 to 2 days following weight training. Research indicates that this may be a result of the muscle-rebuilding process. Proper cool down and adequate stretching are encouraged for prevention of soreness. If the soreness is light, gentle stretching and range-of-motion exercise are beneficial, along with elevation and ice for swelling. If there is no swelling, then a warm bath and massage are beneficial. For severe soreness, it is recommended that one use the RICE method: rest, ice, compression, and elevation.

b. Sample Strength Exercise: Rowing, Low

Sit upright, leaning slightly forward from your hips. Keep your back straight and your shoulders down. Pull your shoulders back. Now, if you're exercising on a machine or are using an exercise band, pull the handles or end of the band back to your upper abdomen over a 2- to 4-second period (in the first 4 weeks, you will not use resistance). Squeeze your shoulder blades together. Hold for 1 to 2 seconds. Now, take about 2 to 4 seconds, return to the starting position, keeping your back stationary. Do 8 to 12 repetitions of this exercise. Be sure to pull back for a full 2 to 4 seconds. Then, take another 2 to 4 seconds to return to the starting position. This exercise works your upper back muscle (rhomboid) and your middle back muscle (latissimus dorsi). Common errors that your child may make include moving shoulders upward, leaning back, moving the head forward, or bending at the wrists.

c. Muscular Strength and Endurance Facts:

Overload and Stress

The body responds to stress in one of two ways: adaptation or breakdown. Muscle adaptation may be referred to as training effect such as an increase in strength, power, endurance or speed. Breakdowns result in overuse syndromes and other injuries. The goal of training programs is to obtain as much training effect as possible without sustaining stress injury.

Training Effect

Muscles are the engines of the body. Their performance is improved when stress is applied in excess of their present capacity. This is referred to as overload, which results in a training effect specific to the exercise.

Injury

If stress is excessive, the body's response is a stress injury or overuse syndrome. This may occur as the result of improper technique, too much force, inadequate rest, poor nutrition, or dehydration.

Frequency and Rest

In weight training more demanding workouts require more recovery time. Research supports two to three nonconsecutive exercise sessions per week with adequate rest in between.

Muscle Specificity

Strength

Strength is defined as the maximum ability of a muscle or group of muscles to apply or resist force. It is a pure and independent factor from endurance and power. Training for strength results in adaptation of fibers within the muscles.

Power

Power is defined as performance of work expressed per unit of time. It is dependent on strength because it is the product of strength and speed. (POWER = FORCE × VELOCITY). Training for power exercises must include a rapid speed component specific to the desired goals.

Size

Increases in muscle area size (hypertrophy) are the result of three factors:

1. Muscle fiber lengthening and widening and possibly an increase in the number of fibers.
2. Increased vascularization (blood flow and capillary development)
3. Fluid retention (edema) in the muscle area due to stress.

Endurance

Endurance is defined as the ability of a muscle to repeatedly develop near maximal force and to sustain repeated contractions. It is dependent on the level of strength and uses mainly aerobic metabolic systems

Physical Make-Up

Muscle Fiber Composition

Muscle fibers are generally classified as slow-twitch or fast-twitch. The percentage of each is genetically determined. Slow-twitch = low intensity, long duration. Fast-twitch = high intensity, short duration.

Balance

The ultimate goal of weight training is a strong, symmetrical, and balanced physique. This is achieved by training muscles anteriorally and posterially with the same intensity as well as left and right sides. Differences in strength leave the weaker muscles more prone to injury.

Speed of Movement

Research supports 60 degrees per second or at least 2 seconds for lifting and 2 seconds for lowering. Controlled movement speeds enhance both training safety and training stimulus.

Sets and Repetitions

Research supports one to three training sets per exercise, dependent on training goals and time availability. Repetitions are dependent to some degree on muscle fiber type. Research supports 8 to 12 repetitions for children < 14 years of age.

How to Plan Your Own Resistance Weight-Training Program

Allow sufficient time in your routine for an adequate warm up and cool down, as recommended by your instructor.

Use this sequence of exercises:

- Start with your large muscle groups, preferably leg muscles, and do abdominal exercises at the end of the routine.
- Follow with exercises that work the upper body muscles in unison.
- Follow these with exercises that isolate specific arm muscles.
- Then do another exercise that works upper body muscles in unison and that is different from the earlier exercise.
- Do another large muscle group, such as abdominal muscles or oblique (waist-line) muscles.
- Finally, do exercises for the calf muscles.

If you feel pain during the performance of an exercise, stop immediately. This might indicate an existing injury, a structural problem, or improper technique. Ask your exercise instructor for assistance.

Remember to monitor your results. This is the only way you can determine whether a particular exercise and its duration and intensity are right for you.

Remember that there are genetic factors that determine the results of your exercise program. Respect your own limitations and avoid comparing your progress with that of others.

When you are doing your exercise routine, be courteous to others who are performing an exercise circuit. Try to organize your workout so that it does not upset the rhythm of the majority.

Methods for Stimulating Greater Muscle Development

The human body experiences several plateaus in improvement when pursuing any physical activity. Individual genetic factors limit the potential for development of strength and size of muscles. An example of this is that fast-twitch muscles have a greater potential for hypertrophy.

At first the body has a "learning effect" caused by nervous system adaptations to strength training. Substantial gains are noticed at this first stage. These gains then level out, and it is necessary to use different methods to develop a greater number of muscle fibers.

The key to greater muscle development during a plateau is change.

- Change your training exercises
- Change your training frequency
- Change the relationship between resistance and repetitions

Increase your training intensity

- "Harder" means "smarter" — not necessarily longer. Strength training is limited by the anaerobic respiratory system (30 to 120 seconds).
- High-intensity training
- Breakdown training
- Assisted training
- Super-slow training
- Negative training
- One-and-one-quarter training

And if all else fails, get more sleep (quality rest). At least 7.5 hours per night are necessary; in children < 14 years, 10 hours per night are recommended.

Drink more fluids — muscles are 75% water.

Obtain better nutrition — a well-balanced diet. Increased protein intake may promote dehydration. Eat smaller meals more frequently.

Your muscles get stronger after your workout — during the rebuilding period. This is when proteins are resynthesized, and when connective tissue is rebuilt.

Your goal is to exercise the greatest number of muscle fibers per movement, and to exercise those fibers in different movement patterns.

d. Creating Indoor Play Areas

Verbal cues: Winter always comes, and in most places, that means staying inside. No problem. A little rearranging will do wonders. Transform your child's bedroom or a room you don't use much into an "imagination station" (see the program book [2] for further details). Enlist your child's help to create a fun atmosphere. Pull a few old mattresses into the room so he can jump from one to the next. Bring in a boom box so he or she has plenty of room to dance. Or, if he or she is younger, designate the area for soft balls, hoola-hoops and jump ropes. No child we know can resist a small, indoor trampoline surrounded by fluffy pillows. Hopscotch is always in vogue. Believe it or not, kids still love the game of Twister. You can play too! Or try a piece of technology that actually gets kids out from behind the computer: a power pad. It is connected to both the child's body and the computer, so when the child moves, it records his actions and shows them on the screen – in the form of abstract images. This can make hours of interesting physical twists and turns, and ends up as techno-art!

Enlist your child's opinions and help and spend as much time as necessary putting the room together so your child wants to be there. Of course, you are invited to do some playing, too, which will invigorate your child to play even more.

Here's an idea to act on sooner rather than later: younger children actually enjoy doing household chores. Ask your youngster to help you make the beds in the house, help you transfer clothes from the washer to the dryer, put the dishes in the dishwasher, or water the plants. Even sweeping and vacuuming have a near mystical appeal to them.

The goal is to provide as much opportunity as possible for your child to play, move, and burn calories. Always be certain to select activities that are safe for your child's age and level of fitness.

Inside adventure: When the weather's bad

Have you refurbished your house yet so your child can stay active during rainy, cold, and snowy months?

There are plenty of places to take your child when cabin fever sets in. Sign him or her up for weekly indoor activities or just go for a 1-day visit when the mood strikes.

Gyms/fitness centers: They offer a variety of calorie-burning fun including gymnastics, tumbling, basketball, wrestling, kick boxing or other martial arts, wall-climbing, track, badminton, volleyball, ping pong, and swimming. Don't forget indoor tennis.

Dance studios: Kids are welcome in all kinds of classes including ballet, tap, modern, jazz, hip-hop, line dancing, ballroom dancing, yoga, free movement classes, and other music/dance combination classes.

Indoor rinks: Ice skating and roller skating can fill hours of fun on a rainy day

Children's museums: They exist in most cities and provide interesting, educational, and fun activities that keep your child on the move!

Indoor nature centers or aquariums offer similar movement opportunities.

Restaurants with games: They are popping up all over. Choose those that offer the greatest energy burners, including laser tag and other fast-paced activities. Most have salad bars, so plan on light meals.

To set up your imagination station, here are some ideas for older children:

- A plastic tub filled with costumes, dress-up clothes, and accessories such as crowns, wands, toy shields, armor, masks, vests, belts, shoes, hats, grass skirts, scarfs, play jewelry, wigs
- Boom box with various dance music tapes or CDs
- Microphone, drums, toy musical instruments, stage curtains
- Puppets, marionettes, magician kits, various stuffed animals
- Batons, small flags, pom poms, streamers, hula hoops
- Foam mats and wedges, indoor tents, large building blocks or cardboard boxes, bean bag chairs, soft pillows, old blankets, sheets
- Hopscotch mat, action games such as Twister, Charades, Simon Says, Follow the Leader
- Paddle balls, indoor ball-toss games, bean bags, juggling balls, hacky sack
- Kid-safe dart boards or other target games
- Indoor basketball hoop and soft foam balls
- Jump ropes, skip-it, small kid-safe hand weights, exercise stretch bands.

For younger children, try:

- Small pull/push toys or plastic wagons
- Toy household cleaning items such as brooms, mops, vacuum cleaners, feather dusters
- Toy kitchen, restaurant, and accessories
- Indoor riding toys.

Meanwhile, when you're gathered in front of the television watching your favorite show, don't forget to stand up and do the "television commercial boogie" whenever the ads come on. You'll be amazed at how much moving you'll do to the soundtracks of those endless commercials! And be sure to engage in collective booing when junk-food ads fill the screen.

5. Lesson 5: Family Field Sports — Aerobic Volleyball; Creating Outdoor Play Areas
   a. Creating Outdoor Fun [2]
   Verbal cues: Take an inventory of your yard. Is there a swing set? Sandbox? A wading pool? A sprinkler with an attachment for playing with water? If not, get busy! Your child can engage in the great outdoors in so many ways. His age will determine his or her interests. Older children love to climb rope swings or ladders leading to a tree fort in which they can play endlessly. They also enjoy competition, sporting games (basketball, baseball, badminton, croquet, miniature golf), and tag, tag, and more tag! Younger children enjoy playing knights-in-shining-armor with an open field for battle. They like balls of all sizes. Building makeshift houses out of cardboard boxes provides endless adventure. Or they'll pull their wagons full of their favorite things.
   Enter into this knowing it may be a process of trial and error. Maybe for your child's first 6 to 8 years, watching television was her idea of fun. She may have to explore different corners of this new world of activity before she finds the right fit. Bear with her. Your patience will pay off enormously.
   If you don't have a yard, find the nearest park. Even older kids enjoy monkey bars, swings, teeter-totters, tunnels, and the wonderful playground equipment so many parks offer. Take her to the grassy area and throw a Frisbee, pitch some baseballs, or ride bikes around the periphery of the park. The only hard and fast rule to all this is to find activities your child likes and do them!

6. Lesson 6: Flexibility, Flex Test I, and Stretch and Flex Class [2]
   a. Verbal cues: A car runs more efficiently when it is in alignment. The same holds true for the human body. The function of flexibility is to maintain balance. When your child was born, he was in perfect proportion and symmetrical—the left side was identical to the right. The front of the body was in balance with the rear. After years of using one part of the body more than another, imbalances occur. This can result in poor posture, unfit appearance, or injury and pain in a bone or joint.
   If you overtrain your chest muscles, undertrain your back, and fail to stretch the chest muscles, you will walk around like a gorilla (Instructor demonstrates). Also, your back will begin to hunch and you will resemble an alien from outer space (Instructor demonstrates). However, if your chest is flexible and your back strong, you will appear taller, trimmer, and stronger (Instructor demonstrates proper alignment).
   Flexibility training, or stretching, is just as important as aerobics and strength training. Inflexible joints and muscles inhibit your child from participating in activities to his or her fullest potential. They can also lead to chronic muscle and joint disorders. If you participate in stretching exercises with your child, you will be helping yourself offset chronic pain and disease, too!
   Stretching can be done often and almost anywhere. We encourage it during television time. Make sure you arrange the room in which your child watches television so that he or she can sprawl on the floor and perform his or her stretches
   Be sure your child always stretches after he participates in aerobic or strengthening exercises. This will prevent soreness and possibly even injury. Stretching is also a great way to unwind at the end of the day.

b. Sample Flex Exercise: Shoulder Stretch

Stand with your feet about 18 inches apart. Now, bend your knees slightly. Push your hips forward just a bit. Keep your stomach muscles tight. Inhale as you raise both arms up above your head with your upper arms just ahead of your ears. Interlock your fingers, and turn your hands inside out. Stretch upward at a slight angle forward. Hold this position for 15 to 30 seconds. Lower arms and relax. Repeat this process one more time, holding this position again for 15 to 30 seconds.

7. Lesson 7: Aerobic Exercise and Cardiopulmonary Endurance, Steady State — Monitoring Heart Rate and Aerobic Circuit

a. Monitoring Heart Rate — Keeping the Best Pace

Verbal cues: Working out at the most efficient and safest pace requires that you monitor your breathing, temperature, and heart rate. While exercising, find a pace at which you can talk without difficulty, your breathing is not too labored, and you don't get overheated—meaning very hot, lightheaded, and weak.

You can monitor your heart rate during an aerobic activity by determining your own individual target heart range (THR) beforehand. Here's how:

1. Subtract your age from 220. 220 – _____ = _____
2. To get the low end of your range, multiply your answer by 55%. _____ × .55 = _____.
3. To figure the high end of your range, multiply your answer by 65%. _____ × .65 = _____.
4. Review how to take your heart rate, and the recommended heart rate ranges, in the program book [2] and on the exercise DVD (see Appendix A3.1.1).

Aim for the low end of your THR when you first begin exercising, and gradually work up to the higher range. Also, if you have an existing medical condition, work with your doctor to determine the best THR.

8. Lesson 8: Exercise Prescriptions; the Fit Kit Walking Program

a. The Fit Kit (Walking for Fun, Health, and Fitness)

The Fit Kit was designed especially for children in level 3 (green) or 4 (blue). Children in level 1 (red) or 2 (yellow) should choose an alternate activity this week such as biking or swimming.

Verbal cues: Work with your child to develop a walking program that will maintain his goal weight and keep him fit. By participating in this, you'll burn lots of calories, train your leg and hip muscles, and improve the efficiency of your heart and lungs. Walking is one of the easiest and most convenient ways you can stay active on a daily basis. There may be times you walk with a friend, while at other times you may prefer to do it alone. Either way is fine as long as you keep on truckin'!

Follow these steps to healthy walking.

• Step 1: Check Up. Check your shoes, clothes, and walking route. Get a new pair of walking shoes about every 6 months. Don't try to save money by wearing them longer. These are your precious feet you're working with!

Clothes: In summer, choose loose-fitting, all-cotton tee shirts and tank tops. In winter, dress in layers of warm, soft, loose-fitting clothes, woolen mittens, and a hat.

Walking Route: Sketch a map of your planned walking route on paper. Make sure to include landmarks, phone locations, water stops, and favorite scenic spots. Post your map on the refrigerator. Always tell someone where you will be walking if it is different from your typical route.

• Step 2: Form a Plan of Action. Write a 1-week walking schedule and put it into your daily calendar.

- Step 3: Get Ready: Choose an appropriate warm up that includes dynamic stretches (Appendix A3.3. Stretch while moving); don't do any static stretches without warming up first. Wait until after your walking to do static stretches.
- Step 4: Put Your Best Foot Forward. Walk slowly at first, swinging your arms naturally. Pick up the pace after a few minutes to a comfortable, moderate level. Remember, if you start to breathe too rapidly, slow down until you are going at the pace that is right for you. Use the chart in the program book [2] to calculate your walking speed.
- Step 5: Cool Down and Stretch (Appendix A3.3). Reduce your pace during the last 5 to 10 minutes of the walk. Finish up with at least one stretch of each major muscle group. Refer to the program book and DVD [2] for proper technique.
- Step 6: Keep a Walking Diary. Use the form located in the program book [2].
- Step 7: Weigh the Outcome of Your Walk. Determine how many calories you burned during your walk by using the chart provided. First, determine the distance you walked. Then figure out your speed (miles per hour) from the "Your Miles-Per-Hour Chart" in the program book [2].
- Step 8: Take the Next Step. Many people find walking enjoyable once they get into the habit. If this is true for you, consider joining a local club or entering a fun walk or run. Check with your local recreation, church, or school organizations for upcoming opportunities. This is a great way to meet new friends who also love to walk and be active.

9. Lesson 9: Review Muscular Strength and Endurance: Pull Your Own Weight Series
   a. Verbal cues: Let's say you are out of town visiting relatives or on a family vacation. By now, you love your new, toned, beautiful body and you are aching to do some strengthening exercises. The "Pull Your Own Weight" exercises work the major muscle groups, and you do not need a gym or special equipment to do them. Instead you will use your own body weight to tone and strengthen your muscles. Be sure to do them slowly, and be sure to fully extend and contract your muscles to get full strengthening and toning benefit.
   b. Sample Exercises
   Modified Standing Push-up
      Stand two to three feet from a wall, sturdy table, or chair, with your feet together and your hands extended forward. Place your hands on the wall or grasp the table or chair, as you lean your body forward at a 45 degree angle to the floor. Slowly, bend your elbows and lower your chest until it touches the edge of the table or chair. Now, push with your hands, extending your arms, and return to the original position. Keep your head in line with your body. Keep your legs straight and extended throughout the exercise. Repeat 8 to 12 times. You are training the chest muscles (pectorals) and the back of the upper arms (triceps).
   Modified Lunge
      Stand with your feet about 6 to 8 inches apart and grasp the back of a sturdy chair with both of your hands. Step forward with your right leg approximately 18 to 36 inches. Keep your head, shoulders, and hips in a straight line. Bend your knees and lower your left knee onto floor. Do not allow the right knee to move in front of your right foot. Push the heel of the right foot into the floor as you lift and return to the starting position. Repeat with your left leg forward. Repeat 8 to 12 times on each leg. You are working the buttocks muscles (gluteus), the back of upper leg (hamstrings), and the front upper leg (quads).

10. Lesson 10: See Park Day — Outdoor Play in Chapter 20.

## A3.4   TABLE OF FOOD PORTION AND UNITS

### YOUR DAILY NUTRITION PLAN

*Verbal Cues*

To make it easier, we have assigned daily food portion guides for each calorie level. Instead of counting calories, all you have to do is eat a specified number of units (or portions) daily from the carbohydrate, meat and protein substitute, and fat food groups — not to exceed your calorie goal. Refer to Chapter 12 by Schumacher et al. and the program book [2] to find the daily portion allowance for your child's calorie goal.

*Daily Food Prescription*

My Daily Calorie Goal:                              _____ calories per day

I am allowed to eat:

_____ Carbohydrate units per day

These include
* Starches/breads
* Fruits
* Milk/dairy


_____ Meat and protein substitutes per day

_____ Fats per day

_____ Unlimited vegetables

*Keeping Track Using the Food Checklist*

*Verbal cues:* To help keep track of your child's daily food intake, use the Aerobic Activity and Food Checklist found in Appendix A3.10. Each small box on the checklist represents one unit. Check the appropriate boxes for every food or drink your child consumes. For example:

**Turkey Sandwich**

| | |
|---|---|
| Two slices wheat bread | Check two carbohydrate boxes |
| 2 ounces sliced turkey | Check two meat/substitute boxes |
| Lettuce/tomato | Check vegetable box |
| 1 cup skim milk | Check one carbohydrate box |

Checking the boxes will help you practice staying within your child's daily recommended portion intake. Don't worry if you have to "guesstimate" at times, especially if your child is away from home. Following a tight calorie level is not the goal, but practicing and "reteaching" the body portion control (until it becomes a habit) is.

*Food Portion and Unit Lists*

Keeping track of portions ensures that your child is eating the right amounts of foods to achieve the weight loss calorie goal. Refer to the chart below for food group portions and their specific food units.

# Food Portion and Unit Lists

| Common Foods | Portion | Carbohydrate Units |
|---|---|---|
| | **Starches** | |
| ***Breads*** | | |
| Bread | | |
| "Lite Bread" | 1 slice (1 ounce) | 1 carb |
| Bagel | 2 slices | 1 carb |
| Bagel | Medium (2 ounce) | 2 carbs |
| English muffin | Large (4 ounce) | 4 carbs |
| Hamburger or hot dog bun | Whole | 2 carbs |
| Dinner roll | Whole | 2 carbs |
| Muffin | 1 (small-1 ounce) | 1 carb |
| Muffin | Small (2 ounce) | 2 carbs |
| Waffle/pancake | Large (4 ounce) | 4 carbs |
| Tortillas | 1 regular | 1 carb |
| ***Cereals*** | | |
| Dry (breakfast) cereal | 1 cup | 1 carb |
| Hot cereal (oatmeal, cream of wheat, grits) | | |
|     Plain | ½ cup (1 packet, instant) | 1 carb |
|     Fruit/flavored | ⅔ cup (1 packet instant) | 2 carbs |
| ***Grains*** | | |
| Pasta | ½ cup (cooked) | 1 carb |
| Rice | ½ cup (cooked) | 1 carb |
| Beans (red, navy, lima) | ½ cup (cooked) | 1 carb |
| Lentils | 1 cup (cooked) | 1 carb |
| Stuffing | ¼ cup (cooked) | 1 carb |
| ***Snacks*** | | |
| Chips (reduced-fat) | 1 ounce (1 small bag) | 1 carb |
| Cereal-fruit bar | 1 | 2 carbs |
| Crackers | | |
|     Animal | 15 | 1 carb |
|     Graham | 3 squares | 1 carb |
|     Wheat/saltine-type | 6 crackers | 1 carb |
| Granola bar | 1 granola bar | 2 carbs |
| Popcorn (reduced-fat) | 3 cups (popped) | 1 carb |
| Pretzels | 1 ounce (small bag) | 1 carb |
| Rice cakes | | |
|     Small | 8 small | 1 carb |
|     Large | 2 large | 2 carbs |
| ***Starchy Vegetables*** | | |
| Corn | ½ cup | 1 carb |
| Peas | ½ cup | 1 carb |
| Potatoes (sweet, white) | 1 medium | 2 carbs |
| Squash (acorn, butternut) | ¼ cup | 1 carb |
| ***Fruits*** | | |
| Fresh fruit | Medium (or about 1 cup ) | 1 carb |
| Canned fruit | ½ cup | 1 carb |

| Common Foods | Portion | Carbohydrate Units |
|---|---|---|
| Dried fruit: | | |
|   Dried apricots | 4 | 1 carb |
|   Dried figs | 2 | 1 carb |
|   Dried prunes | 3 | 1 carb |
|   Raisins | ¼ cup (small box) | 1 carb |
| Fruit juice: | | |
|   Apple juice | 1 cup (8 ounces) | 2 carbs |
|   Cranberry juice | 1 cup (8 ounces) | 3 carbs |
|   Grape juice | 1 cup (8 ounces) | 3 carbs |
|   Grapefruit juice | 1 cup (8 ounces) | 2 carbs |

### Dairy*

| | | |
|---|---|---|
| Milk (skim/reduced-fat) | 1 cup (8 ounces) | 1 carb |
| Soy milk | 1 cup (8 ounces) | 1 carb |
| Yogurt: | | |
|   Plain | 1 cup | 1 carb |
|   Fruit/regular sweetened | 1 cup | 2 carbs |
|   Fruit/artificially sweetened | 1 cup | 1 carb |
| Frozen yogurt | ½ cup (4-ounce "kiddie-size) | 1 carb |
| Reduced-fat ice cream | ½ cup | 1 carb |
| Cheese, reduced-fat | 1-ounce slice | 1 protein (no carbohydrates) |
| Cheese, regular | 1-ounce slice | 1 protein + 1 fat |

*Choose dairy products containing less than 3 to 5 grams of fat per unit.
*Choose dairy products containing less than 25 to 30 grams of "sugar" on the label.

### Vegetables (lower-carbohydrate)
Unlimited

### Meat, Poultry, Seafood and Protein Substitutes

| | | |
|---|---|---|
| Beef: | | |
|   Flank, round, sirloin, tenderloin | 1 ounce | 1 protein |
| Poultry (skinless) | | |
|   Chicken | 1 breast (about 4 ounces) | 4 proteins |
|   Turkey | 1 drumstick (about 2 ounces) | 2 proteins |
| Pork: | | |
|   Canadian bacon, chops (fat trimmed), ham, | 1 ounce | 1 protein |
|   Loin, tenderloin | 1 ounce | 1 protein |
| Seafood: | | |
|   Fish (all) | 1 ounce | 1 protein |
|   Shellfish (all) | 6 shrimp | 1 protein |
|   Tuna fish (canned in water) | ½ cup | 2 proteins |
| Cold cuts (less than 3 to 5 grams of fat per ounce) | 1 ounce | 1 protein |
| Reduced-fat cheese (less than 3 to 5 grams of fat per ounce) | 1 ounce | 1 protein |
| Regular cheese | 1 ounce | 1 protein (+ 1 fat) |
| Eggs: | | |
|   Egg with yolk | 1 whole egg | 1 protein (+ 1 fat) |
|     Egg substitute | ½ cup | 2 proteins |
| Vegetable patties | 1 patty (about 3 ounces) | 2 proteins |
| Peanut butter | 1 tablespoon | 1 protein (+ 1 fat) |
| Tofu | 4 ounces | 2 proteins |

| Common Foods | Portion | Carbohydrate Units |
|---|---|---|
| *Fats* | | |
| Avocado* | ¼ avocado | 2 fats |
| Butter/Margarine (regular) | 1 tablespoon | 3 fats |
| Cream cheese, lite-Neufchatel | 1 tablespoon | 1 fat |
| Cream cheese, fat-free* | No limit | 0 |
| Margarine, reduced-fat | 1 tablespoon | 1 fat |
| Margarine, fat-free* | No limit | 0 |
| Mayonnaise, regular | 1 tablespoon | 3 fats |
| Mayonnaise, reduced-fat | 1 tablespoon | 1 fat |
| Mayonnaise, fat-free* | No limit | 0 |
| Nuts/Seeds:* | | |
|    Peanuts, cashews | About ¼ cup | 3 fats |
|    Almonds | (4 tablespoons) | |
|    Pine nuts, pumpkin, sunflower seeds | 1 teaspoon | 1 fat |
| Oils: | | |
|    Canola, olive, peanut* | 1 tablespoon | 3 fats |
|    Corn, safflower, soybean, sunflower | 1 tablespoon | 3 fats |
| Olives | About 10 olives | 1 fat |
| Salad dressing, reduced-fat | 2 tablespoons | 1 fat |
| Salad dressing, fat-free* | No limit | 0 |
| Sour cream, reduced-fat | 2 tablespoons | 1 fat |
| Sour cream, fat-free* | No limit | 0 |

*Better choices

| Common Foods | Portion | Carbohydrate Units |
|---|---|---|
| *Condiments/Seasonings* | | |
| BBQ sauce | 2–3 tablespoons | 0 |
| Catsup | No limit | 0 |
| Herbs and spices | No limit | 0 |
| Horseradish | No limit | 0 |
| Hot sauce | No limit | 0 |
| Lemon/lime juice | No limit | 0 |
| Mayonnaise (regular) | 1 tablespoon | 3 fats |
| Mayonnaise (reduced-fat) | 1 tablespoon | 1 fat |
| Mayonnaise (fat-free) | No limit | 0 |
| Mustard | No limit | 0 |
| Pickles | No limit | 0 |
| Salsa | No limit | 0 |
| Soy sauce (lower-sodium is better) | No limit | 0 |
| Taco sauce | No limit | 0 |
| Teriyaki sauce | No limit | 0 |
| Worcestershire sauce | No limit | 0 |

| Common Foods | Portion | Carbohydrate Units |
|---|---|---|
| *Entrees/Soups* | | |
| Casseroles: | | |
| Hamburger Helper™, Lasagna, Stew | 1 cup | 2 carbs |
| | | 1 protein |
| | | 2 fats |
| Chili | 1 cup | 2 carbs |
| | | 1 protein |
| | | 3 fats |

| Common Foods | Portion | Carbohydrate Units |
|---|---|---|
| Chinese stir-fry | 1 cup | 2 proteins<br>low-starch vegetables as desired<br>1 to 3 fats |
| Italian meat sauce | 1 cup | 2 proteins<br>2 to 3 vegetables |
| Jambalaya | 1 cup | 2 carbs<br>1 protein<br>2 to 3 fats |
| Macaroni and cheese | 1 cup | 2 carbs<br>1 protein<br>3 fats |
| Ravioli/SpaghettiOs® | 1 cup | 2 carbs<br>1 protein<br>1 vegetable |
| Soups: | | |
|   Chicken noodle | 1 cup | 1 carb |
|   Vegetable | 1 cup | 2 vegetables |
|   Cream or cheese (regular) | 1 cup | 1 carb<br>4 fats |
|   Cream or cheese (reduced-fat) | 1 cup | 1 carb<br>1 fat |
|   Chunky | 1 cup | 1 carb<br>1 vegetable<br>1 fat |
| **Fast Food** | | |
| Chicken nuggets/tenders | 6 nuggets or 4 tenders | 2 proteins<br>1 carb<br>3 fats |
| French fries | "Kids Meal"-size | 1 carb<br>2 fats |
| French fries | Small | 2 carbs<br>3 fats |
| French fries | Medium | 3 carbs<br>4 fats |
| French fries | Large | 4 carbs<br>5 fats |
| Hamburger | Small-"Kids Meal" or "Junior" size | 1½ carbs<br>2 proteins<br>2 fats |
| Hamburger | Regular | 2 carbs<br>3 proteins<br>3 fats |

| Common Foods | Portion | Carbohydrate Units |
|---|---|---|
| Pizza, thin crust | 1 slice, large | 2 carbs<br>2 proteins<br>3 fats |
| Taco | 1, regular | 1 carb<br>2 proteins<br>3 fats |
| Taco | 1, soft | 1 carb<br>2 proteins<br>1 fat |

## A3.5   THE FOOD GROUPS

*Verbal Cues*

The Trim Kids Nutrition Plan teaches portion control by using a food unit or portion-control system*
as the guide. Foods are grouped into different food groups according to their nutrient compositions.
The food groups are

> Meat/protein substitutes
> Vegetables
> Carbohydrates, including starches and breads, fruits, and milk/dairy products
> Fats

Every food falls into one of these groups and is assigned a "unit" or a specified portion. Each
food group unit provides similar amounts of calories. It safe to assume, for instance, that one unit
of any fruit has about 60 calories and contains no fat. Or, one unit of any lean meat has about 25 to
50 calories and 1 to 3 g fat. Knowing this allows you and your child to make informed decisions
about what and how much food he or she can eat. Let's look a bit more closely at each food group
to learn more about their portions and nutritional values.

### Meats and Protein Substitutes

This food group includes most animal products and other foods that are good sources of protein.
In general, these foods contain mostly protein and few carbohydrates. A unit in this food group
generally equals1 ounce or 0.25 cup. One 3-ounce chicken breast, for example, equals three protein
units (we will often refer to this group as "proteins" for short).

Because some animal products can be very high in fat, we divide this group into three parts
based on the number of fat and calories in each: lean proteins, medium-fat proteins, and high-fat
proteins. Take time to review the lean protein choices listed below.

Lean proteins are the best choices. These contain no more than 2 or 3 grams of fat and 25 to
50 calories per ounce. Because they are so low in fat — especially seafood, egg substitutes (whites),
vegetable protein substitutes — consuming a few additional units of these foods, especially if you
are hungry, is allowed. Some examples of lean proteins include

> Lean beef (round, sirloin, flank)
> Vegetable protein substitutes (e.g., veggie or soy burgers), tofu
> Ham or Canadian bacon
> Veal chops or roasts
> Skinless chicken or turkey
> Seafood (the fat in fish and seafood, called omega-3 fatty acids, has been linked to reducing
>   some diseases, especially heart disease)
> Very low-fat cheeses and cold cuts (containing less than three to five grams of fat per ounce)
> Egg whites or egg substitutes

*Sidebar: Soy Protein*

Eating more soy protein helps lower LDL, or bad cholesterol levels. Many soy protein–based foods
are also good sources of dietary fiber, which means they are really healthy food! They also contain
no cholesterol. Replace some animal proteins (meat/poultry and dairy) with soy protein substitutes
as desired. Good sources of soy protein include

---

\* Food groups are based on the American Dietetic Association and American Diabetes Association food exchange lists.
The calorie assignments of some groups have been modified to offer a general calorie range rather than a specific calorie level.

Soy milk
Soy/vegetable meat and cheese substitutes
Soy nuts
Tofu

Medium-fat proteins and meat substitutes contain no more than 5 to 6 g fat and 75 calories per ounce. Eat them less often than lean meats. Examples include

Most beef (ground, roasts, or steaks)
Pork, lamb, and veal cutlets
Low-fat cheeses and cold cuts (containing about 5 g or more of fat per ounce)
Whole eggs (egg yolks are high in cholesterol)

High-fat proteins contain 8 to 10 g fat and 100 calories per ounce. Because of their high fat and caloric content, avoid these foods as much as possible. They include

Deep-fat fried meat or meat substitute
Prime beef (ribs, corned beef)
Pork sausage or spare ribs
Bacon
Regular cheeses
Luncheon meats (bologna, salami, liver, cheese)
Regular hot dogs, Vienna sausages

*Sidebar: Peanut Butter*
Peanut butter is a good protein substitute, although it is fairly high in fat. The good news is that it is a monounsaturated fat and may be eaten in moderation — usually not to exceed 1 or 2 tablespoons. Choose peanut butters that contain no added hydrogenated vegetable oils.

## Vegetables

The vegetable group includes all nonstarchy vegetables and contains on average less than 1 g fat and fewer than 25 calories per serving. These vegetables are also low in carbohydrates (less than 5 g per serving) and, thus, calories. Therefore, your child may usually eat as much of them as desired. These include

Artichokes, asparagus, green beans
Bean sprouts, beets, broccoli
Brussels sprouts, cabbage, carrots
Cauliflower, eggplant, greens, hearts of palm
Okra, onions, pea pods
Peppers, spinach, tomatoes
Tomato sauce
Tomato or vegetable juice
Salad greens
Summer or zucchini squash
Vegetable soup

We recommend that your child consume a minimum of five servings per day of fruits and vegetables. Not only are these foods naturally fat-free and packed with vitamins and minerals, but eating an abundance of them may decrease the risk of certain types of cancer, heart disease, and stroke.

## Carbohydrate-Containing Food Groups: Starches/Breads, Fruits, and Milk/Dairy Groups

The following food groups contain carbohydrates and will be grouped together as "carbohydrate food units." These include starches/breads, fruits, and milk/dairy foods. These food groups may be mixed and matched as desired, but try not to exceed the Daily Food Prescription in the program book [2] for carbohydrate units specified for your calorie level.

### Starches and Breads

In general, one carbohydrate unit of a starch or bread is one-half cup of cereal, grain, or pasta, or a 1-ounce slice of bread, and contains about 80 to 100 calories per unit. Here is a useful portion control hint: An average 9-inch plate equals about 2 cups or four carbohydrate units. If you choose starches or breads with added fat (oil, butter, etc.) make sure to count the fat portions as part of your daily intake, too. Some items in this food group include

> Cereals (those containing greater than 3 grams of fiber are better choices)
> Pancakes, waffles, muffins
> Grains, pasta
> Beans, peas, lentils
> Corn, potatoes
> Breads, bagels, tortillas (whole-wheat/whole-grain choices are better)
> Crackers (wheat), popcorn, pretzels

### Fruits

This group includes fresh fruit and unsweetened canned fruit and fruit juices. (Fresh or canned fruit is a better choice than fruit juice.) One unit is generally equal to one medium-sized piece of fresh fruit or ½ cup of canned fruit or fruit juice. Each unit contains less than ½ g fat and about 60 to 90 calories. Some items in this food group include

> Apple, applesauce (unsweetened), banana, berries (any kind)
> Fruit cocktail, grapes, grapefruit, kiwi
> Mandarin oranges, mango, melons (any kind), nectarines
> Oranges, peaches, pears, pineapple
> Tangerine, watermelon
> Dried fruits such as figs, dates, raisins
> Fruit juices (in moderation)

### Milk and Dairy Products

This food group includes skim and very low fat milk and milk products. One unit generally equals 8 ounces (1 cup) of milk or ½ to 1 cup of milk products and averages 90 to 120 calories per unit. Choose milk and dairy products that are lower in fat (containing less than 3 to 5 g fat per serving) to keep the calories lower. Some items in this food group include

> Skim and very low-fat (1–1½%) milk
> Soy milk
> Nonfat and very low fat yogurt
> Nonfat and very low fat ice cream, pudding, frozen yogurt

## Fats

Foods in this group contain mainly fat and very little carbohydrate or protein. Fats must be counted in addition to carbohydrate and protein units according to the Trim Kids Nutrition Plan Portion

Control Chart in the program book [2]. Each serving in this group averages 50 calories and 5 g fat. Some items in this food group include

Better Choices:
    Oil (olive, canola, peanut), olives
    Nuts
    Avocado

Other Choices:
    Lite margarine (look for liquid vegetable oil as the first ingredient)
    Reduced-fat salad dressings (consume fat-free versions as desired — "free food")
    Reduced-fat mayonnaise (consume fat-free versions as desired — "free food")
    Light whipped topping (2 tablespoons)

Less Healthy Choices (saturated fat):
    Regular margarine (containing hydrogenated or partially hydrogenated vegetable oils)
    Butter
    Bacon
    Sour cream (consume fat-free versions as desired — "free food")
    Cream cheese (consume fat-free versions as desired — "free food")
    Half & half

## Free Foods: "Anytime" Foods and Beverages

When your child focuses on what she can eat rather than on what she cannot, she will be more apt to want and choose those foods. Below is a list of "free foods," which means she can eat them without having to worry about measuring portions. They contain none to very little fat and fewer than 20 calories per serving.

Sugar-free beverages:
    Water — the best beverage!
    Mineral Water
    Club soda
    Sugar-free drink mixes*
    Sugar-free sodas*
    Broth/bouillon

Condiments:
    Fat-free butter substitutes such as butter/olive oil–flavored nonfat, nonstick cooking spray
        and liquid butter substitutes
    Fat-free cream cheese
    Fat-free mayonnaise
    Fat-free salad dressings
    Fat-free sour cream
    Flavoring extracts (vanilla, almond, peppermint, lemon)
    BBQ sauce
    Catsup
    Horseradish
    Herbs/spices/seasoning blends (any kind)**

---

\* Check with your health care team about using artificial sweeteners.
\** Although salt contains no calories, don't go overboard. Substitute lower-sodium versions when possible.

Hot pepper/Tabasco sauce
Lemons/limes
Mustard (any kind)
Pickles (any kind)
Powdered salad dressing/soup packets (mixed with fat-free sour cream to make a dip)
Seasoning (chili, stir-fry, taco, etc.) packets
Salsa
Soy sauce (lower-sodium preferred)
Teriyaki sauce
Taco sauce
Vinegar (any kind)
Worcestershire sauce

Sweet tooth*:
Sugar-free gum
Diet (sugar-free) Jello
Sugar-free popsicles
Low-sugar jelly/jam and fruit spreads
Low-sugar pancake syrup
All vegetables in vegetable category (see vegetable list above)

---

* Check with your health care team about using artificial sweeteners.

## A3.6 FULL MEAL PLANS, RECIPES FROM TRIM KIDS [2]

| | | | | Snacks (one to two choices per day) |
|---|---|---|---|---|
| | Breakfast | Lunch | Dinner | |
| Monday | Cold cereal with fiber (1 cup) <br> Wheat toast (one slice) with low-sugar jelly <br> Banana <br> Milk (1 cup) | Peanut butter (1 tablespoon) sandwich on wheat bread <br> Grapes (1/2 cup) <br> Milk (1 cup) | Roast beef (two to three slices) <br> Mashed potatoes (1/2 cup) with reduced-fat gravy (or one baked potato) <br> Low-fat broccoli and cheese <br> Tossed salad as desired (with 1–2 teaspoons olive oil or reduced-fat salad dressing) <br> Water or calorie-free beverage | Celery sticks with reduced-fat cream cheese (2 tablespoons) or peanut butter (1 tablespoon) <br> Cereal with fiber (1 cup) and skim milk <br> Cereal-fruit bar (1) <br> Reduced-fat chips (about 15 chips or 1 ounce) with fat-free dip or salsa <br> Wheat crackers (6) with reduced-fat cheese (2 slices) |
| Tuesday | One-half English muffin with reduced-fat cream cheese, 1 tablespoon peanut butter, or low-sugar jam/jelly <br> Scrambled egg substitute cooked in nonstick cooking spray (optional) <br> Strawberries (1 cup) <br> Milk (1 cup) | Fast food meal: 6" submarine sandwich (turkey, ham, chicken breast, or tuna with lite mayo) <br> Baked chips (1 single serving bag) <br> Water or calorie-free beverage | Oven-fried chicken (about 1 breast-size) <br> Brown rice (1/2 cup) with fat-free liquid butter substitute <br> Mixed vegetables <br> Fruit cocktail (1/2 cup) <br> Milk (1 cup) | Lite cream cheese (2 tablespoons) <br> Peanut butter (1 tablespoon) <br> Hot cocoa made with skim milk (1 cup) <br> English muffin or bagel "pizza" (1/2 muffin with tomato/pizza sauce and reduced-fat cheese) |
| Wednesday | Oatmeal (1 cup) with raisins and walnuts (2 tablespoons each) and 1 teaspoon brown sugar or honey (or reduced-sugar pancake syrup) if desired <br> Milk (1 cup) | Whole-wheat pita (1/2 pita) with tuna or chicken salad (made with reduced-fat mayo) and vegetables <br> Carrot and celery sticks with fat-free dip <br> Fresh fruit of choice <br> Milk (½–1 cup) | Open roast beef sandwich (leftover roast) made with one to two slices of wheat bread, 2 to 3 slices of roast beef with reduced-fat gravy <br> Cooked/steamed vegetables of choice <br> Tossed salad with 1–2 teaspoons olive oil or reduced-fat dressing <br> Milk (½–1 cup) | Fruit (1 piece fresh, 1/2 cup canned, or 3 tablespoons dried) <br> Frozen fruit bar (1) <br> Fruit juice "spritzer" <br> 3 ounces fruit juice mixed with 5 ounces club soda or sparkling water <br> Graham crackers (3 squares) <br> Teddy Grahams (1/2 cup) |

Table header: **Week 3 Weekly Menu**

| Thursday | Cheese toast:<br>1–2 slices wheat bread<br>  with reduced-fat cheese, melted<br>Fruit yogurt (1/2 cup)<br>Orange juice-calcium fortified (1/2 cup) | Chef salad with ham and/or turkey slices/cubes and reduced-fat dressing (2 tablespoons)<br>Small rice cakes (eight)<br>Milk (1 cup) | Restaurant: Mexican meal:<br>• Soft tacos or fajitas — chicken or beef (2) with salsa<br>• Black beans (1/2 cup)<br>or<br>• Mexican rice (1/2 cup)<br>• Tortilla chips (15) with salsa<br>Water or calorie-free beverage | Nuts (2 tablespoons)<br>Oatmeal (1/2 cup)<br>Oatmeal cookies (2 small)<br>Popcorn (3 to 5 cups)<br>Reduced-fat pudding or ice cream (1/2 cup)<br>Quesidilla (1 tortilla)<br>With melted, reduced-fat cheese, salsa and fat-free sour cream |
|---|---|---|---|---|
| Friday | Wheat toast (one to two slices) with fat-free liquid butter substitute and low sugar jelly<br>Scrambled egg substitute cooked with nonfat butter-flavored cooking spray (optional)<br>Turkey bacon (three) or "veggie" breakfast sausage links (two)<br>Sliced, fresh tomato<br>Milk (1 cup) | Wheat crackers (12) with reduced-fat sliced cheese<br>Vegetable soup<br>Fat-free pudding (1/2 cup)<br>Water or calorie-free beverage | Tuna noodle bake (1 cup)<br>Carrots (cooked with fat-free liquid butter substitute)<br>Tossed salad with 1–2 teaspoons olive oil or reduced-fat dressing<br>Fruit salad (1 cup)<br>Milk (½–1 cup) | Rice cakes (10 small or 2 large)<br>Sandwich on wheat bread (1/2) with turkey, tuna with lite mayo or reduced fat cheese<br>Soup: vegetable or chicken noodle (2 cups)<br>Trail mix (4 tablespoons)<br>Yogurt, regular or frozen (4–6 ounces)<br>Raw vegetables with fat-free dip (unlimited) |
| Saturday | Whole-grain waffle (one) with reduced-sugar syrup<br>Cottage cheese (1/2 cup) and canned pineapple or peaches (1/2 cup)<br>Orange juice-calcium fortified (1/2 cup) | English muffin "pizza" — whole English muffin with tomato sauce (any kind) and reduced-fat cheese<br>Popcorn (about 3 cups popped)<br>Strawberries (1 cup) or grapes (1/2 cup)<br>Milk (½–1 cup) | Seasoned lentils (1 cup)<br>Brown rice (1/2 cup)<br>Creamed spinach<br>Green salad with 1–2 teaspoons olive oil or reduced-fat salad dressing<br>Water or calorie-free beverage | |
| Sunday | Yogurt shake:<br>1 cup yogurt<br>1 cup frozen or fresh strawberries<br>½ banana (optional)<br>ice<br>Skim or soy milk as needed if a "thinner" consistency shake is desired | Low-fat chicken parmesan (about 1 breast-size)<br>Noodles (1/2 cup cooked)<br>Garlic bread (1 slice)<br>Steamed/cooked vegetables of choice<br>Green salad with 1–2 teaspoons olive oil or reduced-fat dressing<br>Water or calorie-free beverage | Leftover night | |

## Week 3 Recipes

### Low-Fat Broccoli and Cheese

2 small (or 1 large) bunches fresh broccoli, cut into bite-size pieces
1 can reduced-fat cream of mushroom soup
½ can skim milk or chicken broth
1½ to 2 cups (6–8 ounces) reduced-fat shredded cheddar or American cheese
Salt, pepper to taste

Preheat oven to 375 degrees. In a casserole dish, combine all ingredients. Bake uncovered for 30 to 40 minutes. Top with bread crumbs and spray with nonfat butter spray prior to baking if desired.

Microwave directions: Microwave the broccoli until just tender (about 3 to 5 minutes). Add remaining ingredients and microwave (on medium-high) for another 5 minutes.

Nutrition Analysis:
    Vegetable Group: No limit (½ cup = 45 calories, 1–3 g fat)

### Oven-Fried Chicken

Chicken breasts, skin removed
Salt or salt substitute and pepper to taste
1 cup egg substitute
Italian seasoned breadcrumbs
Nonfat butter-flavored spray

Preheat oven to 375 degrees. Season the chicken breasts. Dip the chicken breasts into the egg substitute and roll in the bread crumbs (redip and roll in the bread crumbs again for a thicker crust). Spray with the butter-flavored spray and place on a cookie sheet or baking pan. Bake for 45 to 50 minutes.

Nutrition Analysis:
    1 breast: 3–4 protein units, ½ carbohydrate unit (145 calories, 5 g fat)

### Tuna Noodle Bake

3 to 4 cups cooked macaroni (or your favorite type of noodles)
1 can reduced-fat cream of mushroom or celery soup
½ can skim milk
¼ cup fat-free mayonnaise
2 teaspoons mustard
1 cup (4 ounces) reduced-fat shredded American or cheddar cheese
1 to 2 cans water-packed tuna, drained
1 cup reduced-fat potato chips, crushed (optional)

Preheat oven to 375 degrees. In a casserole dish, mix all of the ingredients except the chips. Sprinkle with the crushed chips (or bread crumbs) and spray lightly with nonfat liquid butter spray if desired. Bake uncovered for 40 to 45 minutes.

Nutrition Analysis:
    1 cup: 2 carbohydrate units, 1 protein, 1 fat (200 calories, 7 g fat)

### Seasoned Lentils

1 pound dried lentils, sorted and rinsed
4 to 5 cups water
Chicken, ham, beef or vegetable bouillon cubes (3 to 4)
Bay leaf (2) — optional

In a saucepan, combine lentils, bouillion, and bay leaves. Bring to a boil and simmer (uncovered) for about 15 to 20 minutes, until just tender*. Drain and remove the bay leaves. Salt and season with a little hot sauce as desired. Can also spray with the nonfat butter-flavored pump spray.

Mix with the cooked lentils (optional):

## Mushroom/Onion Sauté

½ pound fresh mushrooms (washed and sliced)
1 medium onion (chopped)
2 teaspoons olive oil
Butter-flavored spray
¼ teaspoon hot sauce (optional)

In a skillet, sauté the mushrooms and onions on medium heat in 2 teaspoons olive oil and butter-flavored spray enough to coat the skillet until tender (about 15 minutes). Hint: Cook the onions for about 5 minutes before adding the mushrooms, as the onions take a bit longer to soften. Toss with the cooked, drained lentils. Season with salt and hot sauce as desired.

* Be careful not to overcook the lentils, as they will become mushy.

OR

## Cheesy Tomato Lentils

1 large can diced tomatoes, drained
2 cups shredded, reduced-fat cheese (we like the American or cheddar flavor)
½ cup of the lentil-broth water
½ teaspoon hot sauce (optional)

In a saucepan, combine these ingredients with the cooked lentils and heat through.
Nutrition Analysis:
    1 cup: 2 carbohydrate units (160–180 calories)

## Creamed Spinach

2 packages frozen spinach, defrosted and drained
1 cup fat-free sour cream (more if you like it creamier)
2 tablespoons fat-free mayonnaise
¼ teaspoon salt or salt substitute
¼ teaspoon hot sauce (optional)
1 to 2 teaspoons finely chopped jalepeno pepper (optional)

In a saucepan, heat the spinach in butter-flavored spray and 2 teaspoons olive oil. Add the remaining ingredients and heat through.

To make a "cheesy" creamed spinach, add ½ to 1 cup reduced-fat shredded cheese (American, cheddar, or mozzarella).
Nutrition Analysis:
    Vegetable group: No limit (1/2 cup = 35–40 calories, 0 g fat)

## Low-Fat Chicken Parmesan

6 skinless, boneless chicken breasts
1 cup egg substitute
Italian-seasoned bread crumbs
Reduced-fat (part-skim) mozzarella cheese slices (6)

1 jar spaghetti sauce (your favorite brand)

½ cup parmesan cheese

Preheat oven to 375 degrees. Dip the chicken breasts in the egg and roll in the breadcrumbs. Lay the breaded chicken breast slices in a baking pan that has been sprayed with olive oil or butter-flavored non-stick cooking spray. Bake uncovered for 20 to 25 minutes*. Remove from the oven and top each chicken breast with one slice of mozzarella cheese. Cover with the spaghetti sauce and sprinkle with Parmesan cheese. Bake for another 15 to 20 minutes or until heated through.

Nutrition Analysis:

1 breast: 4 protein, ½ carbohydrate (180 calories, 7–8 g fat)

* Important: Bake the coated chicken breast first as instructed before adding the cheese and sauce to ensure a chicken coating that is not soggy.

| Week 3 Weekly Shopping List | | | |
|---|---|---|---|
| **Fruits** | **Vegetables** | **Meat/Deli** | **Dry/Can** |
| Apples<br>Banana<br>Grapes<br>Strawberries<br>Misc. fruits for snacks | Broccoli (two<br>  bunches)<br>Carrot/celery sticks<br>Salad greens:<br>  Lettuce, tomato<br>  Cucumbers, etc<br>Misc. vegetables for<br>  snacks | Beef roast<br>Chicken breasts,<br>  skinless, boneless (buy<br>  a "family pack" —<br>  enough to make two<br>  recipes during the<br>  week)<br>Ham (or preferred cold-<br>  cut) slices<br>Turkey bacon | Oatmeal<br>Breakfast cereal (fiber content<br>  should be more than 2–3 g per<br>  serving)<br>Bread crumbs, Italian-seasoned<br>Macaroni (or preferred noodles) for<br>  the tuna noodle casserole<br>Brown rice<br>Lentils (one bag, dried)<br>Beef gravy mix (package)<br>Reduced-fat cream of mushroom<br>  soup<br>Tuna (water-packed) — extra cans<br>Reduced-fat pudding, diet Jello<br>Pineapple, fruit cocktail, or other<br>  fruit (can)<br>Raisins |
| **Dairy Case** | **Frozen Food Section** | **Breads/Misc.** | **Staples** |
| Milk (skim, 1½% or soy<br>  milk)<br>Egg substitute/Eggs<br>Reduced-fat/part-skim<br>  cheese slices (<5 g fat<br>  per ounce/slice)<br>Reduced-fat shredded<br>  cheese (extra)<br>Fruit yogurt<br>Calcium-fortified orange<br>  or fruit juice<br>Cottage cheese<br>Fat-free sour cream | Mixed vegetables<br>Spinach, chopped<br>  (2 boxes)<br>Mashed potatoes<br>Waffle (whole-grain is<br>  better)<br>Frozen strawberries | Wheat bread<br>English muffin<br>Whole-wheat pita bread<br>French or Italian bread<br>  (to make the garlic<br>  bread during the week)<br>Reduced-fat popcorn<br>Baked (less than 3 grams<br>  of fat) chips | Reduced-fat/very low fat (<3 g fat<br>  per serving) mayonnaise<br>Reduced-fat/very low fat (<3–5 g fat<br>  per serving) salad dressings<br>Catsup, mustard, BBQ sauce,<br>  pickles (regular versions OK)<br>Reduced-sugar syrup, low-sugar or<br>  all-fruit jelly<br>Peanut butter (no added<br>  hydrogenated or partially<br>  hydrogenated vegetable oils)<br>Nuts<br>Oil (olive, canola, peanut), Nonfat<br>  cooking spray, Nonfat liquid butter<br>  (dairy section)<br>Lite margarine (first ingredient<br>  should be liquid vegetable oil —<br>  not hydrogenated or partially<br>  hydrogenated oil) |

## Week 3 Portion Control/Food Record Practice

Don't forget to use Aerobic Activity and Food Checklist (Appendix 3.1 and program book [2]) to help keep track of your daily intake. Let's practice portion control checks for 1 day.

| | THURSDAY |
|---|---|
| **Breakfast:** | |
| Cheese toast (1–2 slices): | 1–2 carbohydrates (bread), 2 proteins , 1–2 fats (cheese, 0 fats if using fat-free cheese) |
| Yogurt (1/2 cup or 4-oz.) | 1 carbohydrate |
| Orange juice (1/2 cup) | 1 carbohydrate |
| **Lunch:** | |
| Chef salad: | 2–3 proteins (ham, turkey, reduced-fat cheese), 1–2 fats |
| Vegetables-as desired | |
| Reduced-fat dressing (2 tablespoons) | 1–2 fats (0 if fat-free) |
| Rice cakes (8–10 small) | 1 carbohydrate |
| Milk (1 cup) | 1 carbohydrate |
| **Dinner:** | |
| Soft taco or Fajitas (2) | 2 carbohydrates (tortillas), 2–3 proteins (meat/chicken), vegetables — as desired |
| Black beans (1/2 cup) | 1 carbohydrate + 0–2 fats if oil is used |
| Tortilla chips (15) | 1 carbohydrate + 2 fats |
| Salsa | Vegetable — as desired |
| **Sample Snacks:** | |
| Cherry tomatoes | Vegetable — as desired |
| Reduced-fat pudding cup | 1 carbohydrate |
| | |
| **Total Thursday food units:** | 10 carbohydrates |
| | 7–8 proteins |
| | 6 fats |
| | Vegetables — as desired |

## A3.6.1 Low-Calorie Pizza Recipe

   Light bread (40 calories per slice)
   No-sugar-added tomato sauce
   Fat-free mozzarella cheese
   Italian seasoning
   Low-fat pizza toppings: ground turkey (cooked) or vegetables
   Spread bread with tomato sauce and sprinkle with Italian seasoning to taste. Top each piece of bread with ¼ cup of the cheese and the low-fat toppings. Place pizza on a broiler pan sprayed with nonstick cooking spray. Broil approximately 5 minutes or until the cheese is melted.
   Nutrition Information
   Yield: 1 serving = 1 pizza
   Exchange(s): 1 light bread exchange, 1 meat/protein, 1 vegetable
   Per Serving
   Calories 80
   Protein 8 g
   Carbohydrate g
   Fat 1 g

## A3.7 CALCIUM: THE BONE BUILDER

One of the most important minerals for our bodies — and the one that is most lacking — is calcium. More than half of America's children and adolescents don't consume the calcium they need. Children should consume between 800 and 1300 mg per day, and teenagers need to boost their intake to 1500 mg per day.

Many foods contain calcium, but dairy products supply the most abundant amounts. Dairy products also serve up much-needed vitamin D, which helps the body to absorb calcium. If your child doesn't routinely consume three to four servings of dairy foods daily, chances are good that he isn't meeting his recommended daily allowance. But don't worry — adding calcium doesn't have to mean adding calories or pounds: nonfat, low-fat, and skim versions of dairy products contain similar amounts of calcium as their higher-fat cousins.

Conduct a calcium intake check for your child by referring to the list below. If you realize that your child isn't eating enough calcium-rich foods to meet the minimum requirements, consult your doctor about putting him on a calcium supplement. Remember, without adequate calcium intake, your child could suffer some serious health consequences later in life. Your child's skeletal framework is forming now. Studies indicate that females especially are at risk for developing osteoporosis and related bone fractures later in life unless they consume enough calcium.

### Calcium Content of Common Foods

| Food | Serving | Calcium |
|---|---|---|
| Yogurt | 1 cup | 400 mg |
| Low-fat/skim milk | 1 cup | 300 mg |
| Calcium fortified fruit juice | 1 cup | 300 mg |
| Cheese pizza | 1 slice | 200 mg |
| Cheese | 1 ounce | 200 mg |
| Collard greens | ½ cup | 170 mg |
| Soups made with milk | 1 cup | 160 mg |
| Macaroni and cheese | ½ cup | 150 mg |
| Custard | ½ cup | 150 mg |
| Cottage cheese | 1 cup | 145 mg |
| Pudding | ½ cup | 130 mg |
| Ice cream/frozen yogurt | ½ cup | 125 mg |
| Shrimp | 3 ounces | 100 mg |
| Beans | 1 cup | 90 mg |
| Broccoli | ½ cup | 45 mg |

## A3.8   PROTEIN-MODIFIED FAST DIET

The protein-modified fast diet (PMF) is a high-protein, low-carbohydrate, low-calorie diet designed to promote rapid body fat loss while maintaining lean body mass (muscle mass) when combined with the appropriate exercise prescription. A reduced carbohydrate and fat intake allows for a lower daily caloric intake of 900 to 1100 calories per day while maintaining the required protein prescription. Protein in the diet is derived from lean meat, fish, poultry, egg whites, reduced-fat cheeses, and soy protein substitutes — an average of 13 to 22 ounces per day are needed, depending on the body size. Low-carbohydrate vegetables and very limited quantities of starches, dairy, and fruit will be allowed in addition to the protein food sources. A minimal amount of fat in the diet is derived from the lean protein choices and small amounts of allowed vegetable oils. The PMF diet must be adhered to closely and only under medical supervision to allow for safe and effective weight loss.

Daily vitamin and mineral supplements must be prescribed due to the restrictive nature of the diet. The PMF diet must be medically monitored and followed under physician supervision only.

### DAILY VITAMIN AND MINERAL SUPPLEMENTS

1.  A daily multivitamin containing iron and minerals. One tablet per day.
    Brand: _____
2.  Calcium.
    800 to 1000 mg per day for patients under 10 years of age.
    1200 to 1500 mg per day for patients over 10 years of age.
    Brand: _____
    Amount:_____
3.  Potassium supplement: Morton's Lite Salt
    Under 10 years old: 1½ teaspoon per day (19 mEq)
    Over 10 years old: 1 teaspoon per day (36 mEq)
    OR
    A prescription for potassium as prescribed by your physician

### FLUID INTAKE

Maintaining an adequate fluid intake is very important. A minimum of 8 to 12 cups (64 to 96 ounces) of fluid should be consumed per day. Water is the best choice; however, the allowed (sugar-free) beverages may be also used to meet part of your daily fluid intake goal.

---

### Protein Modified Fast Diet Food List

#### Protein Source: Meat and Substitutes

_____ ounces per day minimum

| Allowed | Restricted |
|---|---|
| Poultry: | Poultry: |
|   Chicken (without skin) |   Chicken with skin |
|   Canned chicken (in broth) |   Fried chicken |
|   Turkey (without skin) | |
|   Ground turkey (lean — less than 3 grams of fat per ounce) | |
| | |
| Beef: | Beef: |
|   Flank, round, chuck, sirloin, tenderloin |   Prime beef, beef ribs, corned beef |
| |   Regular ground beef |

Veal:

   Roast, chop, steaks

Pork:

   Canadian bacon

   Ham

   Roast (loin, tenderloin)

   Chops — fat trimmed

Seafood:

   Fish — all

   Shellfish — all

   Tuna fish canned in water (1/4 cup = 1 ounce equivalent)

Eggs:

   Egg substitute (1/4 cup = 1 ounce equivalent)

   Egg whites (2 whites = 1 ounce equivalent)

**Allowed**

Wild Game:

   Venison, rabbit

Lamb:

   Chops, leg, roast — fat trimmed

Cold Cuts (reduced-fat)*:

   Sliced turkey, ham, roast beef

   Reduced-fat* luncheon meats

   Reduced-fat* hot dogs, sausage

Cheese (reduced-fat)*

Soy "vegetable" meat substitutes

*Read labels: should contain less than 3 grams of fat per ounce.

Veal:

   Veal cutlets — ground and breaded

Pork:

   Pork spareribs, pork sausage

   Ground pork

   Bacon

Seafood:

   Fried fish or shell fish

   Breaded fish such as fish sticks

   Tuna fish canned in oil

Eggs:

   Egg yolks

   Fried eggs in butter, margarine, or oil

**Restricted**

Cold Cuts:

   Luncheon meats — regular bologna, liver, cheese,
     pimento loaf, salami

   Regular hot dogs, sausage

Other:

   Peanut butter

---

## Protein Modified-Fast Diet Food List

### Vegetables: Four to Six Servings per Day

### 1 Serving = 1/2 Cup Cooked or 1 Cup Raw

**Allowed (low-starch vegetables)**

Artichokes, asparagus

Bean sprouts, broccoli, Brussels sprouts

Beets

Cabbage, carrots, cauliflower

Eggplant

Greens (collard, mustard, turnip)

Green beans

Hearts of palm

Mushrooms

Okra, onions

Pea pods, peppers (green, red, or yellow)

Salad greens — all

Sauerkraut, spinach

Squash (zucchini, yellow, or spaghetti)

**Restricted**

Beans (red, lima, kidney, white)

Corn

Peas (green, split, black-eyed)

Potatoes

Pumpkin

Squash (winter or acorn)

Yams

Vegetable casseroles made with restricted ingredients

Tomatoes (fresh or canned)
Tomato juice
Tomato paste, tomato sauce (no added sugar)
Turnips
Water chestnuts
Vegetable juice
Vegetable soup

## Protein Modified-Fast Diet Food List
### Fruits

One choice per day:                      Fruit juice
1 piece fresh fruit
2 tablespoons dried fruit
½ cup canned, no added sugar canned fruit

## Protein Modified-Fast Diet Food List
### Dairy (should contain less than 3 grams of fat per ounce; 1 ounce = 1 ounce protein equivalent)

Reduced-fat cheese                       Milk (whole, low-fat, or skim)
                                         Yogurt, ice cream, ice milk, frozen yogurt
                                         Regular cheese

## Protein Modified-Fast Diet Food List

### "Free Foods" — As Desired

#### Beverages

Plain broth/bouillon (beef or chicken)
Carbonated water, club soda
Decaffeinated coffee, tea (unsweetened)
Sugar-free drink mixes
Sugar-free sodas (caffeine-free is preferred)
Diet snowballs

#### Salad Greens

Lettuce, endive, romaine, spinach
Celery, cucumber
Onions, peppers, radishes
Mushrooms

#### Snacks and Sweet Substitutes

Sugar-free gelatin
Sugar-free gum
Sugar-free popsicles (3 per day)
Artificial sweeteners (check with your healthcare team for the preferred brand)

#### Condiments

Catsup, mustard
Fat-free or very low-fat (less than 3 grams fat) mayonnaise or salad dressing
Fat-free or very low-fat (less than 3 grams fat) salad dressings
Fat-free "butter substitutes" — liquid and pump spray
Nonstick cooking sprays

Horseradish

Taco sauce, salsa

Vinegar — all flavors

Lemon, lime juice

Salt or salt substitute, pepper, seasonings, and spice blends

Soy sauce

Worcestershire sauce

Hot sauce

Barbecue sauce (2 tablespoons)

Dill pickles

Seasoning packets (e.g., taco seasoning packet, chili seasoning packet, stir-fry seasoning packet, etc.)

## Protein Modified-Fast Diet Food List

### Breads and Starches

| Allowed | Restricted |
|---|---|
| After 1 to 2 weeks: Two choices per day*: | Other than the allowed amounts of: |
| One choice equals: | Hot cereal |
|    Whole wheat bread — 1 slice | Regular bread-all types |
|    Beans — 1/2 cup | Biscuits, muffins, dinner rolls |
|    Dry Cereal (low sugar) — 1 cup | Rice |
|    Oatmeal, Cream of Wheat — 1/2 cup | Pasta, spaghetti, macaroni |
|    Wheat crackers — 6 | Pancakes, waffles |
|    Pasta (wheat is better) — 1/2 cup | Cold cereal |
|    Popcorn — 3 cups | Crackers, pretzels, popcorn, potato chips |
|    Potato — 1 small or 1/2 cup mashed | Stuffing (bread) |
|    Brown rice — 1/2 cup | Taco shells |
|    Soup (chicken noodle) — 1/2 cup | |
|    Tortilla — 1 | |
|    Waffle/pancake — 1 medium | |

*Check with your physician and/or dietitian prior to adding.

### Fats

| Allowed | Restricted |
|---|---|
| Up to 2 teaspoons per day: | Butter, lard |
|    Oils — olive, canola, peanut, cottonseed, safflower, sunflower, sesame, sunflower | Margarine |
| | Olives |
|    Nuts — all types | Regular mayonnaise or salad dressing |
| | Regular sour cream |
| | Regular cream cheese |

## A3.9   FILLING UP WITH FIBER

*Verbal Cues*

It is important to introduce more fiber into your child's diet. Fiber is found in whole-grain bread and grain products, beans, fruits, and vegetables. By definition, "fiber" is the part of these foods that we cannot digest or absorb. There are a host of benefits to eating it, including:

- Stabilizing blood sugar fluctuations. The carbohydrates in many high-fiber and whole-grain foods are metabolized more slowly than those in other foods. This slow metabolizing can also decrease post-meal cravings.
- Constipation relief. Fiber draws water into the digestive tract, resulting in softer stools that are easier to pass.
- Lowering the LDL cholesterol level in the blood. Consuming foods containing soluble fiber can literally help the body absorb cholesterol.
- Promoting a feeling of fullness. Fiber is bulky, making you feel fuller. This can help reduce overeating.

To determine how much fiber your child should eat, add five to the age of your child. So, if your child is eight years old, she should be consuming 13 grams of fiber. Most adults should consume at least 20 to 30 grams of total fiber per day. If you have not been doing this, you should work up to it gradually, as the body must become accustomed to processing larger amounts of fiber.

Good sources of soluble ("cholesterol-lowering") fiber include oatmeal, oat bran, barley, avocado, broccoli, Brussels sprouts, carrots, collard greens, sweet potatoes, beans (any kind), split peas, lentils, apricots, figs, prunes, flax seeds, and sunflower seeds.

### High-Fiber Food Choices
**Average Fiber Grams**

| | |
|---|---|
| Beans | 6–8 |
| Bran/oat cereals | 3–11 |
| Brown rice/pasta | 4 |
| Whole grain bread products | 2–6 |
| Oatmeal | 4 |
| Fruits and vegetables | 2–3 |

Average serving size: 1 cup where applicable.

## A3.10 AEROBIC ACTIVITY AND FOOD CHECKLIST

You will need to have 12 copies of this form on hand — one for every week. Complete one form during each week, whenever you exercise or whenever you are going to have something to eat.

### Week No. _____ Date:_____

| Day | *My goal this week is this many minutes: | This is the type of physical activity I did each day: | This is how long I did it: | My heart rate was (see program book [2]): |
|---|---|---|---|---|
| Sun | | | | |
| Mon | | | | |
| Tue | | | | |
| Wed | | | | |
| Thu | | | | |
| Fri | | | | |
| Sat | | | | |

\* Refer to the recommendations for your child's color level listed in each week. Ask your child to select activities she enjoys from the list for her color level in in the program book.

1. Fill in your daily portion units.
2. As you consume each unit/portion, place a check mark in the box.
3. Try to stay within your daily allowances.
4. Remember: your Calorie Level is :_____ (see program book)

| | I can have ___ Carbohydrate Units each day | | | | | | | I can have ____ Meat/Protein Substitute Units each day | | | | | I can have ___ Fat Units each day | | | I can have Unlimited Vegetables! |
|---|---|---|---|---|---|---|---|---|---|---|---|---|---|---|---|---|
| Sunday | | | | | | | | | | | | | | | | |
| Monday | | | | | | | | | | | | | | | | |
| Tuesday | | | | | | | | | | | | | | | | |
| Wednesday | | | | | | | | | | | | | | | | |
| Thursday | | | | | | | | | | | | | | | | |
| Friday | | | | | | | | | | | | | | | | |
| Saturday | | | | | | | | | | | | | | | | |

Refer to the recommendations for your child's color level listed [2].

## A3.11  INITIAL GROUP CHECK-IN FORM

Hello, my name is _____.

I am _____ years old. I attend _____ school and am in _____ grade.

Some things I do really well (or am proud of) include

_____

_____

Some things I would like to do to be healthier include

_____

_____

## A3.12  WEEKLY GROUP CHECK-IN FORM

Hello, my name is _____.

This week I: (check one below)

☐ Lost _____ pounds.

☐ Gained _____ pounds.

☐ Stayed the same.

Since beginning the program I have: (check one below)

☐ Lost _____ pounds.

☐ Gained _____ pounds.

☐ Stayed the same.

My accomplishments for the week are

_____

_____

_____

My questions or problems this week are

_____

_____

_____

## A3.13  COMMITMENT RATING FORM

Parents and Children: Rate yourself on the scale below from 0–100. Circle the number that describes how you feel right now.

How badly do you want to lead a healthier lifestyle?

| 0 | 25 | 50 | 75 | 100 |
|---|---|---|---|---|
| Not At All | A Little | Somewhat | A Lot | Very Much |

Do you think you will feel the same way in 6 months? YES or NO

Do you think you will feel the same way a year from now? YES or NO

## A3.14 BENEFITS AND SACRIFICES FORM

Make a list of the benefits and sacrifices of leading a healthier lifestyle.

| Sacrifices | Benefits |
| --- | --- |
| | |
| | |
| | |
| | |

## A3.15  THE ABCs OF THE BEHAVIOR CHAIN — VIGNETTE

Shelly is trying to lose weight by making healthier food choices and by becoming more active. On her way to recess to play softball, she meets up with three friends. She follows her friends to the snack shack, where they all sit at a picnic table gossiping and munching on chips, candy bars, and sodas. Shelly realizes as she finishes a can of soda and a chocolate bar that she slipped off her diet, and begins feeling down, while her friends gossip on.

Antecedent:

What happened first?

_____

Behavior:

Did the kids make a healthy, unhealthy, or questionable food choice?

_____

Consequence:

How did the kids feel?

_____

Think of a time when you had a tough decision to make about what to eat, and write it down:

Antecedent:

What happened first?

_____

Behavior:

Did you make a healthy, unhealthy, or questionable food choice?

_____

Consequences:

How did you feel afterwards?

_____

## A3.16  SHORT-TERM AND LONG-TERM GOALS FORM

### SHORT-TERM GOALS

My Short-Term Goals are:

_____

_____

Examples: Drop one size, lose 10 pounds, walk ½ mile without resting, try 3 to 5 new fruits and vegetables, set and try to meet weekly goals

### LONG-TERM GOALS

My Long-Term Goals are:

_____

_____

Examples: Reduce my waistline by 5 inches, walk a 10K race, eat 3-5 fruits and vegetables a day, set and try to meet weekly goals

## A3.17  WEEKLY GOAL SETTING AND ACTION PLANNING FORM

My GOAL this week is to

_____

_____

1.  Does it say what you WILL do (NOT what you WON'T do this week)?
2.  Do you have control over it?
3.  Is it easy to do?

Steps and reminders (include who, when, where, or how)

_____

_____

My reward for accomplishing my goal is

_____

## A3.18  COGNITIVE RESTRUCTURING TECHNIQUES FORM

1. Avoid allowing participants to set unreasonable, nonspecific, or unattainable goals.
2. Encourage participants to think about, embellish, and discuss their progress, not short-comings.
3. Enforce that participants avoid imperatives such as "always" and "never." Also, disallow the use of adjectives such as "good" or "bad" when referring to food or activity—instead, encourage participants to use the adjectives "healthy" or "unhealthy."
4. Instruct participants to counter negative thoughts with rational, positive restatements.
5. Encourage participants to set easy, realistic, specific, and attainable weight loss goals that focus on healthier eating and activity.

## A3.19  GOAL ASSESSMENT FORM

List the GOALS you have set to become more active and eat more healthfully below.

_____

_____

_____

_____

List the GOALS you have accomplished below. Place a (+) next to those you have been able to keep doing every week.

_____

_____

_____

List the GOALS you have been unable to accomplish below.

_____

_____

_____

List the GOALS you still want to achieve or that you may want to set in the future.

_____

_____

_____

## A3.20  BEHAVIOR SUBSTITUTION OR RESTRUCTURING FORM

This week I will (to be more active)

_____

_____

Instead of

_____

_____

This week I will try (to eat more healthfully)

_____

_____

Instead of

_____

_____

## A3.21  RELAPSE ROAD MAP

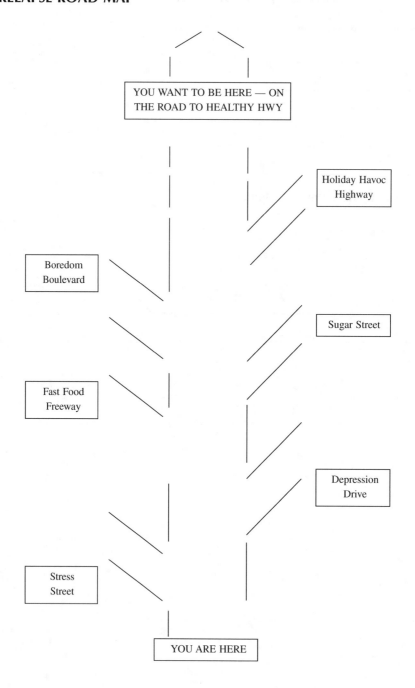

## A3.22 RULES FOR EATING FORM

1. Ask participants to chew more (15 to 30 per bite) and try to eat more slowly. Encourage family members to engage in conversation and discussions during meals to decrease their speed of eating.
2. Encourage participants to take smaller bites.
3. Discourage participants from "taking seconds" (except for vegetables)!
4. Encourage participants to leave some of every type of food on their plate (explain why this is OK).
5. Ask participants to take smaller portions and leave the serving bowls of food in the kitchen.
6. Encourage participants to use a smaller plate.
7. Suggest that participants put their forks down between every bite.
8. Enforce that participants eat ONLY at the table, NOT in front of the television, at the kitchen counter, or while engaged in other activities.
9. Encourage participants to eat three bites of every food. Participants should "grade" the new foods that are served and decide whether they are acceptable to continue serving on a regular basis.
10. Have participants drink a large glass of water or sugar-free beverage 15 minutes before every meal.
11. Encourage participants to eat with their other (nondominant) hand.
12. Ask participants to eat their meals with chopsticks for an entire day or week!

## A3.23  BEHAVIORS FOR CONTROLLING EATING HABITS FORM

Here are four useful behaviors:

1. Follow an eating schedule and don't eat at other times. Plan your schedule for eating:

   Breakfast        time _____
   Morning snack    time _____
   Lunch            time _____
   Afternoon snack  time _____
   Dinner           time _____

2. Eat in one place, for example, at home, in the kitchen at the table, for all meals and snacks.
3. Don't do anything else while eating. Don't eat while you are studying, watching TV, reading, or doing other activities.
4. Make your list of alternative activities. These should be practical as well as enjoyable.

   What I Can Do Instead of Eating (Alternative Activities): _____

   _____

   _____

   _____

   _____

(Make sure you include some activities that you can do inside and some that you can do outside. Keep this list handy so that you can consult it when you feel tempted to eat between your scheduled meals.)

## A3.24  SOCIETAL TRIGGERS FORM

Name the people, places, times, or events that tempt you to overeat or to be less active.

_____

_____

What can you do to change or avoid these temptations?

_____

_____

List the people and places where it is easiest for you to stay on your program.

_____

_____

List the times and events when it is easiest for you to stay on your program.

_____

_____

List the people and places where it is hardest for you to stay on your program.

_____

_____

List the times and events when it is hardest for you to stay on your program.

_____

_____

Next, what can you do to change or to avoid these situations (people, places, times, or events)?

_____

_____

## A3.25  TEMPTATIONS AND POSITIVE SELF-STATEMENTS FORM

To begin, identify the situations that tempt you to eat and what you usually say to yourself when you feel unable to resist. Have your parents help you identify these associated negative thoughts.

Tempting Situations:

_____

_____

Associated Negative Thoughts:

_____

_____

After identifying these tempting situations, practice responding to them with positive self-statements that allow you to react in a positive way. Your parents will help you.

Tempting Situations:

_____

_____

Positive Self-Statements:

_____

_____

## A3.26 ADDITIONAL ROLE PLAYS, VIGNETTES OR SCENARIOS TO CONSIDER USING

### WHEN WORKING WITH OVERWEIGHT CHILDREN AND FAMILIES

Teasing and Bullying
Not Wanting to Be Different
The Usual Suspects of Overeating and under Activity
Peer Pressure to Overeat or Be under Active
Temptation (Home, School, Peer, Societal)
Sabotage (Home, School, Peer, Societal)
Expect the Unexpected

## A3.27  WEIGHT-O-RAMA

Game rules: All players place one forearm flush on the table. If you are ready to answer, raise your hand and keep your elbow on the table. The first player to raise a hand gets a chance to answer a question. If that player gives an incorrect answer, the other players can try to answer the same question. Players get 1 point for each correct answer. The player with the last correct answer picks the next category. The youngest player starts each game. The first player to score 5 points chooses one of the incentives available. Play continues as long as there is time.

The five categories are: Food Labels, Holidays, About Foods, Funnies, About Me

### FOOD LABELS

1. True or False: Foods or ingredients are listed from the least amount (first) to the most amount (last) on a food label.
2. How many grams of fat per 1 ounce make a meat low fat?
3. Name a food that has no label.
4. Name a brand of hot dog that is low in fat.
5. Does "no cholesterol" or "cholesterol free" mean a product is low in calories?
6. Name a brand of cold cut that is low in fat.
7. Name a product that contains lard.
8. Which type of fat is bad for your heart?
9. A particular candy bar you like has 15 calories per 1 ounce. If your candy bar weighs 6 ounces, how many calories does it contain?
10. Name a brand of cheese that is low in fat.

### HOLIDAYS

1. How can you make brownies so that they are low in fat and calories?
2. What can you do to reduce the caloric content of a school holiday party full of high-calorie snacks?
3. When dashing through the snow, how many horses are pulling the "open sleigh"?
4. How could you enjoy watching the Super Bowl and also be more active?
5. What are Santa's helpers called?
6. What is Frosty's nose made of?
7. Give an example of one small change you could make while out of school over the holidays, which could become a habit when you start back to school next year.
8. Name a holiday tradition that will also increase your activity level?
9. What day is Independence Day?
10. What is your favorite activity?

### ABOUT FOODS

1. High-fat meats provide how many calories per 1-ounce serving?
2. What would ensure that your fast-food chicken sandwich was low in calories?
3. How many calories in a typical slice of pepperoni pizza?
4. The Sta-Puff Marshmallow Man belongs in which food group?
5. How many peanuts make up one serving? BONUS: This represents how many calories?
6. One serving (1 cup raw, 1/2 cup cooked) of vegetables contains how many calories?
7. One slice of bread (2 slices of diet bread) contains how many calories?
8. Which ingredient in tuna salad is most likely to increase its caloric value?
9. Cranberries belong to which food group?
10. Name three high-calorie and three low-calorie toppings for a salad or baked potato.

## FUNNIES

1. Which burns more calories: sleeping or skiing?
2. Tell a funny Knock-Knock joke.
3. What is your doctor's last name? BONUS: What is the clinic phone number?
4. The Pillsbury Dough Boy belongs to which food group?
5. What is the funniest movie you've ever seen?
6. What was Bill Cosby's profession on *The Bill Cosby Show*?
7. What is Charlie Brown's dog's name?
8. What is your favorite comic strip or comic strip character?
9. Name the rock star that has the same name as a ground meat dish.
10. Name the four Beatles.

## ABOUT ME

1. Name a brand of low-fat cheese that you have tried and liked.
2. Would you rather walk, roller skate, or ride a bike?
3. Name one thing you have changed since coming to this program.
4. If you could have any three things you wanted for your holiday presents, what would they be?
5. Name three low-calorie snack foods you've tried. Did you like them?
6. What is the best thing about coming to this program?
7. What is the worst thing about coming to this program?
8. If you could make your favorite high-calorie food low in calories, which food would you pick?
9. What high-calorie food is hardest for you to resist?
10. Name a sport you've tried? Do you like it?

## APPENDIX REFERENCES

1. Ogden, C. L., K. M. Flegal, M. D. Carroll, and C. L. Johnson. Prevalence and trends in overweight among US children and adolescents, 1999–2000. *JAMA.* 288:1728–1732, 2002.

2. Sothern, M., Von Almen, TK. & Schumacher, H. Trim Kids: The Proven Plan that has Helped Thousands of Children Achieve a Healthier Weight. New York, NY: Harper Collins Publishers, 2001.

3. CDC. Available at: http://www.cdc.gov/growthcharts/ (accessed April 2005) Accessed.

4. Lohman, T., Roche, AA, Martorell, R., Eds. Anthropometric standardization reference manual. Champaign, IL: Human Kinetics., 1988

5. Roche, A., Heymsfield, SB, Lohman, TG., Eds. *Human Body Composition.* Champaign, IL: Human Kinetics., 1996

6. Durnin, J. V. and J. Womersley. Body fat assessed from total body density and its estimation from skinfold thickness: measurements on 481 men and women aged from 16 to 72 years. *Br J Nutr.* 32:77–97, 1974.

7. Jackson, A. S. and M. L. Pollock. Generalized equations for predicting body density of men. *Br J Nutr.* 40:497–504, 1978.

8. Lohman, T. G. Skinfolds and body density and their relation to body fatness: a review. *Hum Biol.* 53:181–225, 1981.

9. Sloan, A. W. Estimation of body fat in young men. *J Appl Physiol.* 23:311–315, 1967.

10. Goran MI, D. P., Johnson R, Nagy TR, Hunter G. Cross-calibration of body-composition techniques against dual-energy X-ray absorptiometry in young children. *Am J Clin Nutr.* 63:299–305, 1996.

11. Cameron, N., Griffitns, PL, Wright, MM, Blencowe, C, Davis, NC, Pettifor, JM Norris, SA. Regression equations to estimate percentage body fat in African prepubertal children aged 9 y. *Am J Clin Nutr.* 80:70–75, 2004.

12. Bray, G., DeLaney, JP, Volaufova, DW, Harsha, DW, Champaign C. Prediction of body fat in 12-y-old Arican American and white children: evaluation of methods. *Am J Clin Nutr.* 76:980–990, 2002.

13. Gutin, B., M. Litaker, S. Islam, T. Manos, C. Smith, and F. Treiber. Body-composition measurement in 9-11-y-old children by dual-energy X-ray absorptiometry, skinfold-thickness measurements, and bioimpedance analysis. *Am J Clin Nutr.* 63:287–292, 1996.

14. Slaughter, M. H., T. G. Lohman, R. A. Boileau, C. A. Horswill, R. J. Stillman, M. D. Van Loan, and D. A. Bemben. Skinfold equations for estimation of body fatness in children and youth. *Hum Biol.* 60:709–723, 1988.

15. Friedl, K. E., J. P. DeLuca, L. J. Marchitelli, and J. A. Vogel. Reliability of body-fat estimations from a four-compartment model by using density, body water, and bone mineral measurements. *Am J Clin Nutr.* 55:764–770, 1992.

16. Mazess, R. B., H. S. Barden, J. P. Bisek, and J. Hanson. Dual-energy x-ray absorptiometry for total-body and regional bone-mineral and soft-tissue composition. *Am J Clin Nutr.* 51:1106–1112, 1990.

17. Ellis KJ, S. R., Pratt JA, Pond WG. Accuracy of dual-energy x-ray absorptiometry for body-composition measurements in children. *Am J Clin Nutr.* 60:660–665, 1994.

18. Godin, G. and R. J. Shephard. Gender differences in perceived physical self-efficacy among older individuals. *Percept Mot Skills.* 60:599–602, 1985.

19. Sallis, J. F. Epidemiology of physical activity and fitness in children and adolescents. *Crit Rev Food Sci Nutr.* 33:403–408, 1993.

20. Sallis, J. F., C. C. Berry, S. L. Broyles, T. L. McKenzie, and P. R. Nader. Variability and tracking of physical activity over 2 yr in young children. *Med Sci Sports Exerc.* 27:1042–1049, 1995.

21. Crespo, C. J., E. Smit, R. P. Troiano, S. J. Bartlett, C. A. Macera, and R. E. Andersen. Television watching, energy intake, and obesity in US children: results from the third National Health and Nutrition Examination Survey, 1988–1994. *Arch Pediatr Adolesc Med.* 155:360–365, 2001.

22. Parcel, G. S., E. Edmundson, C. L. Perry, H. A. Feldman, N. O'Hara-Tompkins, P. R. Nader, C. C. Johnson, and E. J. Stone. Measurement of self-efficacy for diet-related behaviors among elementary school children. *J Sch Health.* 65:23–27, 1995.

23. Edmundson, E., G. S. Parcel, C. L. Perry, H. A. Feldman, M. Smyth, C. C. Johnson, A. Layman, K. Bachman, T. Perkins, K. Smith, and E. Stone. The effects of the child and adolescent trial for cardiovascular health intervention on psychosocial determinants of cardiovascular disease risk behavior among third-grade students. *Am J Health Promot.* 10:217–225, 1996.

24. Edmundson, E., G. S. Parcel, H. A. Feldman, J. Elder, C. L. Perry, C. C. Johnson, B. J. Williston, E. J. Stone, M. Yang, L. Lytle, and L. Webber. The effects of the Child and Adolescent Trial for Cardiovascular Health upon psychosocial determinants of diet and physical activity behavior. *Prev Med.* 25:442–454, 1996.

25. McMurray R., W. Guion, B. Ainsworth, and J. Harrell. Predicting aerobic power in children: a comparison of two methods. *Med Sci Sports Exerc.* 38:227–233, 1998.

26. Loftin, M., M. Sothern, L. Trosclair, A. O'Hanlon, J. Miller, and J. Udall. Scaling $VO_2$ peak in obese and non-obese girls. *Obes Res.,* 9:290–296, 2001.

27. *American College of Sports Medicine (ACSM)'s Guidelines for Testing and Prescription,* 6th ed. Baltimore, MD: Lippincott, Williams & Wilkins, 2000.

28. Achenbach, T. M. Manual for the Child Behavior Checklist/ 4-18 and 1991 Profile. Burlington, VT, 1991.

29. Achenbach, T. M. Integrative Guide to the 1991 CBCL/ 4-18, YSR and TRF Profiles. Burlington, VT, 1991.

30. Kovacs, M. *Children's Depression Inventory.* San Antonio, TX: Multi-Health Systems, 1981.

31. Olson, D. H., Porner, J., Lavee, Y. Family Adaptability and Cohesion Evaluation Scales (FACES III). In: F. S. Science. Ed. *Handbook of Measurements for Marriage and Family Therapy.* New York: Brunner Mazel, 1985, pp. 180–185.

32. Piers, E., Harris, D. *The Piers-Harris Children's Self-Concept Scale.* Los Angeles, CA: Western Psychological Services, 1969.

33. Piers, E. V. *Piers-Harris Children's Self-Concept Scale: Revised Manual.* Los Angeles, CA: Western Psychological Services, 1984.

34. Piers, E., Harris, D., Herzberg, D. *The Piers-Harris Children's Self Concept Scale.* 2nd ed. Los Angeles: Western Psychological Services, 2002.

35. Falkner F, Tanner J. *Human Growth.* London, UK: Baillier Tindall, 1979.

36. Strong, W. Physical fitness of children: mens sana in corpore sano. *Am J Dis Child.* 141:488–496, 1987.

# Index

## A

Abdominal adiposity, exercise and, 196
Absentees, 240
Academic performance, 60, 173
Acanthosis nigricans, 84, 101
Achenbach Child Behavior Checklist (CBCL), 106
Adolescent bariatric surgery, *See* Bariatric surgery
Aerobic exercise
    activity and food checklist, 371
    field sports, 239, 259–260, 337, 345
    interdisciplinary, interactive approach, 256, 261, 346
Aerobic performance, 68–69, 113–114, *See also*
        Cardiopulmonary fitness
    ventilatory anaerobic threshold, 115
Aerobic volleyball, 239
"A" factors, 237, 245
Age-specific BMI criteria, 46
Alanine aminotransferase (ALT), 36
American Heart Association guidelines, 127
Amphetamines, 211
Anorexia nervosa, 56, *See also* Eating disorders
Anthropometrics, 45, 100–101
Antidepressants, 56
Anxiety, 56, 107
Arthritis, 10, 89
Aspartate aminotransferase (AST), 36
Asthma, 37
"At risk of overweight," 46
    dietary prevention and treatment recommendations, 125
Attention deficit disorder, 37
Audience segmentation, 15
Autonomic function, 114–115
Awards, 23

## B

Bardet–Biedl syndrome, 32, 86
Bariatric surgery, 4, 81, 223–231
    behavior modification component, 4
    cautions, 230
    contraindications, 225
    efficacy, 230
    indications and referral guidelines, 223–225
    nutritional considerations, 226–230
    postoperative management, 228–230
    preoperative team assessment, 226–228
Beckwith–Wiedeman syndrome, 32
Behavioral assessment tools, 106
Behavioral counseling, 62, *See also* Behavioral therapy
Behavioral theories and models, 175–177, 244–246

Behavioral therapy, 3, 61, 82, 147–167, 2443–246, *See also*
        Eating behaviors, behavioral modification
        techniques; Pediatric weight management
        programs; *specific approaches, programs*
    adolescent studies, 164–165
    bariatric surgery and, 4
    behavior chain ABCs, 376
    cognitive restructuring form, 379
    component analysis, 165
    contingency management, 149
    contingent reinforcement, 150
    counseling, 62
    dietary approaches and, 122
    eating and activity patterns, 148–149
    efficacy, 42, 148
    family-based counseling interventions, 150
    family-based studies overview, 149–165
    family-centered approach, 3
    family-therapist relationship, 243
    goal setting and action planning, 148, 239, 249,
        377–378
    individual treatment approaches, 166–167
    interdisciplinary interactive approach, 235–240,
        243–265, *See also* Interdisciplinary, interactive
        pediatric weight-management program
    knowledge and, 61–62
    motivational interviewing, 63
    multicomponent approach, 148
    parent-focused treatment, 165–166
    program objectives, 13
    psychosocial factors, 55
    relapse prevention, 148, 250, 382
    role plays, vignettes or scenarios, 387
    self-efficacy and, 62–63
    self-monitoring, 148–149
    social reinforcement and modeling, 149
    societal triggers form, 385
    stimulus control and cue elimination, 149, 248–249
    temptations and positive self-statements, 386
    transtheoretical approach, 244
    treatment techniques and strategies, 148–149
Behavior change, environmental barriers to, 62
Behavior-modification skills instruction, 236, 238
Behaviors for controlling eating form, 384
Behavior specialist, 17–18
Behavior substitution or restructuring form, 381
Benefits and sacrifices form, 375
Beverages, 3, 99
    sugar-free, 357
Biliopancreatic bypass, 228
Binge eating, 56, 57, 58, 89, 98
Bioelectrical impedance, 47, 318
Blood pressure, 88